AF520583

SETHI'S
HPTLC

High Performance
Thin Layer Chromatography

Quantitative Analysis of Pharmaceutical Formulations

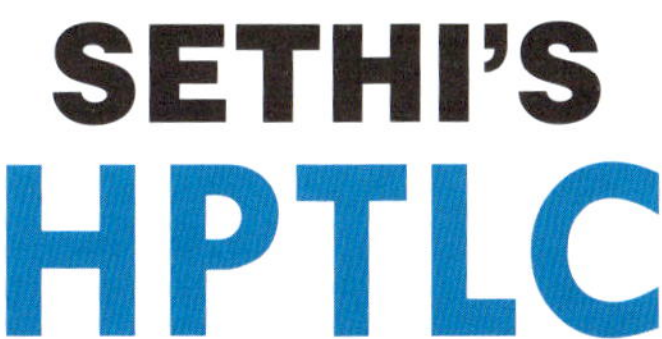

High Performance Thin Layer Chromatography

Quantitative Analysis of Pharmaceutical Formulations

Volume 1

Dr. P.D. Sethi
M.Pharm., Ph.D.

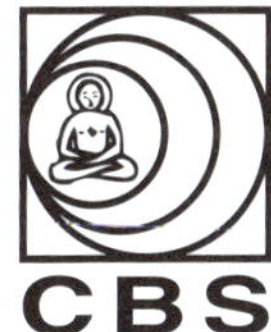

CBS PUBLISHERS & DISTRIBUTORS PVT. LTD.
New Delhi • Bengaluru • Pune • Kochi • Chennai

ISBN : 978-81-239-2279-9

First Edition : 2013

Published by:
Satish K. Jain and produced by Vinod K. Jain for CBS Publishers & Distributors Pvt. Ltd.,
4819/XI Prahlad Street, 24 Ansari Road, Daryaganj, New Delhi - 110002 (India)
E-mail: cbspubs@airtelmail.com, delhi@cbspd.com • www.cbspd.com

Branches:
- ***Bengaluru:*** 2975, 17th Cross, K.R. Road,
  Bansankari 2nd Stage, Bengaluru - 560070
  Ph.: +91-80-26771678/79
  E-mail: cbsbng@gmail.com, bangalore@cbspd.com
- ***Pune:*** Bhuruk Prestige, Sr. No. 52/12/2+1+3/2,
  Narhe, Haveli (Near Katraj-Dehu Road By-pass), Pune - 411051
  Ph.: +91-20-64704058/59, 32342277 • E-mail: pune@cbspd.com
- ***Kochi:*** 36/14, Kalluvilakam, Lissie Hospital Road, Kochi - 682018, Kerala
  Ph.: +91-484-4059061-65 • Fax: +91-484-4059065
  E-mail: cochin@cbspd.com
- ***Chennai:*** 20, West Park Road, Shenoy Nagar, Chennai - 600030
  Ph.: +91-44-26260666, 26208620 E-mail: chennai@cbspd.com

Printed at :
Aegean Offset Printers, Greater Noida (UP)

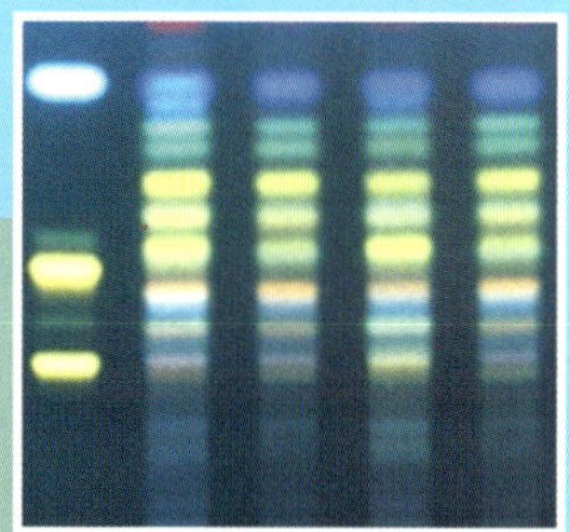

TLC / HPTLC

- VERSATILE ANALYTICAL TECHNIQUE
- UNRIVALED IN RAPID & ROBUST SCREENING OF MANY SAMPLES IN PARALLEL.
- POWERFUL, FAST & INEXPENSIVE ANALYTICAL TECHNIQUE WITH PROVEN SEPARATION EFFICIENCY.
- DOCUMENTATION OF SEPARATION RESULTS & EXTENSIVE PUBLISHED DATA AVAILABLE

FLEXIBILITY (APPLICATIONS)

- QUALITY CONTROL (IDENTIFICATION, ASSAY, CONTENTS UNIFORMITY & STABILITY)
- PRODUCTION CONTROL
- SYNTHESIS MONITOR & CONTROL
- IMPURITY PROFILING
- HERBAL ANALYSIS
- FINGER- PRINT PROFILING
- MARKERS ISOLATION
- COSMETICS ANALYSIS
- FOOD ANALYSIS
- FORENSIC CHEMISTRY
- CLINICAL STUDIES

FLEXIBILITY (METHOD DEVELOPMENT)

- STATIONARY PHASES (NORMAL & MODIFIED)
- MOBILE PHASE CHOICE
- DEVELOPMENT METHODS
- DIFFERENT DEVELOPMENT CHAMBERS
- SEVERAL DETECTION METHODS (DESTRUCTIVE / NON-DESTRUCTIVE)

SIMPLICITY

- SAMPLE PREPARATION MINIMAL
- STEPWISE PROCEDURE
- MOBILE PHASE OPTIMIZATION
- EASY TO LEARN & OPERATE
- EASY TO MAINTAIN

ECONOMICS

- HIGH SAMPLE THROUGHPUT
- RAPID SCREENING
- SHORT ANALYSIS TIME
- LOW SOLVENT CONSUMPTION
- PRE-COATED LAYERS

An essential condition for all fruitful research is to have at one's disposal a satisfactory technique.

M.S. Tswett

HPTLC Applications

Process monitoring in organic synthesis

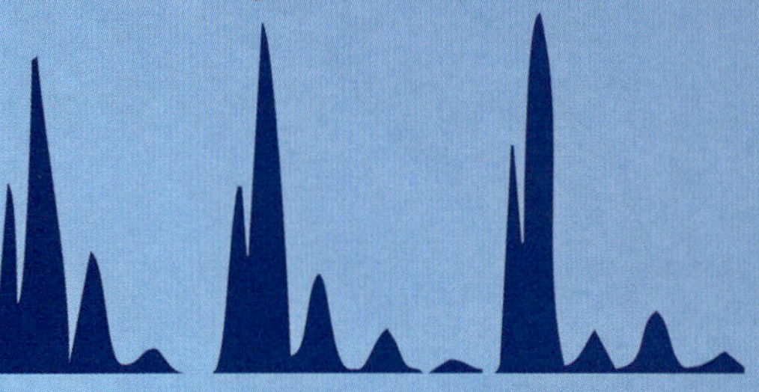

After 1 Hours. After 2 Hours. After 4 Hours.

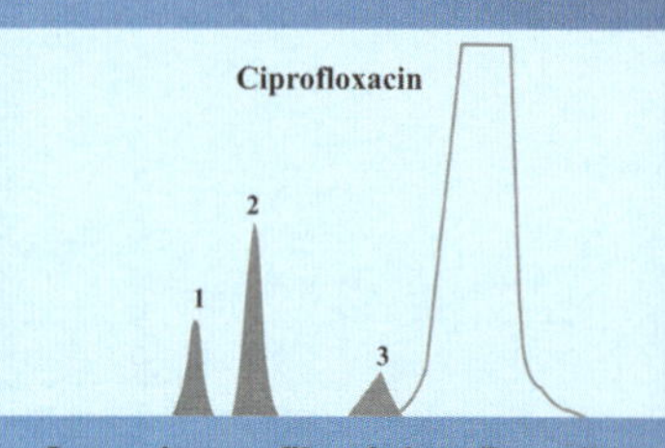

Impurity profile of ciprofloxacin

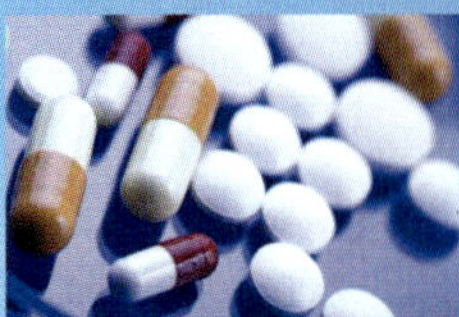

Analysis of pharmaceutical formulations

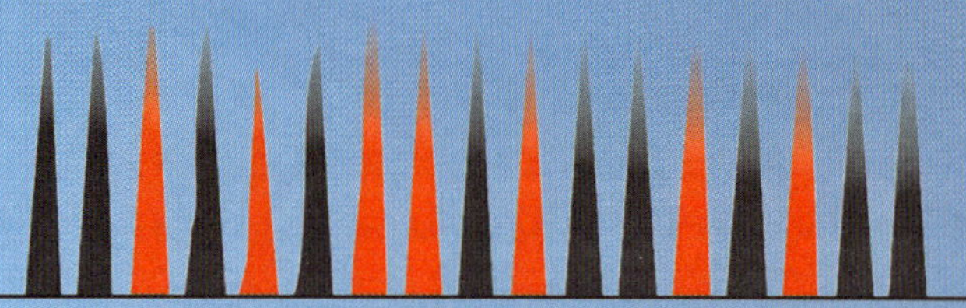

Content Uniformity Test

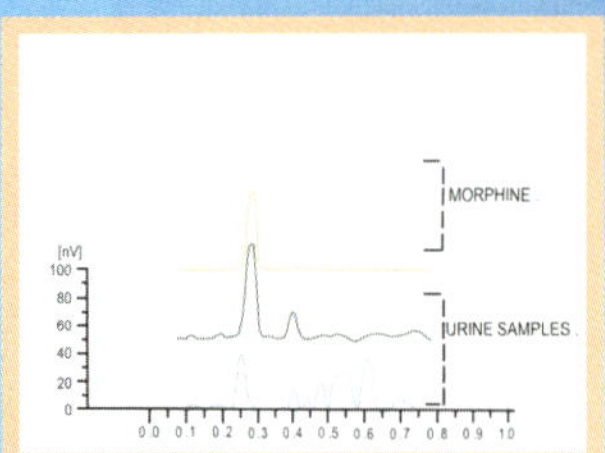

Forensic

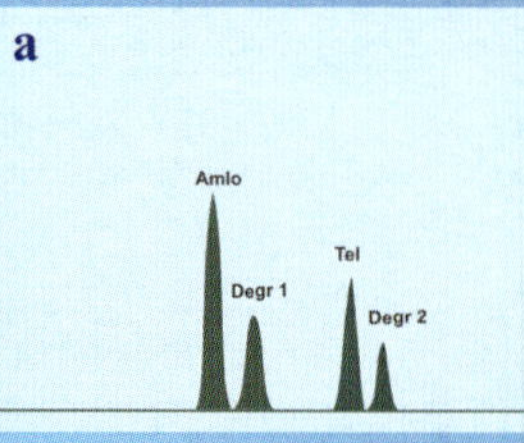

Stability profile of amlodipine & telmisartan under stress conditions, a-base, b-oxidative (Reproduced with permission, A.B. Thomas et. al. J Pharm. Res., 10 (2), 66 - 72, 2011

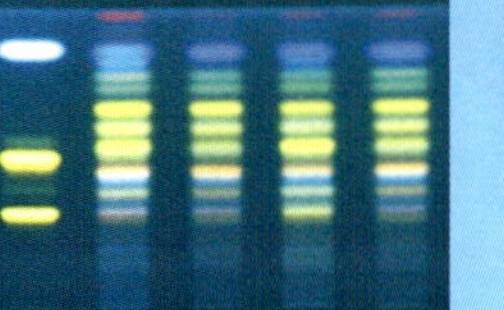

Finger-printing, herbal identification

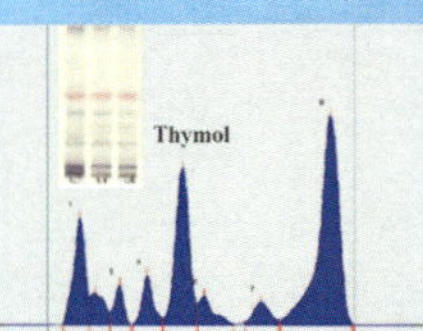

Quantification of Thymol in Trachyspermum ammi (Ajowan) Herbal Standardization

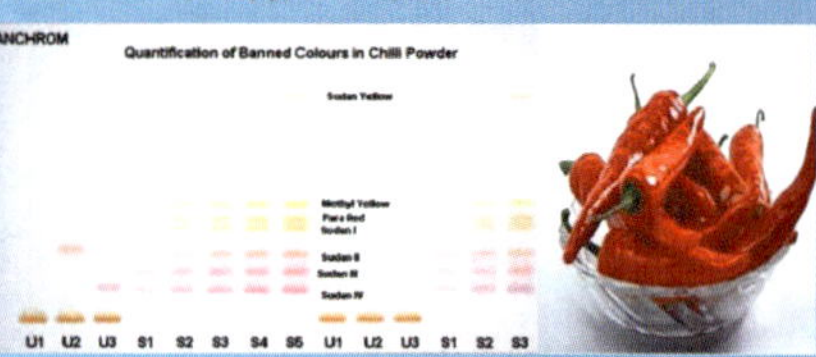

Banned dyes in chilli (Food)

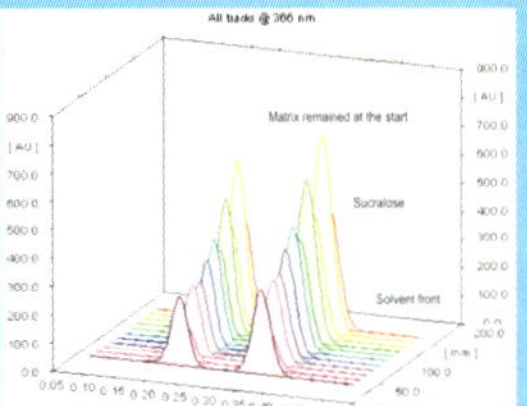

Analysis of sucralose in waste water (Reproduced with permission, Camag, CBS - 106) Environments

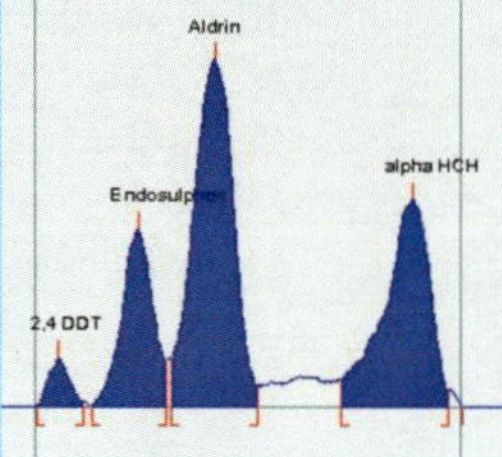

Analysis of pesticides in poultry feed

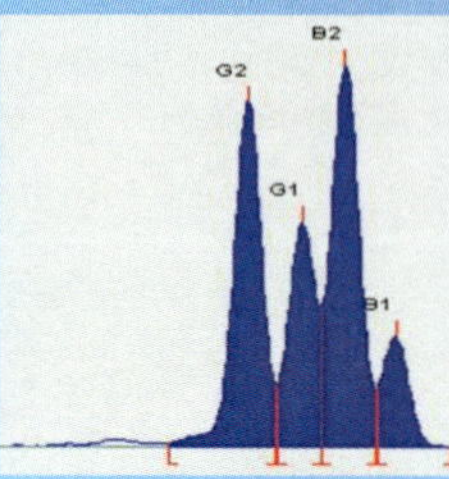

Analysis of aflatoxins in groundnut

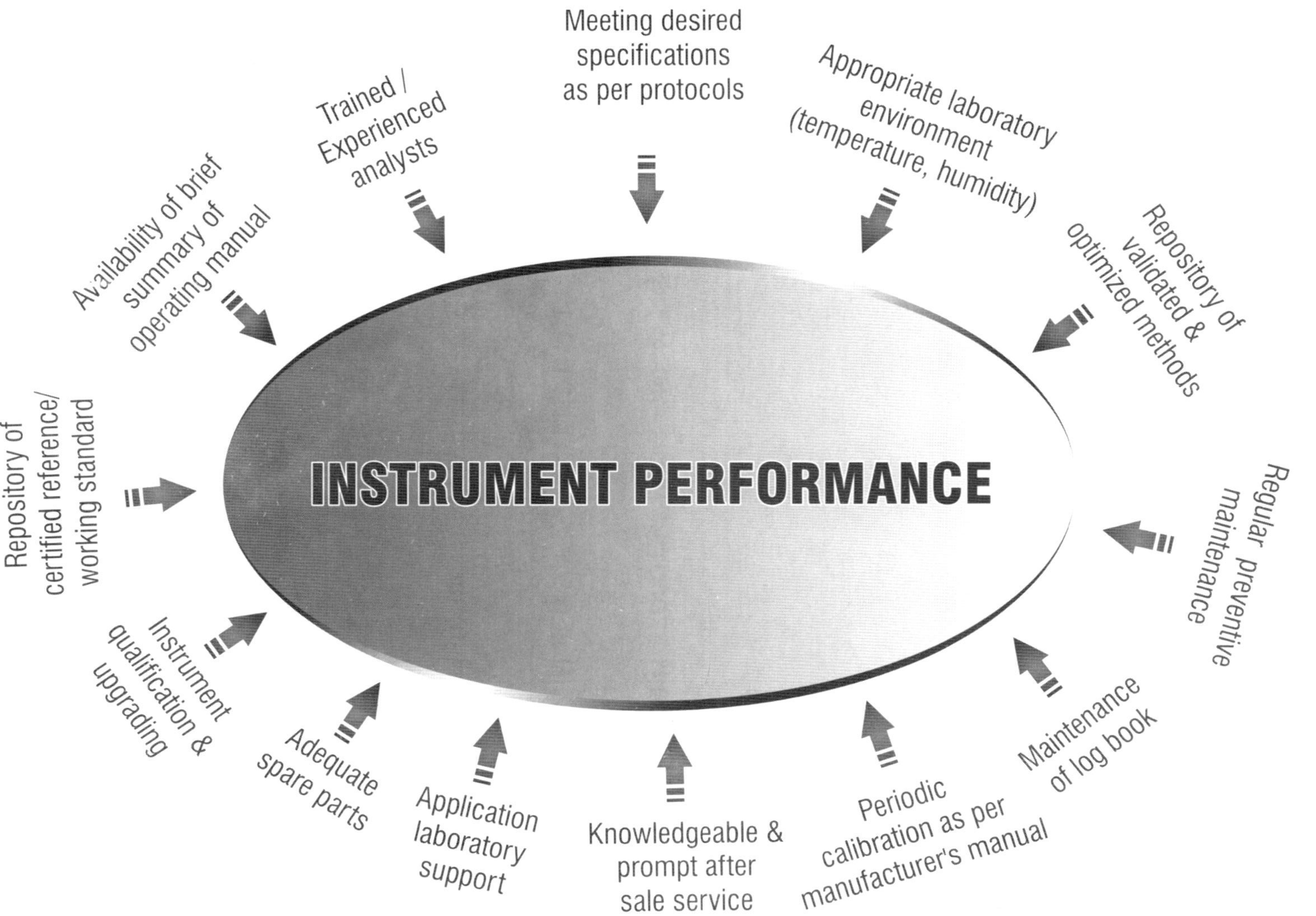

INSTRUMENT PERFORMANCE
Meeting desired specifications as per protocols
Appropriate laboratory environment (temperature, humidity)
Repository of validated & optimized methods
Regular preventive maintenance
Maintenance of log book
Periodic calibration as per manufacturer's manual
Knowledgeable & prompt after sale service
Application laboratory support
Adequate spare parts
Instrument qualification & upgrading
Repository of certified reference/ working standard
Availability of brief summary of operating manual
Trained / Experienced analysts

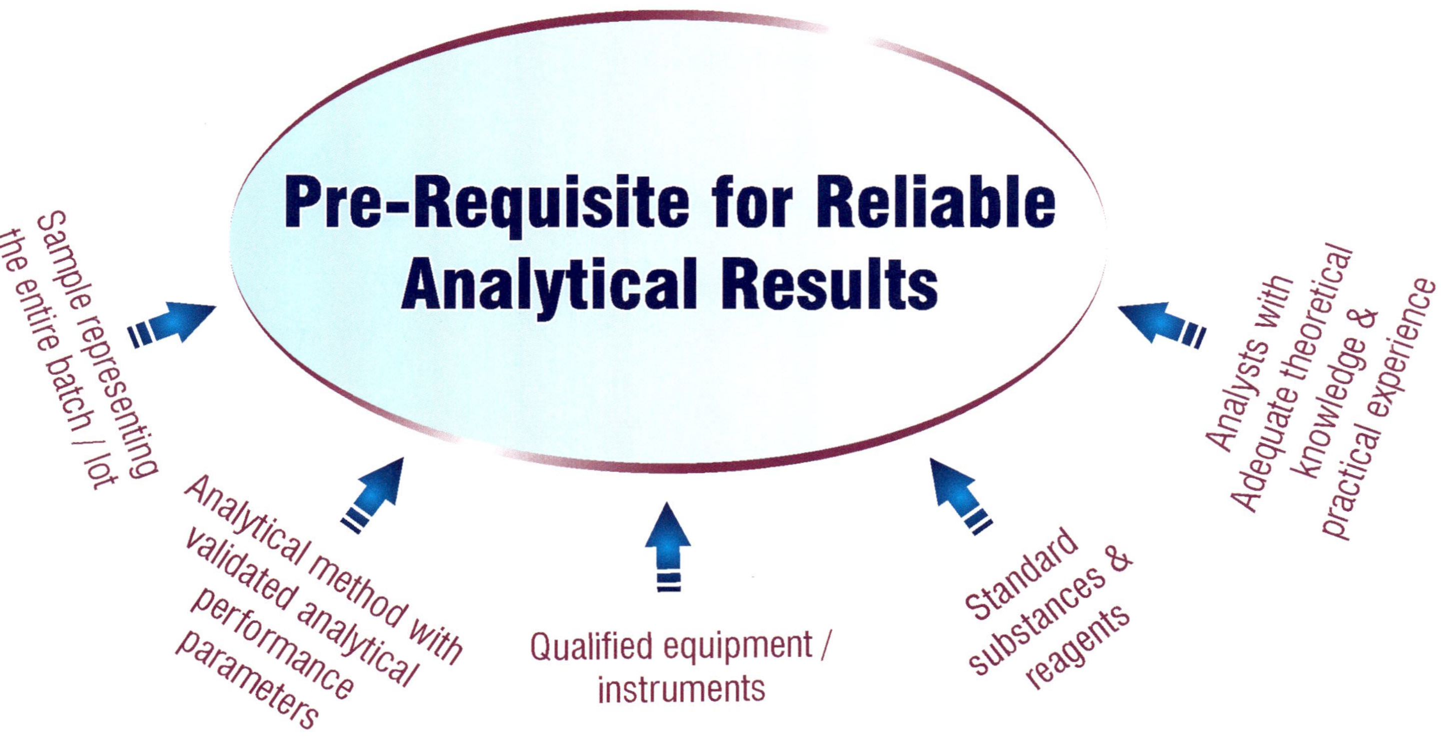

Method's real uncertainity need to be ascertained to avoid unrealistic expectations on reliability and validity of results.

To

The woman, USHA,
my wife, my friend
who stood by me all the time.

Life is all about aspiration, struggle, failures, triumph and achievement.

Dedicated to fellow analysts exploring wider application of TLC/HPTLC, a versatile analytical technique.

Please remember, how good analyst you may be but one can't do inspired analysis without aesthetic qualities, the gift possessed by relatively very few like skill of a musician or a painter but one can emulate their mentors, teachers/gurus.

"Guru/teacher/mentor is like a live-map; if you can read the map, you know the right path to go, without map it may take life-time to find the right path."

Preface

Quality level of any analytical work depends on appropriate analytical method, performance of analytical instruments, certified standard substances, reagents, suitable sample preparation and analysts having adequate scientific knowledge of the analytical chemistry and practical experience. The analytical data so generated for any decision-making process must be technically sound, defensive and with very low level of uncertainty. Please remember, analytical data may be dealt with computers and human intellect but intuition is exclusively human.

High performance thin layer chromatography (HPTLC) works on the same principles as other chromatographic techniques such as HPLC/GC with added advantages of fastness, high sample throughput analysis, less labour intensive sample cleanup procedures, and simultaneous parallel analysis of several samples under identical conditions avoiding system suitability test (SST), disposable stationary phase, and static detection. Now HPTLC system is fully automated thus enhancing the system reproducibility allowing reliable, accurate and precise analytical results. These advantages have made HPTLC a comprehensive analytical technique for application in different fields (pharma and herbal analysis, food, cosmetology, environmental analysis, clinical laboratories, forensic and biochemistry) providing same level of quality results as that of HPLC/GC. However, there are many challenges which the analyst shall often face while working with this technique successfully as HPTLC being an open system method, is highly affected by experimental and environmental conditions which need to be controlled and regulated for reproducible results in each chromatoplate. It need to be borne in mind that consistency of performance of each application shall squarely depend on controlling various influencing factors. This compilation is an attempt to demonstrate how HPTLC fits in a well-managed analytical laboratory as an independent analytical technique on its own merit.

There is no contemporary monograph on application of HPTLC in analysis of multi-component pharmaceutical formulations except the one authored by

Acknowledgement

I place on record my gratitude to analytical fraternity, students, teachers and professionals for their support and inspiration in my entire analytical career.

I am extremely obliged to all TLC/HPTLC practitioners for sharing analytical data (published and unpublished) without which this compilation would never have been possible. I am thankful to Dilip Charegaonkar, CMD, M/s Anchrom Enterprises (I) Pvt. Ltd., Mumbai, India, for extending facilities in HPTLC application laboratory for verification of several reported methods and scientific support in compilation of this monograph. Valued advice by Mr. Dilip Charegaonkar for practically-oriented presentation of the subject matter is highly appreciated.

Merck Specialities Private Limited, Mumbai, India was kind enough to provide pre-coated plates for analytical work and also permission to reproduce data and figures required. I am thankful to M/s Camag, Switzerland for permission to reproduce different figures related to their HPTLC system.

I am thankful to Prof. Nitin Dubey and his team for contributing an exhaustive chapter on validation of HPTLC method and sharing their knowledge and experience with analytical fraternity. This should help analysts in planning validation of chromatographic methods. Sharing knowledge and experience with bench-analysts for the last 35 years for ultimate successful application has been source of unmatched happiness for me. At the end, I place on record my most sincere appreciation for Mr. Dharmvir for his dedicated support not only in compilation of this monograph but also giving practical shape to many of my ideas.

New Delhi, India

P.D. Sethi, M.Pharm, Ph.D.
Pharmaceutical Analyst

"Have creative mind, evaluate critically and logically."

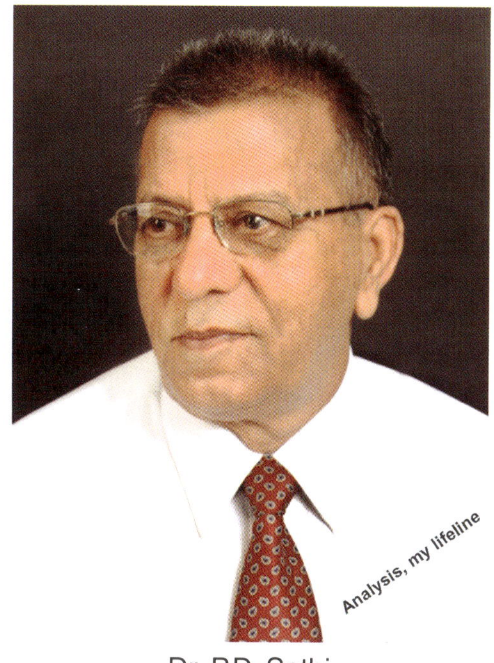

Dr. P.D. Sethi
(1936 –)

Making of An Analyst & The Author (My Story)

"Practical experience is mastered in the laboratory; scientific knowledge is mastered in the library."

Dr. C.K. Atal, my guide for M. Pharm at Punjab University, Chandigarh, now residing at Delhi often asks me, in spite of majoring in pharmacognosy both in M. Pharm. & Ph.D. programmes, how I became a pharmaceutical analyst. This prompted me to pen down my journey towards being an analyst & the author. This is what my story is all about.

I obtained my M. Pharm. (1962) and Ph.D. (1973), both in Pharmacognosy. During my Ph.D. programme, I worked on isolation and characterization of withanolides and physalins from Solanaceous plants. After a short stint at BHU, Varanasi, I joined Central Indian Pharmacopoeia Laboratory (CIPL), Ghaziabad in Sept. 1975 as Senior Scientific Officer (Gr-I). The main function of the laboratory was to update Indian Pharmacopoeia (IP) in addition to analysis of drug samples received from CDSCO and drugs control departments of some States. Being next to the Director, I was entrusted with overall charge of the chemistry division, the major division of the laboratory. The chemistry division had two officers (SSO-II) and few SSA's in addition to about 30 bench analysts.

Before joining CIPL, I had practically no experience in analysis of drugs, thus interacting with analysts during routine rounds of the laboratory was quite embarrassing. I stopped taking rounds of the laboratory and decided first to update my scientific knowledge in the field.

Mr. N.C. Dhawan, then SSA, was the immediate supervising officer responsible for assigning samples to different analysts for testing and guiding them in routine analytical work. During lunch hours, I started discussing with him common analytical methods being followed in the laboratory. However it was felt that both scientific knowledge of the methods and practical experience are very much essential.

Fortunately, the laboratory had a good collection of Indian and foreign analytical journals and books. I started spending most of my free time in the library collecting references and cataloguing them. Occasionally, I visited National Medical Library (NML) New Delhi for the purpose This helped me to a great extent in knowing the scientific as well as practical aspect of different methods. For practical experience, I set up a separate bench-space in the laboratory and started parallel analysis of samples, comparing the assay results with that of the analysts who had been initially assigned the samples for analysis. Limited practical experience along with scientific knowledge of the methods gave me adequate confidence. After about three months, I started taking rounds of the laboratory and interacting with bench-analysts. Whenever draft test reports were submitted to me for scrutiny, I started calling the concerned analyst in my room and discussed the nitty-gritty of each step involved in the analysis, difficulties encountered and how they were solved. These practical tips were regularly recorded and were incorporated as foot notes in my first book "Quantitative Analysis of Pharmaceutical Formulations" published in 1985. I continued the practice of interacting with bench analysts at their working benches and having a separate bench-space for experimental work till my retirement.

Dr. P.R. Pabrai, the director gave me a free hand in organising the laboratory. I constituted a separate R&D group and started working on development of analytical methods on problems often encountered by the industries. Our work was published in important journals and presented at annual Indian Pharmaceutical Congress and much appreciated. Soon our laboratory became the leading centre for R&D work in pharmaceutical analysis with excellent standing among analytical fraternity.

In 1976, during my visit to State Drugs Laboratory, Baroda, Gujarat, I had a chance to study working of their repository for working/reference standards and protocols for analysis of patent and proprietary formulations. I set up a separate section at CIPL for maintaining working/reference standards and analytical protocols and started obtaining protocols for different formulations from the manufacturers. Soon the section developed into a full-fledged division (Repository) with good collection of protocols and working/reference standards. While analysing samples as per protocols received, practical difficulties encountered and changes made were recorded.

In view of contradictory test reports often emanating from different laboratories mainly due to different protocols being followed, to bring uniformity, Drugs Controller of India (DCI) constituted a committee with Director CDL, Calcutta as its chairman, government analysts of Maharashtra, Karnataka and Gujarat as its members and myself as convenor. The methods being followed in different laboratories in respect of certain common formulations were obtained and after comparative evaluation, final methods to be followed were circulated to all laboratories. This exercise gave me several alternate methods for significant number of formulations.

While analysing samples, compendial identification tests, usually based on test tube tests, were being followed. Analysts had then very limited experience in application of thin layer chromatography (TLC). Realizing the practical importance of this technique, I encouraged analysts in the use of this technique, trained them in preparation of laboratory hand-made TLC plates. We locally got fabricated the entire plate-coating assembly suitable for 20 × 10, 10 × 10, 5 × 10 and 2.5 × 10 cm plates and soon TLC was routinely used as an alternative analytical technique for identification. Later on, we could develop semi-quantitative assay method by TLC “Quick Assessment System” for several dosage forms and an analyst could analyze 40-50 samples of such formulations everyday. The use of TLC was further extended to identification of individual component in multi-component formulations. Each densitogram so obtained was traced on paper and attached with analytical data along with detailed chromatographic conditions as a permanent record. Salient feature of this study was that we could work out a single solvent system, so called “Universal Solvent System”, which could separate different ingredients for identification in more than 80 formulations of divergent combinations. TLC data based on actual laboratory experiments was latcr on compiled and published as a book “Identification of Drugs in Pharmaceutical Formulations by TLC” in 1992.

In 1977, our laboratory was approved by Meerut University as a R&D centre and my name was only approved as guide for the Ph.D program. Probably due to my increasing popularity as an analyst because of my professional competency and the university not approving the name of Dr. P.R. Pabrai as guide due to his fewer research publications, created a wedge between us and our relations started drifting. Though there were some administrative reasons, but it will not be appropriate to discuss them. He divested me of all my official responsibilities and withdrew all the facilities including my office room, telephone, peon etc. I was made to sit in the laboratory alone with no staff member allowed to interact with me. All possible efforts were made on daily basis to humiliate and demoralize me. Initially I was quite depressed but with confidence in my professional knowledge and being a **Scorpio** (hindrance and obstacles bring out the best), I decided to accept the situation and make best use of adversity to my advantage. Now when I look back I realize that adversity had in fact been the major driving force for me to be an analyst & the author, for this I am extremely obliged to Dr. P.R. Pabrai. I started spending most of my time in the library, collecting published literature on analytical methods. It was observed that some of the most popular books in pharmaceutical analysis were quite old and not of much use for analysis of currently available formulations, except the book by Hashmi, "Assay of Vitamins". Considering the challenge being faced by analysts for analysis of fixed-dose multi-component formulations due to mutual interference of different ingredients present in the formulations, I decided to explore the possibility of compiling available analytical methods and sharing my practical experience with fellow analysts.

Since I was not allowed to use any of the office facility, I hired a typewriter and requested Mr. V.K. Arora, P.A. to the director to type the draft manuscript of the book at his home. As the subject was very new, no publisher was prepared to take the risk of publishing the book. Ultimately with the help of a friend dealing with sale of scientific books, I decided to get the book published at my own level. In December 1984, during IPC at Bangalore, I circulated a brief synopsis of the proposed book. I was rather thrilled and surprised with the response. Orders for more than 200 copies were received within a week with advance payments.

Believe me, not even a single page of the final manuscript of the proposed book was ready at that stage. I took two months leave and worked for 12-14 hrs a day to complete the manuscript. In those days hand composing was done for final printing. My publisher was based in East Delhi. Daily I used to visit him every evening on my way back home from Ghaziabad to hand over fresh manuscript and collect proof of the earlier part and reach home after 10 pm. The efforts put in by my wife, Usha in managing the home and education of the children is hard to ignore, in fact nothing would have been possible without her full support. When the book ultimately appeared in mid-1985, the entire stock (1000 copies) was sold out in few weeks. The book ultimately established me as an analyst & the author. Although this book was revised in 1992 (2nd ed.), & 1997 (3rd ed.), the first edition (1985) even today is prized possession of analysts and is considered the most popular practical compilation ever published in the field.

After Dr. Pabrai retired in August 1983, in spite of being senior most officer in the laboratory, I was not promoted as director due to some adverse remarks recorded in my ACR by Dr. P.R. Pabrai. Dr. S.C. Sharma was transferred from CDL, Calcutta to CIPL as director on ad hoc basis. After my repeated representation to the authorities of the fact that as per ruling of SC, adverse remarks in the ACR are to be communicated to the officer concerned, which was never done in my case. The authorities, taking a view that sudden sharp fall in the skill of the officer being suggestive of bias, stroke off the adverse remarks and I was promoted as director CIPL in February 1986.

On the special request of Ministry of Health and Family Welfare, the laboratory started the testing of oral contraceptive pills. The analysis of ethinyl estradiol, the minor component required 5 cm glass cell for colorimetric analysis. Most of the laboratories in the country were not equipped with this facility, hence unable to analyse such samples. Although our laboratory was testing the samples the method being tedious and lengthy, only 4-5 samples could be analyzed in a day. Having adequate experience in application of TLC/HPTLC and the laboratory having HPTLC system (Camag), we validated HPTLC method for simultaneous estimation of both ethinyl estradiol and norgestrel and could analyse 20-25 samples each day. The credit for this entire work goes to Dr. Murugesan, then JSA at CIPL and now Director RDTL, Chennai.

In February 1992, I was transferred to Bombay as director CDL. In fact there was no functional laboratory and I was not provided even a chair to sit which had to be borrowed from CDSCO (WZ). Ministry of Health had just taken over possession of part of 4th floor of ESI hospital at Thane. There was hardly any work done on alteration of different wards into the laboratory. Though my office was situated at Antop Hills along with the office of the CDSCO but I was spending most of my time at site coordinating with CPWD who was entrusted with completion of entire project. As the work on the project started progressing satisfactorily, I initiated the process of procurement of laboratory equipments and instruments and recruitment of sanctioned staff. By September 1992, the laboratory was handed over to us and by that time most of the technical and administrative staff was in position. I shifted my office to the laboratory at Thane. All equipments such as IR, HPLC, UV, balances were in position. Microbiology and Pharmacology divisions along with animal house were fully functional. In mid November 1992 the functioning of the laboratory was inaugurated. Within a period of 6-8 months I could establish a well equipped laboratory from scratch with excellent facilities. Leading analysts from the Industries and institutions frequently visited the newly established laboratory to see the set-up and discuss their analytical problems.

Since the analysts were not having adequate work and with past experience in the application of HPTLC, I decided to extend R&D work on the application of HPTLC in analysis of fixed-dose multi-component formulations. Since, CDL was not equipped with HPTLC system, Mr. Charegaonkar, MD, Anchrom Enterprises (I) Pvt. Ltd., Bombay was kind enough to extend all the facilities available at his analytical laboratory in Mulund. Within 2 years, we could develop and standardize HPTLC methods for more than 150 divergent fixed-dose formulations. This project would not have been completed without the support of Ms. Virinda, then JSA, CDL and Sujata of Anchrom. Entire analytical data as obtained in the laboratory and information retrieved from published literature was compiled and published as a book "Quantitative Analysis of Drugs in Pharmaceutical Formulations by HPTLC" in 1999. This book proved to be the ultimate guide for all HPTLC practitioners and even today is cited as reference almost in every publication related to application of HPTLC in pharmaceutical analysis. Chromatographers started associating me with TLC/ HPTLC technique.

HPLC, then another up-coming analytical technique, was gaining popularity. Dr. Vaibhav working as JSA in the laboratory had earlier worked for his Ph.D under Dr. R.T. Sane on application of HPLC in pharmaceutical analysis, I assigned him the job of screening published literature on application of HPLC in analysis of fixed-dose formulations. After getting permission from libraries of IIT, BARC and Bombay college of pharmacy, Dr. Vaibhav regularly visited these libraries and collected copies of published papers. By the time I retired in 1994, I had fairly good collection of published literature on the subject which I continued to update. After I was free from revision of other titles I started work on the compilation of all available data on HPLC and finally volume 1 was published in 2001. In sequence to volume 1, volume 2 appeared in 2006 and volume 3 & 4 in 2010. I intend to continue the series if health and life permits.

During one of my visit to the office of my publisher at Delhi in 1992, I purchased one book Pharmaceutical Analysis (volume 2) by H.J. Roth for our CDL Library. This book contained detailed chemical reactions of drugs based on their functional groups. Since analytical methods described in 1st & 2nd editions of my book "Quantitative Analysis of Pharmaceutical Formulation" were primarily based on colour reactions of the functional groups with specific reagents, I realized that for proper understanding of the methods, chemistry involved i.e. "Reaction Mechanism" need be provided along with the methods.

It is how the idea of this project was conceptualized. I discussed this subject with Ms. Padma, one of the JSA in the laboratory who had just obtained her M.Sc. in organic chemistry. She readily agreed to take up the project and could write down reaction mechanism for almost all the methods included in 1st & 2nd edition of my book as well as in respect of published methods. When I retired, the literature on HPLC collected by Dr. Vaibhav and reaction mechanism compiled by Ms. Padma was the only treasure I carried home and left behind a fully equipped functional laboratory with well trained analysts.

During the first APA convention held at Bombay in 1997, I presented "Reaction Mechanism" of some important pharmacopoeial identification tests. The presentation being unique was well appreciated. I made up my mind to revise the 3rd edition of my book giving reaction mechanism for each method included in 1st, 2nd, 3rd, editions of the book. In view of complexity of the subject, I initially did harbour some doubts about its ultimate completion. Since it was my **DESIRE** to complete the project before I close my shop, knowing fully well that nothing can be achieved without dedication, and it shall need constant adaptation, definite level of discipline and above all hunger to keep going, I decided to accept the challenge with **SELF BELIEF**.

It gives me pride to record that 4th edition of my book *Quantitative Analysis of Pharmaceutical Formulations – Methods with Reaction Mechanism*, a 4-volume series, has just been published. It took me about 20 years to complete – my ultimate dream.

The books authored by me so far in the field of pharmaceutical analysis using different analytical techniques (UV-Vis spectrophotometry, TLC, HPTLC, HPLC) continue to have excellent response and have proved to be a cradle for my success. How useful these books have been to analysts in discharging their analytical functions; I leave the decision to them. Although I can claim being an analyst by virtue of my professional contribution, but what standing I enjoy among pharmaceutical analysts of the country, let the present and future generation of analytical fraternity take a view. However today whatever I possess i.e. name, fame and money, it is simply because of my being an analyst & the author.

"No one is ever born talented nor talent obtained as a gift or lucky coincidence. It is a resource acquired through ones own endeavour, in this process, others may provide some help, inspiration and guidance."

"DESIRE is perhaps the starting point of achieving something."

"Belief is the knowledge that we can do some thing. It is the inner feeling that what we undertake, we can accomplish."

I am deeply indebted to Mr. Dilip Charegaonkar, M.D. Anchrom Enterprises (I) Pvt. Ltd. Mumbai for extending every possible support for me to be a sound HPTLC practitioner. I express my gratitude to Anchrom Enterprises (I) Pvt. Ltd., Mumbai and KONGPOSH Publication Pvt. Ltd. New Delhi for independently establishing lifetime annual awards for Best Research Papers in HPTLC Analysis & Pharmaceutical Analysis respectably in recognition of my contribution in the field.

I humbly bow my head before the temple (Central Indian Pharmacopoeia laboratory), where I started my analytical career and which provided me all the facilities and inspiration to be an analyst. I express my gratitude to all the bench analysts of CIPL particularly N. C. Dhawan and Ms. Savita Devi from whom I learnt basics of analysis. In my becoming an analyst & the author, Dr. Y.K.S. Rathore, Dr. N. Murugesan and Dr. S.C. Mathur had played major role, thanks to them for giving practical shape to my ideas.

Before I close my story I would like to share one important aspect of my being an author. I had no access to any of the modern gadgets i.e. Computer, Internet, E-mail, etc. All the published literature on different subjects was surveyed by frequent personal visits to different libraries. The manuscript of all books authored by me had been handwritten and given to the publisher for publication. It was only the **passion** to achieve something that kept me performing.

At the end I would like to express my sincere gratitude to fellow analysts, students, researchers, teachers, professionals and mentors for their continuous support and inspiration in shaping my analytical career spanning about four decades.

With a pledge to dedicate my knowledge and experience to the fellow analysts, I end my story with the hope that it will inspire some to be analyst.

P.D. Sethi

"Nothing dies faster than the idea kept in closed mind, so share your knowledge and experience and let the world be richer."

Brief Contents
(Volumes 1 – 3)

VOLUME 1

VOLUME 2

VOLUME 3

CHAPTER 3

Introduction

- Hand-made layers
- Pre-coated plates
- Different support surfaces
- Code letters and numbers for product identification
- Comparative specifications of TLC, HPTLC and UTLC pre-coated plates
- Common commercially available pre-coated plates
- Commonly available sorbents for TLC and preparative layers
- Plate sizes (formats)
- Pre-washing of pre-coated layers
- Activation of pre-coated layers
- Sample preparation
- Sample application
- Mobile phase (MP)
- Relative humidity of saturated salt solutions
- Processing in developing chamber
- Development
- Parameters affecting HPTLC performance
- Detection and visualization
- Post-chromatographic derivatization by spraying
- Quantitative evaluation
- Selection of suitable wavelength for densitometric scanning
- Reversed-phase TLC/HPTLC

Various steps involved in TLC/HPTLC/Planar chromatography

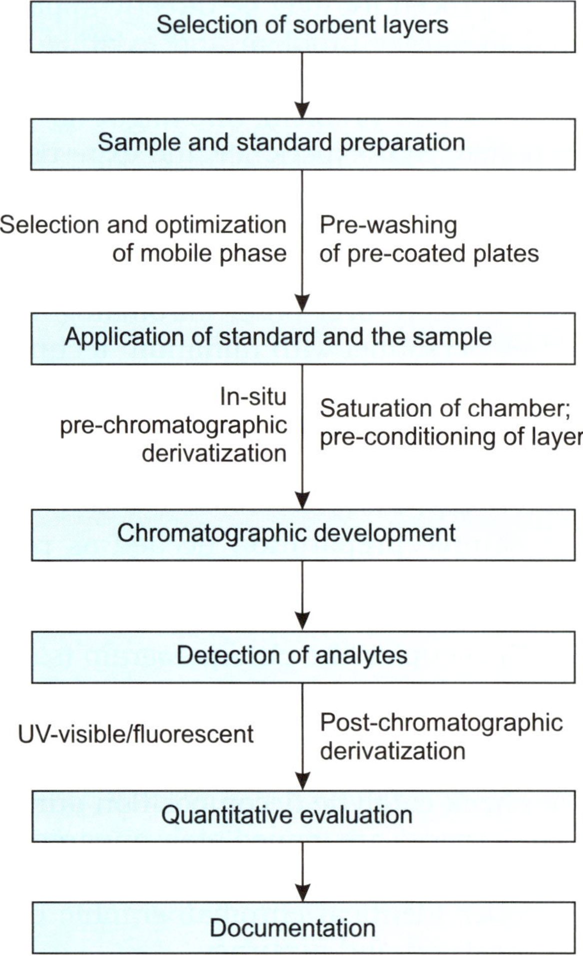

for stability testing. These advantages offered by HPTLC add up to compelling reasons for choosing it as a sound analytical technique.

You can rely on TLC and HPTLC solutions to reach your analytical goal faster and easier.

Plates

Hand-made layers (self-prepared layers)

In view of easily available TLC/HPTLC pre-coated plates, it is not commercially viable to prepare the plates in the laboratory. Further, for consistent chromatographic behaviour with respect to different chromatographic formulations, surface homogeneity and uniform layer thickness being important, the use of hand-coated plates is on the decline except in very specific cases. However, it was felt that to be a sound TLC/HPTLC practitioner, the chromatographer ought to have some basic experience of preparing plates in the laboratory to meet any exigency. Therefore, brief procedure for preparing the slurry of different sorbents for coating and important general precautions have been described. The amount of sorbent indicated in each case is sufficient to coat 5 plates of 20 × 20 cm.

Hand-made layers can be prepared by using suitable apparatus (spreader and aligning tray) for coating the glass plate with suitable sorbent. Since commercially available coating apparatus is suitable for coating only 20 × 20 cm and 10 × 20 cm plates, to meet the frequent demand of the laboratory for plates of different formats, the author got fabricated spreaders along with aligning trays suitable for coating plates of different formats, i.e., 10 × 10 cm, 5 × 10 cm, 2.5 × 10 cm for routine use.

The following precautions must be taken while coating the plates:

1. All the plates should be of same dimensions (length, breadth and thickness), preferably cut from single glass sheet.
2. Surface of the glass plates should be absolutely even, smooth and without scratches.
3. Clean the plates with water, followed by acetone.
4. Handle the plate with gloves so that no grease is transferred from the fingers on to the plates, otherwise adhesion of the sorbent layer shall be reduced.
5. Freshly coated plates should be left on the stand/tray till transparency of the layer has disappeared.
6. The layer should appear homogenous in transmitted light and show no unevenness or streaks and no large grains should be visible in reflected light.
7. Adhesiveness of the layer can be tested by gentle rubbing of fingers across the surface of the sorbent layer.
8. The layer on the edges of the plate which is under the base of spreader is thinner. About 1–2 cm of sorbent layer is removed with the help of thumb and index finger before application of samples. This is to avoid boundary/ edge effect.

Procedure for preparing different hand-made layers

1. *Cellulose (native):* To 15 g of native fibrous cellulose, add about 100 ml of distilled water, mix with an electric stirrer for 1 min to produce a homogeneous

slurry. Spread the slurry with an applicator set at 250 mm. Allow the plates to dry in air and then dry at 110°C for 15 min.

Note: Amount of water can be varied depending upon the thickness of slurry.

2. *Cellulose with starch as binder:* Suspend 0.4 g of starch in about 10 ml of water, pour the suspension into 90 ml of boiling water. Boil the suspension for 60 s, add 20 g of acid-washed cellulose. Homogenize the slurry with the help of electric stirrer (30 s). Plates are immediately coated while the slurry is still hot. Allow the plates to dry in air or by heating at 110°C for 45 min. Activation at elevated temperature is avoided. Usual layer thickness so obtained is 200 μm.

3. *Cellulose (microcrystalline):* Suspend 20 g of cellulose (microcrystalline) in 60 ml of water. Stir in an electric mixture exactly for 30 s to homogenize the slurry. Plates are coated with spreader. Dry the plates in air or by heating at 110°C for 30 min. No activation at elevated temperature is required. Layer thickness is about 100 μm.

4. *Cellulose (microcrystalline) with fluorescent indicator:* Suspend 25 g of cellulose (microcrystalline) in 40 ml of methanol (this will ensure uniform distribution of indicator), add 20 ml of water. Homogenize in electric stirrer exactly for 30 s. The plates so prepared are dried in the air or by heating at 110°C for 30 min. No activation is necessary at elevated temperature. Layer thickness is about 100 μm.

5. *Acetylated cellulose + $CaSO_4 \cdot ½H_2O$:* Suspend 30 g of acetylated cellulose and 4.5 g of $CaSO_4$ in a mixture containing 60 ml of water and 10 ml of methanol. Stir in an electric stirrer for 30 s to get homogeneous slurry. Sometimes air bubbles get trapped which can be removed by pouring 2–3 ml of methanol over slurry, followed by shaking. Use the slurry thus prepared within 30 min for coating the plates. Dry the coated plates in air or by heating at 110°C for 30 min, layer thickness is about 130 μm.

6. *Silica gel or silica gel G:* Suspend 30 g of silica gel or silica gel G in 60–65 ml of water, mix in an electric stirrer to get homogeneous slurry. The plates so coated may be dried in air or by heating for 45 min at 110°C. In case of silica gel G, the slurry must be used within 2 min. Activation of plates can be carried out by heating at 110°C for 30 min. Layer thickness is usually 250 μm.

7. *Silica gel with starch:* Suspend 1 g of starch in about 10 ml of water, pour the suspension into 90 ml of boiling water, boil for 60 s, add 30 g of silica gel, shake to get homogeneous slurry. The plates so coated are dried in the air or by heating at 110°C for 45 min. For activation of the plates, heating at 110°C for 45 min is adequate. Usual layer thickness is 250 μm. Not suitable for charring reaction and also with iodine (universal detection reagent).

8. *Silica gel 60 PF_{254} and Silica gel 60 $PF_{254+366}$ (layer thickness – 1.5 mm):* Suspend 200 g of sorbent in 50–520 ml of water in 2 L round bottom flask, swirl gently without shaking. Allow the suspension to stand for 1 hr and then spread quickly on grease-free plates with coating machine. Adjust to 2.0 mm. Store the prepared plates at room temperature for 2 days in order to dry and then activate at 120°C in drying cupboard for 2 h.

Note:

- 200 g of sorbent is sufficient to coat 5 plates of 20 × 20 cm to give final layer thickness of 1.5 mm.
- To produce layers free from cracks, it is important that plates be dried on an even surface in a small draft-free room, no entry being allowed during drying process.
- In some cases, it can be advantageous to adjust the quantity of water.

9. *Silica gel 60 PF_{254} containing gypsum (layer thickness – 10.0 mm):* Suspend 400 g of sorbent in 650 ml of water in 2 L round bottom flask, shake for 1 min. Immediately pour the suspension onto clean grease-free plates placed in casting frame. After about 30 min, when the mass is solidified, remove the plates from the frame and allow them to dry at room temperature for 3 days. Place the pre-dried plates in a cold drying cupboard and heat to 60°C for 1 hr.

Note: 400 g of the sorbent is sufficient to give one plate of 40 × 20 cm or two plates of 20 × 20 cm.

Precautions while handling hand-made layers

- Silica gel G contains gypsum as binder which is totally inert. It contains about 13% calcium sulphate. Such layers are quite soft and get easily damaged, however, while mobile phase is travelling, the layer gets stuck to the plate allowing chromatographic separation to proceed smoothly. Such plates being softer, it is easier to scrap the sorbent, extract the analyte for quantitative analysis.
- Handle the plates with rubber gloves so that no grease is transferred from fingers to the glass plates as it will result in reduced adhesion of the layer.
- Volume of water indicated for suspending sorbents is approximate, may need slight alteration.
- Setting time for gypsum-containing sorbents is 2–4 min, operation to be carried out quickly, increasing the amount of water increases setting time.

Important conditions for preparation of some hand-made TLC layers

	Amount of sorbent	*Amount of water*	*Adjusted layer thickness*	*Layer thickness after drying*	*Drying time in the air*	*Activation Time*	*Activation Temp.*	*Notes*
	(g)	(ml)	(μm)	(μm)	(min)	(min)	(°C)	
Aluminium oxide 60 G	30	40	300	250	60	30	120	
Aluminium oxide 60 GF_{254}	30	40	300	250	60	30	120	
Cellulose	25	100	250	100	60	30	120	60–90 s electric mixer at slow stirring rates
Florisil®	25	60	300	250	60	30	120	
Silica gel 60 G	30	60	250	200	30	30	105	Setting time of gypsum: 2–4 min!
Silica gel 60 GF_{254}	30	40	250	200	30	30	105	Setting time of gypsum: 2–4 min!
TLC-Silica gel 60 G	30	65	250	200	120	30	105	Setting time of gypsum: 2–4 min!
TLC-Silica gel 60 GF_{254}	30	65	250	200	120	30	105	Setting time of gypsum: 2–4 min!
Silica gel 60 H	30	65–70	250	200	120	60	120	
Silica gel 60 HF_{254}	30	65–70	250	200	120	60	120	
Silica gel 60 $HF_{254 + 366}$	30	65–70	250	200	120	60	120	
TLC-Silica gel 60 H	30	65	250	200	120	30	105	
TLC-Silica gel 60 HF_{254}	30	65	250	200	120	30	105	
Kieselguhr G	40	100–110	300	250	60	30	120	

***Courtesy:* Merck Specialities Private Limited, India.**

Note:

- Amount of water indicated is approximate and may be altered slightly as necessary.
- The layer thickness setting for coating apparatus and layer thickness obtained after drying are only approximate.
- Drying time in the air and activation time are approximate.
- Usually setting time for gypsum-containing sorbents is 2–4 min, so coating operation need to be carried out briskly.
- Increasing the amount of water for gypsum-containing sorbents increases the setting time.
- Camag and Desaga are the most popular commercial suppliers of coating machines.
- Although predominantly gypsum ($CaSO_4$) has been used as binder, organic binders such as carboxymethyl cellulose, starch (1–2%), polyvinyl alcohol (1–5%) have also been used. Although these binders gave stronger binding to the layers but had disadvantage of being soluble in aqueous-based solvents and detection was not possible by charring with sulphuric acid followed by heating.

Pre-coated plates

With the availability of pre-coated plates commercially, the use of laboratory hand-made plates is on decline. The pre-coated plates with different support material (glass, aluminium, plastic) and with different sorbent layers are available in different formats and thickness by various manufacturers [Merck, Germany; Whatman International Ltd., England; Macherey-Nagel (M&N), Germany; Schleicher & Schuell, Germany; and Analtech, USA]. Usually plates with sorbent thickness of 100–250 μm are used for qualitative and quantitative analysis. However, for preparative TLC work, plates with sorbent thickness of 0.5–2.0 mm are available in addition to chemically modified layers. Although label on the box of pre-coated plate shall indicate type of plate (TLC/HPTLC), fluorescent indicator and layer thickness, but it is likely that plates of different manufacturers may provide different separation results. The reason for this can be particle size or pore size of silica gel as well as amount and type of binder which may vary from manufacturer to manufacturer. Further, surface smoothness and homogeneity of the layer is an important factor for considering the quality of the pre-coated plates. It is therefore advised that for developing and regular use of a method, plates of one manufacturer may be employed. However the suitability of plates of other manufacturers may be examined during validation of the method. Incidentally, close review of the published work as embodied in this text reveals that chromatographers are predominantly using Merck's pre-coated plates probably due to easy availability and economically priced.

Commercially available pre-coated plates contain 1–2% organic polymeric binder. These binders provide smooth abrasive-resistant surface and effectively ensures binding of even smallest particles of silica gel to different back-material i.e. glass, aluminium and plastic. Quality of chromatographic separation is very superior and provides more reproducible results as compared to hand-made plates.

Different types of support surface

Glass support: It is resistant to heat and chemicals, easy to handle and always offers superior flat and smooth surface for chromatographic work; disadvantage being fragility, relatively high weight (plate is usually 1.3 mm thick), additional packing material and higher production cost. The pre-coated plates with glass support are therefore most expensive ready-to-use layers. Do not place glass plates directly on hot plate. It can cause uncontrolled and irregular breaking of plates.

Code letters and numbers used in product designation

G	= Gypsum ($CaSO_4 . ½H_2O$) used as a binder
S	= Starch, used as a binder (not suitable for detection with iodine)
O	= Organic binder (polymeric organic compounds); organic binders impart mechanical strength, durability and abrasion resistance to layers, hence least damaged during shipping and handling
H	= Containing no foreign binder
R	= Specially purified layers
W	= Water wettable layers; water-tolerant
F	= Layers containing fluorescent indicators
$F_{254+366}$	= Fluorescent indicators with respective excitation wavelengths
P	= Layers for preparative chromatography (thickness 0.5–2 mm)
F_{254}	= Indicator which produces green fluorescence at an excitation wavelength of 254 nm
F_{254s}	= Layers with acid-stable fluorescent indicator that is stimulated to pale blue fluorescence on emission at 254 nm, usually used in reversed-phase layers
C	= Channelled layers (layers divided into lanes), prevent cross-contamination while separating multiple samples
RP	= Reversed-phase
RP-8	= Reversed-phase with C_8 hydrocarbon chain
RP-12	= Reversed-phase with C_{12} hydrocarbon chain
RP-18	= Reversed-phase with C_{18} hydrocarbon chain
RP-2	= Reversed-phase with dimethylsilyl modification
NH_2	= Hydrophilic layers with amino modification
CN	= Hydrophilic layers with cyano modification
CHIR	= Chiral layers for separation of optically active isomers based on ligand exchange
DIOL	= Hydrophilic layers with DIOL modification
40, 60	= Mean pore size in Å

Polyester (plastic) sheets (0.2 mm thick): More economical as they are produced even in roll forms, unbreakable, less packing material, less shelf space for storage, can be cut to any required format. Spots can be cut and eluted, thus eliminating dust due to scraping of layer. Charring reactions are possible but temperature should not exceed 120°C as the plates are dimensionally unstable (lose shape) beyond this temperature. Thus rarely used because of their poor thermal stability.

Aluminium sheet (0.1 mm thick): Aluminium sheets as support offer the same advantage as polyester support but with increased temperature resistance. However, with eluents containing high concentration of mineral acids or concentrated ammonia, one may find problem as they will chemically attack aluminium. Aluminium sheets are otherwise compatible with organic solvents and organic acids such as formic acid and acetic acid.

In HPTLC, the smaller particle size, narrow particle size distribution, higher packing density, hence better surface homogeneity, provide several advantages:

- Smaller compact zones, better resolution, increased separation efficiency.
- Shorter analysis time as migration distance is almost half as compared to that of classical TLC layer.
- Increased detection sensitivity because of higher surface concentration of sample.

Comparative specifications of HPTLC, TLC and UTLC

Specifications	*HPTLC*	*TLC*	*UTLC*
Mean particle size (μm)	5–6	10–12	Monolithic layer (no particle, no binder, no indicator)
Particle size distribution (μm)	4–8	5–20	—
Layer thickness (μm)	200 (100)	250 (200)	10
Pore diameter	60 Å	40 Å, 60 Å, 80 Å, 100 Å	Mesopores 3–4 nm Macropore 1–2 μm
Typical plate height (μm)	12	30	—
Band size (mm)	5–10	10–15	—
Spot size (mm)	≤ 1	2–5	—
Sample volume	0.1–0.5 μl	1–5 μl	Spot 5–20 nl Band ≥ 100 nl
Mobile phase volume (ml)	20	100	1–4
Plate format (cm)	As required	As required	6 × 3.6
Number of samples per plate (20 × 20 cm)	< 36 (72)	< 20	< 10
Typical migration distance (mm)	30–60	100–150	10–30
Typical separation time (min)	3–20	20–200	1–6
Detection limits (absorption)	100–500 pg	1–5 ng	10 pg
Detection limits (fluorescence)	5–10 pg	50–100 pg	1 pg

Courtesy: **Merck Specialities Private Limited, India.**

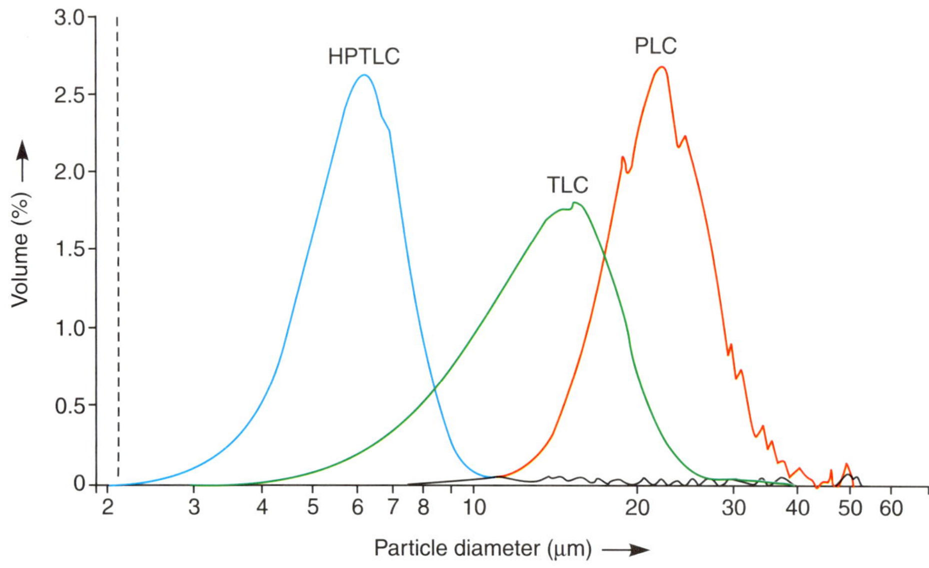

Comparative particle size distribution of TLC, HPTLC and PLC (Preparative layer chromatography).

Courtesy: **Merck Specialities Private Limited, India.**

- Low signal-to-noise ratio, hence suitable for in situ quantitative analysis.
- Efficiency decreases with increasing solvent migration, shorter development distances are mandatory in HPTLC but not in conventional large particle TLC layers.
- Additional sample loading: In HPTLC, the distance between spots, from starting line and bottom or from side edges of the plate is 0.5 cm compared to 1–2 cm for TLC, resulting in increased space for accommodating additional samples.

Common commercially available pre-coated plates and their application

Silica gel 60 and 60 F_{254}: More than 80% analysis is done on this layer. Silica gel 60 has pore diameter of 60 Å, pore volume of 0.8 ml/g and specific surface area 520 m^2/g. Unique organic polymers used as binder have very adherent and hard surface which does not crack or blister. These plates are suitable for adsorption and partition chromatography. These plates are available as glass-, aluminium-, plastic-backed in broad range of sizes to suit application. Aluminium-/plastic-backed plates, being flexible, can be cut to the required format for specific application. For detection of colourless substances, plates with two levels of fluorescent indicator are available – green fluorescence F_{254} (manganese activated zinc silicate or blue fluorescence F_{254s} (magnesium

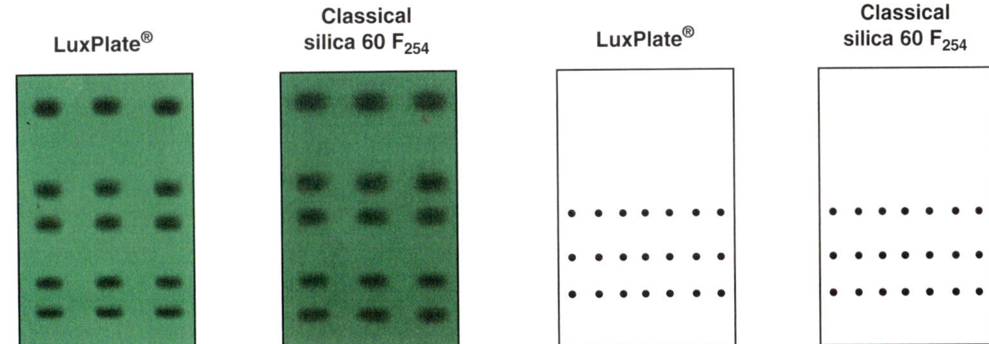

Comparative brightness of Lux silica gel 60 F_{254} plate and classical silica gel 60 F_{254} plate.

***Courtesy:* Merck Specialities Private Limited, India.**

wolframate). Both indicators fluoresce in UV light when excited at 254 nm and detected by fluorescence quenching. Specially developed high fluorescence Lux Plates® contain higher content of fluorescent indicator for improved identification of separated compounds and also contain higher level of binder to provide robust and abrasion-resistant surface. Allows separation of large range of different substances such as aflatoxins, benzodiazepines, carbohydrates, fatty acids, glycosides, mycotoxins, sulphonamides, surfactants and tetracyclines.

High purity silica gel 60: Suitable for analysis of aflatoxins.

Aluminium oxide: Aluminium oxide (basic or neutral) of 60 Å or 150 Å pore size with or without fluorescent indicator is utilized. Basic substances such as alkaloids are best separated on basic aluminium oxide plates, whereas neutral aluminium oxide is best suited for substances such as steroids.

Kieselguhr: A natural diatomaceous earth is best suited for separation of polar or moderately polar substances.

Kieselguhr + Silica gel 60 (mixed layers): These mixed layers are suitable for certain special applications such as separation of inorganic ions, pesticides and some steroids. Other mixed layers available are of aluminium oxide + acetylated cellulose, cellulose + silica gel.

LiChrospher®: Special spherical-shaped silica gel with small particles of 7 µm and narrow particle size distribution as used in HPLC. Such plates offer the ultimate in TLC to provide high throughput, 20% reduced running time, highly compact zones and lower detection limits.

Cellulose and cellulose F: Suitable for separation of hydrophilic substances by partition chromatography. Classical TLC plates use microcrystalline cellulose whereas HPTLC plates use high purity rod-shape microcrystalline cellulose resulting in reduced diffusion of analytes. Both fluorescent indicators – shortwave UV-254 nm and longwave UV-366 nm – are used. Suitable for separation of amino acids, sugars, antibiotics and other labile substances which cannot be chromatographed on silica gel layer.

PEI cellulose: It is polyethylenimine modified cellulose layer. It acts as strongly basic anion-exchanger, suitable for analysis of amino acids, peptides and nucleotides or nucleosides. Such plates should be stored at 0–4 °C to avoid deterioration.

Silica gel G (gypsum as binder): These plates have recently been introduced by Merck-Millipore. These plates are required to be employed in certain monographs official in Indian Pharmacopoeia and are available in 20×20 cm format.

Silica gel, chemically modified (NH_2, CN, Diol): These modified silica layers are less polar and are well suited for separation of hydrophilic substances. CN-modified layers are silica gel 60 modified with cyano propyl group, whereas diol-modified layer uses vicinal diol alkyl ether. Both these layers are moderately polar, hence with their intermediate properties these can be used both for normal and reverse-phase chromatographic separation whereas amino-modified layer provides basic ion-exchange characteristics. This property allows separation of charged compounds such as nucleotides, purines, pyrimidines and phenols. In addition, NH_2-modified layers allow reagent-free detection of certain compounds by thermochemical fluorescence activation such as sucralose. Since most of the compounds separated on these layers are colourless, so they contain fluorescent acid-stable UV indicator UV F_{254s}. The substances are detected by fluorescent quenching.

CN (cyano): Plasticizers, pesticides, tetracyclines, benzodiazepines, gallic acid esters, steroids, pharmaceutical preservatives.

Diol: Antibiotics, steroids, glycosides, aromatic amines.

NH_2: Carboxylic acids, phenols, vitamins (B_1, B_6, B_{12}) and sucralose.

CHIR: Resolution of enantiomeric substances for optical purity such as amino acids, dipeptides and lactones. These plates are coated with reversed-phase silica gel and then impregnated with a chiral selector (a proline derivative) and copper (++) ion. The separation of optical isomers is based on ligand exchange, the chiral selector (on the plate) and the enantiomer to be separated. The mixed chelate-complex of diastereomeric substances with transition element (Cu^{++}) have different stabilities which results in chromatographic separation. For optimal separation and reproducibility of Rf values, activation prior to spotting (100°C for 15 min) and chamber saturation may be required.

Application of chiral plate in separation of amino acids, dipeptides, lactones and thiazolidine derivatives has been reported.

RP-modified plates (RP-2, RP-8, RP-12, RP-18): These layers are suitable for separation problems that cannot be satisfactorily solved by normal silica gel layers. Such layers are less dependant on atmospheric humidity, suitable for separation of compounds which are labile to oxidative degradation. Such layers provide good correlation with HPLC RP-columns and allows TLC for method development as pilot method for HPLC. Since aliphatic hydrocarbons are used as modifier, therefore hydrocarbon chain length in combination with degree of modification strongly affects retention characteristics. Retention of sample and migration time increase in order of RP-2, RP-8, RP-12, RP-18 using the same solvent composition and other chromatographic conditions. Increase in retention means decrease in Rf value. RP-2 layers can tolerate upto 80% water in solvent system; tolerance to water contents decreases as the carbon chain increases from RP-2 to RP-18.

Chemical reaction of the polar silanol group of silica gel with alkyl silanes of different chain lengths yields reversed phases. Hydrophobic character increases with increasing chain lengths of hydrocarbon. Low degree of modification means weak interaction between the sample molecule and the stationary phase, thus leading to higher Rf values as HPTLC plates with silica gel 60RP-18W with low degree of surface modification can be wetted and developed even with water. Show higher Rf values than HPTLC with RP-C18 modification.

Applications: Non-polar substances (lipids), fatty acids, carotenoids, steroids, cholesterol and its esters. Polar substances, basic and acidic drugs which are likely to decompose on active layers, vitamins, antibiotics, amino acids, chloroplast pigments, phenothiazine tranquilizers, cannabinoids, preservatives, sulphonamides, insecticides (DDT, endrin, eldrin), alkaloids (ephedrine, atropine, scopolamine, codeine, morphine), barbiturates, analgesics, cardiac drugs, sweeteners, food dyes, tranquilizers and antioxidants.

Multiformat plates (pre-scored): These plates are pre-scored and can be snapped with fingers to smaller size. Number of possible plates depend on scoring such as 20 × 20 cm plate is normally scored upto 7 different formats such as 15 × 20, 10 × 20, 5 × 20, 10 × 15, 10 × 10, 5 × 10, 5 × 5.

GLP plates: These plates comply with GLP, available in various formats with or without fluorescence indicators. Each GLP plate carries item No., batch No., individual plate No. for traceability and documentation. These plates provide separation profile as per TLC or HPTLC plates.

Preparative layer plates (PLC): Layer thickness ranges from 0.5–2 mm with or without fluorescent indicator. These layers are available as silica gel,

Possible modifications

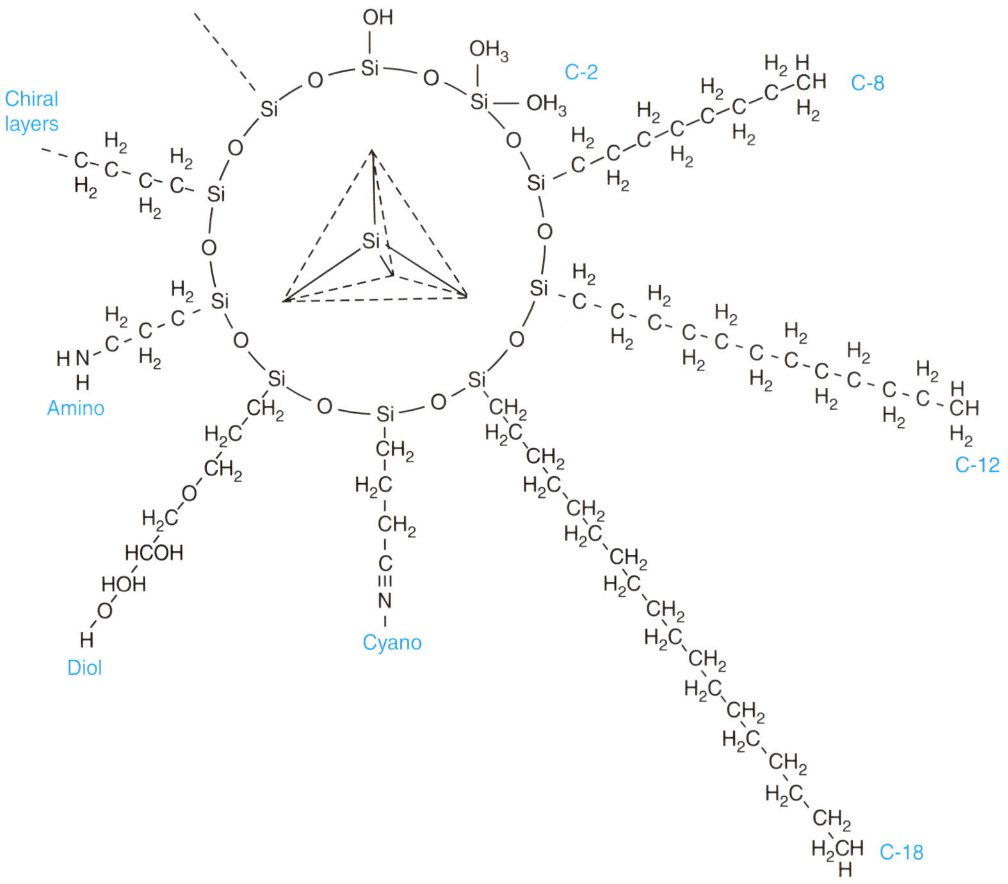

Chemically modified silica gel layers (CN, NH_2, Diol, C-2, C-8, C-12, C-18 and Chiral).

RP-18 modified silica or aluminium oxide. In such plates, samples are applied as band across the whole width of the plate and substances are usually detected by UV. These are usually available as pre-coated soft layers, to be used when separated substances are to be recovered, usually give less sample resolution than analytical plates. These plates are preferred to column chromatography due to ease in recovery of separated zones; sample volume should be moderate.

Note: Suitable for cleaning and enrichment synthetic reaction mixtures, natural products, plant extracts and biological products.

Hybrid plates (RP-18WF$_{254s}$): These plates are suitable both for reversed-phase and normal-phase chromatography. They can be developed using aqueous mobile phases as well as mixture of aqueous-organic solvents. HPTLC grade silica gel 60 (mean pore size 6 nm) forms the basis for these plates. Controlled reaction conditions ensure that certain portion of available silanol groups are chemically bonded with octadecyl chain whereas the remaining silanol groups remain non-bonded, thus giving hybrid (hydrophobic and hydrophilic) character to the plates. Conventional reversed-phase plates resist the flow of eluent considerably and sometime completely depending on the proportion of water present in the mobile phase. To avoid this limitation, the partial chemical bonding of silanol groups results in the hybrid nature of the plate, which makes the plates wettable (W) depending on the residual hydrophilicity of layer. In such plate, the development time is significantly reduced for strongly polar eluents. As untreated silanol groups are blocked by water in the eluent, this type of incompletely silanized RP coating along with high water contents reversed-phase eluents, demonstrates strong reversed-phase characteristics as compared to fully silanized RP layers, conventionally used. Such hybrid plates have application in chromatographic separation of preservatives, barbiturates, analgesics, phenothiazines, amino acids and flavonoids.

Prescreen TLC plates: RPTLC C18 plates in the size 5×7.5 cm are available for quick and inexpensive preview of separation traits prior to HPLC analysis. This can be of help in optimizing sample preparation parameters for use in HPLC.

Proteochrom® silica gel 60F$_{254s}$ HPTLC plates: These plates employ extra thin layer (100 μm), extra smooth layer of silica gel 60F$_{254s.}$ Due to special binder composition, these plates are highly stable in water whereas Proteochrom® cellulose HPTLC plates also use high density extra fine layer (100 μm) of high performance microcrystalline cellulose These should be stored between 0–4°C to avoid deterioration. These plates are suitable for analysis of peptides and protein digests. These layers are highly stable in water, hence suitable for use of aqueous solvent systems.

Dual phase plates: There are two distinct stationary phases on the plate. Most commonly two phases are normal phase and reversed phase, other combinations are also possible. Such plates are used for two-dimensional chromatography. In one phase, silica gel is commonly used for normal phase whereas for silica gel RP-18 is the other phase. With such plates using two-dimensional chromatography, large number of components can be resolved as compared to normal linear chromatography. This is also called two-dimensional mapping.

Concentrating zone plates: TLC, HPTLC concentrating zone plates provide 2.5 cm zone whereas PLC plates provide zone of 4 cm. In fact, concentrating zone has large pore silica gel where sample is initially applied and then a selective separation layer. Irrespective of shape, size and position of the sample spot, it gets concentrated as band at the interface of two adsorbents and then the separation starts. Specially RP-18 modified layers are also available for PAH (polycyclic aromatic hydrocarbons) analysis.

Ultra-thin monolithic silica gel plates (UTLC): These are thin layer chromatography plates with layer thickness of 10 μm and has mesopores of 3–4 nm and macropores of 1–2 μm. These layers provide increased sensitivity and separation is complete in 5 min. UTLC layers bring miniaturization in TLC. It is suitable for low analyte concentration and can be used for analysis of steroids, amino acids, phthalates and phenols.

Pre-coated plates (20 × 20 cm) of silica gel (250 μm) impregnated with ammonium sulphate for separation of detergents and polymide-6 (100 μm) with or without fluorescent indicator (UV 254) in different format for separation of dansylamino acids, antioxidants, optical brighteners, dyes and pesticides are commercially available (Macherey-Nagel, Germany).

Preparation of modified layers by impregnation

1. **Impregnation of sorbent before coating:** While preparing hand-made layers, the slurry of the sorbent is prepared in aqueous solution of acid, base, salts, buffers and complexing agents instead of water. The modified slurry is used for coating the glass plates as usual. The coated plate is dried and activated prior to use. Impregnating agent has to be non-volatile. Boric acid, oxalic acid, phosphate buffers, silver nitrate and EDTA are used as modifying agents. This technique is limited to water-soluble agents only.
2. **By treating the pre-coated plates:**
   (a) By dipping the pre-coated plate in suitable concentration of impregnating agent in volatile solvent. The solvent is then allowed to evaporate, the impregnated layer is activated and used.
   (b) By blank development of the pre-coated plate in solution of impregnating agent in volatile solvent to a pre-specified distance, dried and used.
   (c) By spraying the solution of impregnating agent uniformly on the pre-coated plate, dried to remove solvent and used.

Note: Silicon oil (5% in pet. ether) and liquid paraffin (5–10% in pet. ether) have been used as impregnating agents to give hydrophobic character to the silica gel layer. These have been successfully used as substitute for RP C-18 layers by the author for separation of several multi-component formulations.

No interference was observed in densitometric scanning of such impregnated plates, however, while eluting the analyte, the contamination with impregnating liquid does exist.

Note:

- Not more than one pack of same product should be kept in the laboratory.
- For rarely used pre-coated plates, the label of the manufacturer should not be removed for correct identity at later date and should not be stored in the laboratory to avoid contamination.
- Once the plate is removed from the pack, write the item No. on the right-hand edge of the plate for correct identification at later date.
- Pre-coated plates should be stored with sorbent layer underneath and covered with plastic to avoid depositing laboratory contaminants on the active layers.
- The plates should be touched with fingertips preferably of both hands on the cut edges.
- Transportation of the plates should always be done in drying racks, commercially available or home fabricated.
- Avoid leaving fingerprints on the plates, they are likely to be visible after derivatization by some reagent such as ninhydrin, methanolic sulphuric acid.
- Perspiration is likely to appear as unknown extra spot/zone and can interfere in the quality of the chromatogram.

Phosphorescent and fluorescent indicators

For detection in absorbance mode, many commercially available pre-coated plates contain inorganic phosphorescent indicators designated by F_{254}. They exhibit yellow, bright green or blue phosphorescence when excited by UV light at 254 nm. Most commonly used indicators are uranyl acetate, magnesium wolframate (acid-resistant), manganese zinc silicate, zinc cadmium sulphide, activated zinc silicate, alkaline earth metal silicates and tin strontium phosphate. The detection by absorbance is due to quenching of phosphorescence by sample components. Pink or violet spots/bands may be observed due to quenching on green phosphorescent background. Most of these inorganic indicators do not get eluted with mobile phases and are also not affected by detection reagents. Organic fluorescent indicators used are optical brighteners, hydroxypyrene sulphonates, fluorescein and rhodamine dyes. For detection, these indicators fluoresce when excited at UV 366 nm.

Commonly available sorbents for thin layer chromatography (TLC) and preparative layer chromatography (PLC)

Sorbent	*Particle size* (μm)	*Application*	*Usual packing* (kg)
Silica gel 60 G and 60 GF_{254}	5–40	TLC	1, 5, 25
Silica gel 60 GF_{254}	15	TLC	1
Silica gel 60 H	5–40	TLC	1, 2.5, 25
Silica gel 60 H	15	TLC	1
Silica gel 60 HF_{254}	5–40	TLC	1, 2.5, 25
Silica gel 60 HF_{254} + F_{366}	5–40	TLC	1
Silica gel 60 PF_{254}	5–40	PLC	1, 2.5, 25
Silica gel 60 PF_{254} + F_{366}	5–40	PLC	1, 2.5
Silica gel 60 PF_{254} with gypsum	5–40	PLC	1, 2.5, 25
Aluminium oxide 60 G (neutral)	5–40	TLC	2.5, 25
Aluminium oxide 60 GF_{254} (neutral)	5–40	TLC	0.5
Cellulose microcrystalline (Avicel)	< 20	TLC	0.5
Kieselguhr G	5–40	TLC	0.5

$F_{254:}$ Green fluorescent indicator; $F_{254s:}$ Acid-resistant blue fluorescent indicator

***Courtesy:* Merck Specialities Private Limited, India.**

Common commercially available PLC pre-coated plates (glass-backed) with different sorbents

Sorbent layer	*Layer thickness* (mm)	*Format* (cm)
PLC Silica gel 60	0.5, 2.0	20 × 20
PLC Silica gel 60 F_{254}	0.5, 1.0, 2.0	20 × 20
PLC Silica gel 60 F_{254} + F_{366}	2.0	20 × 20
PLC Silica gel 60 F_{254} (with concentrating zones – 4 × 20)	0.5, 1.0, 2.0	20 × 20
PLC Silica gel RP-18 F_{254s}	1.0	20 × 20
PLC Aluminium oxide 60 F_{254}	1.5	20 × 20
PLC Aluminium oxide 150 F_{254}	1.5	20 × 20

F_{254} = Green fluorescent indicator, F_{254s} = Acid-resistant blue fluorescent indicator

***Courtesy:* Merck Specialities Private Limited, India.**

Common commercially available classical pre-coated TLC plates with different types of sorbents including mixed sorbents

Sorbent layer	*Layer thickness* (μm)	*Support*	*Format* (cm)
Silica gel 60	250	Glass	2.5 × 7.5, 5 × 20, 10 × 20, 20 × 20
Silica gel 60 G & GF_{254} (gypsum)	250	Glass	20 × 20
Silica gel 60	200	Aluminium	5 × 10, 20 × 20
Silica gel 60 F_{254}	250	Glass	2.5 × 7.5, 5 × 10, 5 × 20, 10 × 20, 20 × 20
Silica gel 60 F_{254}	200	Aluminium	500 × 20 (roll)
Silica gel 60 F_{254}	200	Plastic	4 × 8, 20 × 20
Silica gel 60 F_{254}	200	Plastic	500 × 20 (roll)
Silica gel 60 W	200	Aluminium	20 × 20
Silica gel 60 WF_{254}	200	Aluminium	20 × 20
Silica gel 60 WF_{254s}	250	Glass	20 × 20
Lux Plates (R) (Silica gel 60 F_{254})	250	Glass	2.5 × 7.5, 5 × 10, 10 × 20, 20 × 20
Aluminium oxide 60 F_{254} (basic)	250	Glass	5 × 20, 20 × 20
Aluminium oxide 60 F_{254} (neutral)	200	Aluminium, plastic	20 × 20
Aluminium oxide 150 F_{254} (neutral)	200	Aluminium	20 × 20
Kieselguhr F_{254}	200	Glass, aluminium	20 × 20
Silica gel 60 + Kieselguhr F_{254}	200	Aluminium	20 × 20
Cellulose, Cellulose F	100	Glass	10 × 10, 10 × 20, 20 × 20
Cellulose	100	Aluminium	20 × 20, 500 × 20 (roll)
Cellulose F	100	Aluminium	20 × 20
Cellulose, Cellulose F	100	Plastic	20 × 20
Cellulose F_{254}/F_{366}	100	Glass	10 × 20, 20 × 20
Cellulose F_{254}/F_{366}	100	Aluminium, plastic	20 × 20
PEI Cellulose F (to be stored at 0–4°C)	100	Glass, plastic	20 × 20

W = Water-resistant, F_{254} = Green fluorescent indicator, F_{254s} = Acid-resistant blue fluorescent indicator

***Courtesy:* Merck Specialities Private Limited, India.**

Common commercially available pre-coated HPTLC plates with different sorbents

Sorbent layer	*Layer thickness* (mm)	*Support*	*Format* (cm)
Silica gel 60	200	Glass	10 × 10, 20 × 10
Silica gel 60	200	Aluminium	20 × 20
Silica gel 60 F_{254}	200	Glass	5 × 10, 10 × 10, 20 × 10
Silica gel 60 F_{254}	200	Aluminium	5 × 7.5, 20 × 20
Silica gel 60 F_{254s}	200	Glass	20 × 10
Silica gel 60 (pre-scored)	200	Glass	10 × 10 (4 plates of 5 × 5)
Silica gel 60 WR F_{254s}	200	Glass	20 × 10
Silica gel 60 AMD (extra thin layer)	100	Glass	20 × 10
Silica gel 60 AMD WR F_{254s} (extra thin layer)	100	Glass	20 × 10
Silica gel 60 (premium purity layer)	200	Glass	20 × 10
Cellulose and Cellulose F_{254}/F_{366}	100	Glass	10 × 10, 20 × 10
Cellulose	100	Aluminium	20 × 20
LiChrospher® Silica gel 60 F_{254}	200	Glass	20 × 10
LiChrospher® Silica gel 60 F_{254s}	200	Aluminium	20 × 10, 20 × 20
LiChrospher® Silica gel 60 AMD WR F_{254s} (extra thin layer)	100	Glass	20 × 10
Proteochrom® Silica gel 60 F_{254s} (suitable for analysis of peptides and protein digests)	100	Glass	20 × 10
Proteochrom® Cellulose (suitable for analysis of peptides and protein digests)	100	Aluminium	20 × 10

W = Water-resistant, F_{254} = Green fluorescent indicator, F_{254s} = Acid-resistant blue fluorescent indicator

***Courtesy:* Merck Specialities Private Limited, India.**

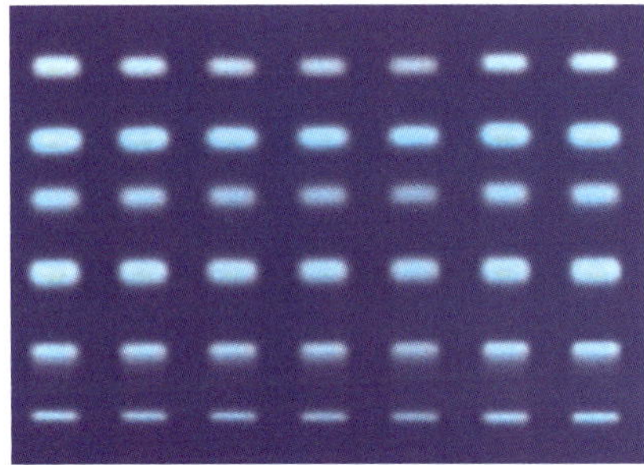

TLC silica gel 60 plate (A)

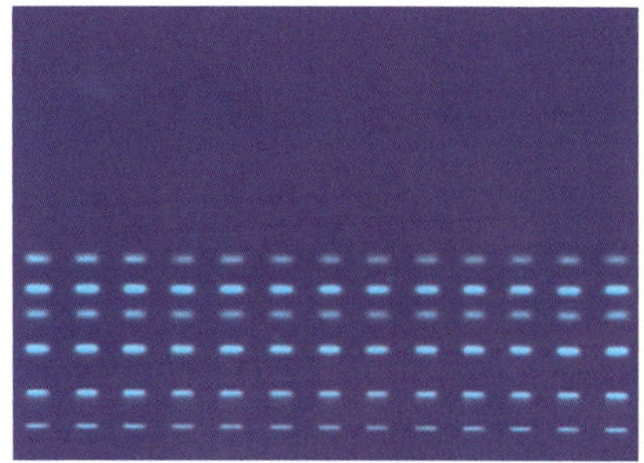

HPTLC silica gel plate (B)

Comparative separation of dansyl amino acids on TLC plate (A) and HPTLC plate (B) under identical conditions. HPTLC plates provide sharper zones in shorter migration distance (50 mm) and shorter time (14 min) as compared to TLC plates i.e. 100 mm and 42 min.

Courtesy: **Merck Specialities Private Limited, India.**

Commercially available TLC/HPTLC GLP plates (glass-backed)

Sorbent	*Layer thickness* (mm)	*Type*	*Format* (cm)
GLP Silica gel 60 F_{254}	250	TLC	10 × 20, 20 × 20
GLP Silica gel 60	250	HPTLC	10 × 20
GLP Silica gel 60 F_{254}	250	HPTLC	10 × 10, 10 × 20

Courtesy: **Merck Specialities Private Limited, India.**

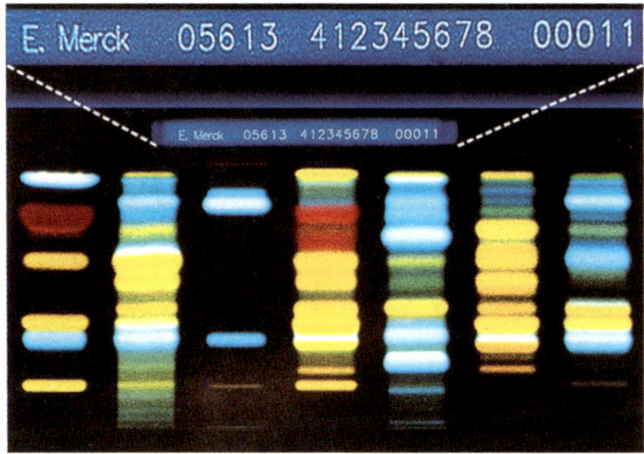

Laser-coded TLC/HPTLC GLP plate with individual plate number

(*Courtesy:* Merck Specialities Private Limited, India)

Commercially available multiformat TLC/HPTLC plates, glass-backed			
Sorbent	*Layer thickness* (mm)	*Type*	*Format* (cm)
Silica gel 60 F_{254} (20 × 20)	200	TLC	5 × 10, 5 × 20
Silica gel 60 F_{254} (10 × 10)	200	HPTLC	5 × 5

Note: 20 × 20 cm plate is suitably scored to give 7 possible formats.

***Courtesy:* Merck Specialities Private Limited, India.**

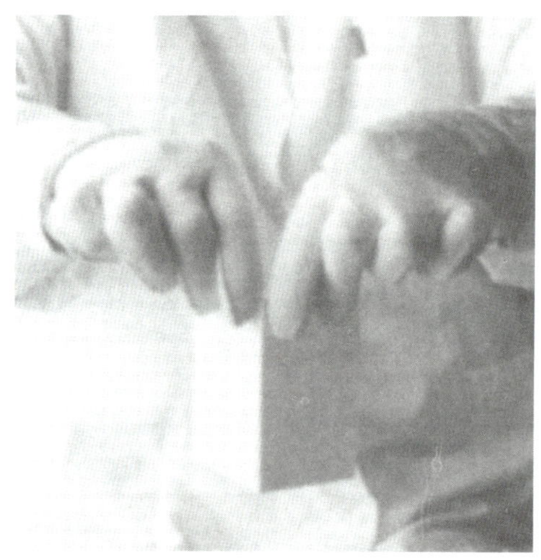

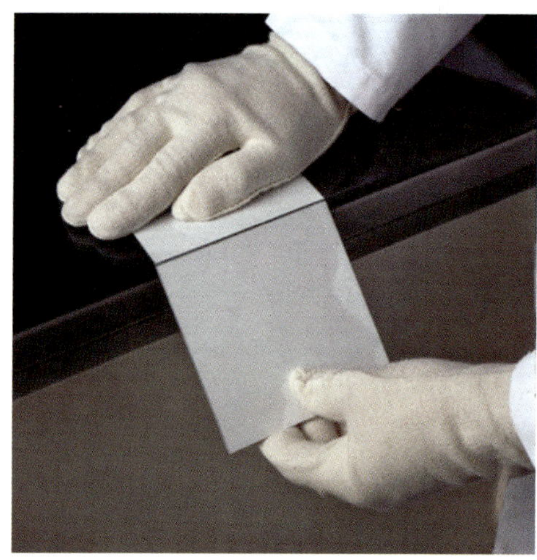

Multiformat TLC/HPTLC plate, pre-scored for easy snapping

(*Courtesy:* Merck Specialities Private Limited, India)

Common commercially available RP-modified and chemically-modified TLC and HPTLC plates

Modified sorbent layer	*Layer thick-ness* (mm)	*Type of plate*	*Support*	*Format* (cm)
Silica gel 60 RP-2 & RP-2 F_{254s} (silanized)	250	TLC	Glass	20 × 20
Silica gel 60 RP-2 F_{254s}	200	HPTLC	Glass	10 × 10
Silica gel RP-8 F_{254s}	250	TLC	Glass	5 × 10, 10 × 20, 20 × 20
Silica gel RP-8 F_{254s}	200	HPTLC	Glass	10 × 10
Silica gel RP-18 F_{254s}	250	TLC	Glass	5 × 10, 5 × 20, 10 × 20, 20 × 20
Silica gel RP-18 F_{254s}	250	TLC	Aluminium	5 × 7.5, 20 × 20
Silica gel 60 RP-18	200	HPTLC	Glass	20 × 10
Silica gel 60 RP-18 F_{254}	200	HPTLC	Glass	20 × 10
Silica gel 60 RP-18 F_{254s}	200	HPTLC	Glass	10 × 10
Silica gel 60 RP-18 W	200	HPTLC	Glass	10 × 10
Silica gel 60 RP-18 W F_{254s}	200	HPTLC	Glass	20 × 10
LiChrospher® Silica gel 60 RP-18 W F_{254s}	200	HPTLC	Glass	20 × 10
Silica gel 60 NH_2	200	TLC	Aluminium	20 × 10
Silica gel 60 NH_2 F_{254s}	200	TLC	Aluminium	10 × 10, 20 × 10
Silica gel 60 NH_2 F_{254s}	200	HPTLC	Glass	20 × 20
Silica gel 60 CN F_{254s}	200	TLC	Aluminium	10 × 10
Silica gel 60 Diol F_{254s}	200	TLC	Aluminium	10 × 10, 20 × 10

F_{254} = Green fluorescent indicator, F_{254s} = Acid-resistant blue fluorescent indicator; W = Water-resistant (fully wettable with water)

***Courtesy:* Merck Specialities Private Limited, India.**

Commercially available TLC, HPTLC and PLC concentrating zones plates

Sorbent layer	*Layer thickness* (mm)	*Type of plate*	*Support*	*Format* (cm)
Silica gel 60 (concentrating zones 2.5 × 10, 2.5 × 20 cm)	250	TLC	Glass	10 × 20, 20 × 20
Silica gel 60 (concentrating zones 2.5 × 20 cm)	200	TLC	Aluminium	20 × 20
Silica gel 60 (concentrating zones 2.5 × 10, 2.5 × 20 cm)	200	HPTLC	Glass	10 × 10, 20 × 10
Silica gel 60 F_{254} (concentrating zones 2.5 × 10, 2.5 × 20 cm)	250	TLC	Glass	10 × 20, 20 × 20
Silica gel 60 F_{254} (concentrating zones 2.5 × 20 cm)	200	TLC	Aluminium	20 × 20
Silica gel 60 F_{254} (concentrating zones 2.5 × 5, 2.5 × 10, 2.5 × 20 cm)	200	HPTLC	Glass	5 × 10, 10 × 10, 20 × 10
Silica gel 60 RP-18 F_{254s} (concentrating zones 2.5 × 20 cm)	200	HPTLC	Glass	20 × 10
Silica gel 60 RP-18 (concentrating zones 2.5 × 20 cm) (for PAH detection)	200	HPTLC	Glass	20 × 10
Silica gel F_{254} (concentrating zones 4 × 20 cm)	0.5, 1, 2	PLC	Glass	20 × 20

F_{254} = Green fluorescent indicator, F_{254s} = Acid-resistant blue fluorescent indicator

***Courtesy:* Merck Specialities Private Limited, India.**

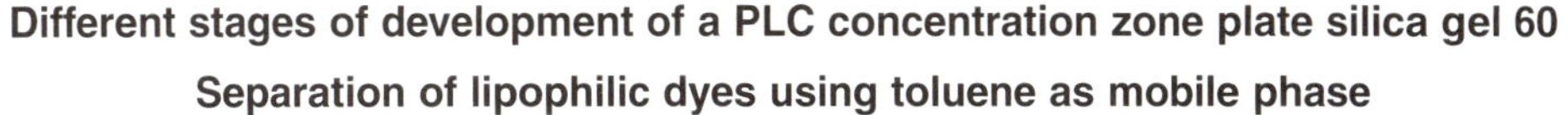

Different stages of development of a PLC concentration zone plate silica gel 60
Separation of lipophilic dyes using toluene as mobile phase

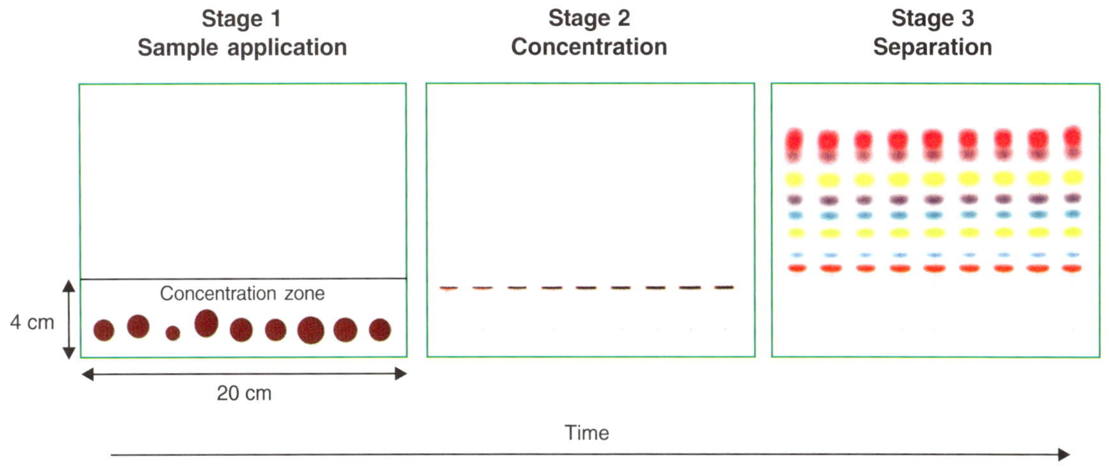

***Courtesy:* Merck Specialities Private Limited, India.**

Plate size (Format)

Pre-coated TLC/HPTLC plates in size of 20 × 20 with aluminium or polyester support are usually procured mainly for economic reasons. These plates can be cut to size and shape (format) to suit a particular analysis. Before handling pre-coated plates for any experimental work or cutting to size it is important to know the direction in which the layer of the sorbent has been applied. Abrasion marks produced on the back of aluminium foil during production stage of pre-coated plates are clearly visible. It may be noted that ultimate chromatographic procedure has to be carried out in the same direction.

Note: Ensure that even when plates are cut into small size, the chromatographic separation is performed in the direction in which sorbent is applied. It is advisable to use gloves while cutting to avoid damage to the hand and contamination of the layer. Glass TLC/HPTLC plates can be cut with a glass cutter. For plastic and aluminium sheet, a pair of scissors with long sharp blades shall be sufficient. The angle of scissors' blades is extremely important. Care has to be taken to avoid any damage to the sorbent layer. Good cuts are obtained if scissors blades are sharp. To avoid minimum damage to the layer, the blades should be inclined to the right at approximately 35–40°. It is important that scissors should never be inclined to the left as it may cause flaking off of layer at one or both sides of cut edges. In case of poor cuts, capillary cracks shall form between the layer and the foil; thereby the mobile phase shall migrate faster at the edge as compared to centre of the layer and

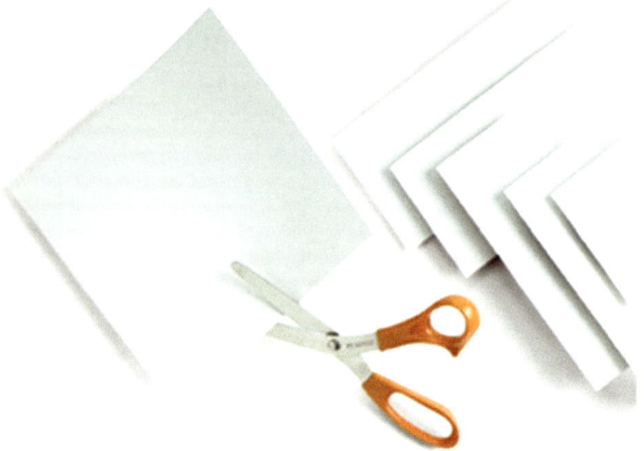

Inclination of scissors blades by 35–40° for proper cutting of a TLC plate of a particular size (format).

also the mobile phase moves from cut edge to the centre of the chromatogram leading to spot deformation and distorted chromatogram not suitable for evaluation.

Note:

- Cutting of plate is sometime required when the band or spot could not be applied properly. The portion is cut and the sample applied again or it may be necessary to cut the plate into several portions after development for trying different methods of identification.
- Any sorbent layer which has loosened as a result of cut should be gently wiped off by lightly moving spatula over the cut edge. This will ensure constant Rf values over the entire width of the layer.
- Blades of the scissors should be long to give fewer cuts.

Plate and Chamber Formats

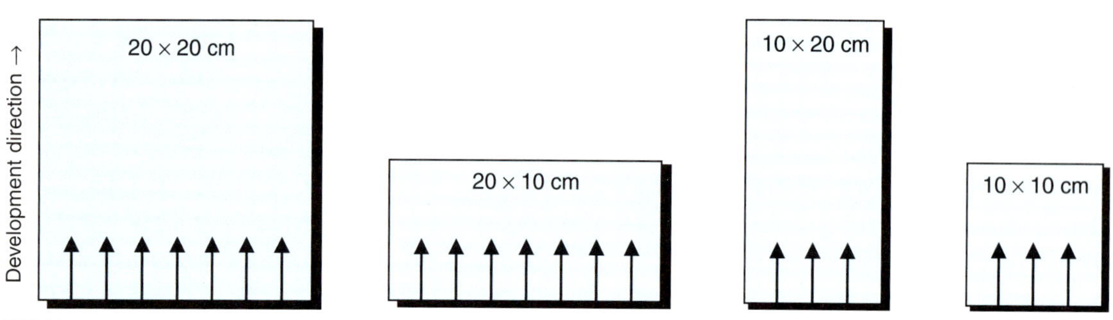

***Courtesy:* Camag, Switzerland.**

Common commercially available plate sizes (cm)			
Backing	*TLC*	*HPTLC*	*PLC*
Glass	20 × 20 10 × 20 5 × 20 5 × 10 2.5 × 7.5	20 × 10 10 × 10 5 × 10 5 × 5	20 × 20
Aluminium	20 × 20 10 × 20 5 × 20 5 × 10 5 × 7.5 500 × 20 (roll)	20 × 20 5 × 7.5	
Plastic	20 × 20 500 × 20 (roll) 4 × 8		

Pre-washing of pre-coated plates

Sorbents with large surface area absorb not only water vapours and other impurities from atmosphere but other volatile substances often condense particularly after the packing has been opened and exposed to laboratory atmosphere for a long time. Such impurities including elutable components of the binder usually give dirty zones and fail to give reproducible results. It is only for these reasons that pre-coated plates are always packed with the glass or foil side upward (coated layer downward). To avoid any possible interference due to impurities with the chromatographic separation particularly in case of quantitative work, it is always recommended to clear the plates before actual chromatography. This process is called pre-washing of plates. Ascending, dipping, continuous mode are the common methods of cleaning the plates. Ascending (blank chromatography) technique takes somewhat longer time but cleaning effect is superior; however, active dirt gets accumulated at solvent front. Therefore compounds of interest that migrate at the rear end of solvent front are partially obscured by overlapping fluorescence of the surface contamination. Thus compounds with HRf value of 75 and above will be difficult to scan particularly under fluorescent mode. This difficulty is often overcome by cutting 5–10% of the upper portion from solvent front of pre-washed plate before proceeding with chromatographic development. This step shall remove the dirt which had accumulated as a result of cleaning of the plate.

The other most commonly employed method for pre-washing is dipping. Quicker dipping process yields rather uniform clean layer but cleaning effect is often not as good as with ascending technique. Maxwell et al. (*J. Liquid Chromatogr.*, **13** (10), 2001–2011, 1990) have suggested the use of specially designed chambers designated as A, B, C, each containing about 10 ml of the cleaning solvent. For pre-washing, the plates are first dipped into chamber marked 'A' for one minute, then taken to chamber 'B'. The chamber can easily clean 20 plates (10 × 10 cm). After initial cleaning process, the chamber marked 'A' is rejected and chamber 'B' serves as initial cleaning chamber, while chamber 'C' is used for secondary cleaning.

Excellent results are obtained if the plates are subjected to pre-washing by continuous mode for some time, i.e., in a chamber closed by a lid having a slit.

After washing, the plates must be dried for a sufficient time to ensure complete removal of the washing liquids (usually for methanol 30-60 min. at 105° are required). If the drying time is too short or the temperature is too low, it will result in incomplete removal of solvent used for pre-washing leading to poorly defined conditions thus change in Rf values. Use of hot or cold air (hair drier) should be avoided as laboratory air which is usually contaminated is blown over the layer and purpose of cleaning the layer is defeated. The washed plates should always be stored in a dust-free atmosphere under ambient conditions. Preferably desiccators of suitable dimensions should be used for storing both cleaned and uncleaned plates till they are used. No grease should be used for sealing the desiccator. Use of drying agents is also not necessary.

Pre-washing of plates must be done to at least 1–2 cm longer than the subsequent actual chromatographic development so that any dirt accumulated at the front does not interfere in densitometric scanning. As a result of pre-washing, signal to noise ratio is substantially low and base lines are straighter, both these steps essential for quantitative analysis by in-situ densitometry. Reduction in signal-to-noise ratio as a result of pre-washing improves the limit of detection (LOD) of the procedure.

Note:

- As after pre-washing, activation of the layer in drying cupboard to remove the washing solvent is essential; analysts often experience difficulty in drying aluminium-backed layers as the foil tends to lose shape during drying/ activation. Obviously any distortion of the layer will make remaining steps of separation more difficult and often impossible. It is, therefore, suggested that aluminium-backed pre-coated plates should be dried by keeping it between two blank glass plates.
- As application of sample(s) usually takes several minutes, the activity of the sorbent layer even after activation is likely to correspond to the relative humidity of the experimental room. Prior activation may therefore not be

required as layer in fact adapts to the relative humidity of the room. An air-conditioned room with air lock system is usually effective in maintaining the humidity and temperature at reasonably constant level.

- After the plates are removed from pre-wash chambers, they should always be dried in vertical position as in horizontal position, drops of solvent may fall on the plate as a result of condensation, thus damaging the layer.

Even for routine analysis (qualitative), one must use pre-washed plates, otherwise, the dirt front will interfere in the detection of substances with high HRf values, i.e., more than 70. Methanol is the most commonly employed solvent for pre-washing but its cleaning power is not good particularly when lipophilic mobile phases are to be used for subsequent chromatographic development. In such cases, it is preferable to carry out pre-washing process with mobile phase in question. However, mobile phase containing acid or alkali should be avoided as they may not be completely removed during subsequent activation, thus impregnating the stationary phase. Mixtures of chloroform in methanol (1 : 1); ethyl acetate-methanol (1 : 1); chloroform-methanol-ammonia (90 : 10 : 1) have been used as solvents for pre-washing. Methylene chloride-methanol (1 : 1) is best suited for removing any impurity picked up during storage in laboratory atmosphere. One may also try pre-washing with 1% ammonia solution or 1% acetic acid in methanol.

Caution:

- Pre-washing is essential if the detection reagent is sensitive to atmospheric impurities or fluorescence quenching is being employed as detection method.
- The direction in which pre-washing is done should be especially marked as for sample analysis, chromatographic development has to be done in that direction only.
- While cutting a pre-washed 20 × 20 cm plate into smaller format, direction of pre-washing must be kept in mind.
- Pre-washing front in blank chromatogram should be marked to avoid rotation of the plate through 90° while carrying out actual chromatography.
- Pre-washing of pre-coated plate is must for stability testing and trace analysis.
- If the pre-washing solvent has poor elution strength, it may not remove all the dirt, leading to poor results. Polar solvent causes concentration of impurities at the solvent front. As the resolution of analytes present in the sample is usually poor near the solvent front, the impurities are not the problem in such cases.
- Pre-washing may be done by dipping technique to save time. However, its effectiveness needs to be experimentally verified.
- Pre-washing by blank chromatography method should always be preferred.
- The best solvent for pre-washing of plates is the mobile phase to be actually used for chromatographic separation provided it has no non-volatile component.

Activation of pre-coated plates

Freshly opened box of TLC/HPTLC plates usually does not require activation. However, plates exposed to high humidity or kept on hand for long time may have to be activated by placing in oven at 110–120°C for 30 minutes prior to sample spotting (aluminium-backed plates should be activated by keeping between two glass plates). This step removes water that has been physically absorbed on the surface of the sorbent.

Activation at higher temperature and for longer time should be avoided as this shall cause release of chemically absorbed water causing irreversible changes in chromatographic properties of the silica gel layer. With such highly active layers, there is risk of sample being decomposed or artifact being formed. Further, such an active sorbent layer shall have high retardation properties i.e. shorter migration distance of the sample components as compared to less active layer. Under these circumstances, for reproducible Rf values, the activity level of layers has to be well-defined.

Note:

- The conditions (time and temperature) described above and pre-washing of layers is suitable for silica gel and aluminium oxide pre-coated layers. For other sorbent layers manufacturers may be consulted for suitable activation conditions.
- For sample containing sensitive analytes, the use of layers with lipophilic modification i.e. RP C-8, 12, 18 shall be suitable.

Sample preparation

The sample preparation is not as demanding as for other chromatographic techniques, however, several steps for sample pretreatment may be necessary such as sampling, mechanical crushing, extraction, filtration and enrichment of minor compounds. Proper sample preparation is an important pre-requisite for success of thin layer chromatographic separation. The sample preparation procedure is to dissolve the dosage form with complete recovery of intact compound(s) of interest and minimum of matrix with a suitable concentration of analyte(s) for direct application on the HPTLC plate. Besides maximizing the yield of analytes in the selected solvent, stability of analytes during extraction and analysis must be considered and ensured. Therefore, the choice of a suitable solvent for a given analysis is very important. For normal-phase chromatography using silica gel pre-coated plates (more than 80-90% of TLC analysis is done using silica gel as sorbent), solvent for dissolving the sample should be non-polar and volatile as far as possible, since polar solvents are likely to induce circular chromatography at origin, particularly when sample is applied in increment on top of each other, leading to spreading of spot, thus loss of separation efficiency. For reversed-phase chromatography, usually polar solvents are used for dissolving the sample; however, such polar solvents must wet the sorbent so that sample penetrates the layer uniformly.

Clean-up steps in the sample preparation, if necessary, must be optimized. Sufficient quantity of sample should be initially taken for clean-up steps. Once the sample is cleaned up, one must ensure that it is subjected to chromatographic separation as quickly as possible particularly while dealing with labile substances. Storage, if necessary, should only be in refrigerator.

It is preferable to keep the solvent as simple as possible and quantity employed be limited to ensure complete extraction of analytes and minimum of extraneous component. Sample and reference substances should be dissolved in the same solvent to ensure comparable distribution at starting zones.

Choice of solvent for the sample

- It should dissolve the analytes.
- It should be reasonably volatile.
- It should have low viscosity.
- It should wet the sorbent layer.
- It should be a weak chromatographic solvent for the analyte.

For TLC on silica gel, the use of weakest (least polar) solvent which allows quantitative dissolving and spotting of sample and there is no preliminary development and separation within the initial spot at the origin, is recommended. Rf values of the components of interest in the selected solvent for preparation of the sample should be less than 0.1%.

Evaporation of solvent

Whenever sample requires concentration, use of rotary evaporator with attached round bottom flask is recommended. The solution should be first evaporated completely to dryness and then the residue is dissolved in same or different solvent for application to the TLC layer. Use of non-polar solvent to dissolve the residue will help to remove polar impurities which will remain undissolved. Solvents with high boiling point or polarity are difficult to remove from sorbent layers during application. If a small amount of solvent is left after application, it can cause serious effects on the separation by causing zone spreading or deformation. Use of hot air to dry the solvent at origin should normally be discouraged as it can cause decomposition of heat labile substances on the surface of an active sorbent.

Note:

- If a sample solvent is predominantly aqueous or viscous, then dilution with polar organic solvent such as methanol is necessary as it will help in application to the layer, shall also wet the layer and penetrate effectively resulting in spots of spherical shape and sharp well-defined lines in case of bands.
- Filtration of sample solution improves the quality of chromatogram.

Sample application

This is the most critical step for obtaining good resolution for quantification by HPTLC. The sample should be completely transferred to the layer, however, under no circumstances, the application process should damage the layer, as damaged layer results in unevenly shaped spots. Wherever possible, use of automatic application devices is recommended for quantitative analysis. While using graduated capillaries, one must ensure that they fill and empty completely.

The sample solution should be applied through clean upper end of the capillary and for that after filling the capillary to marked point, reverse the capillary for applying the sample.

Note: Sample solution in high density solvents such as chloroform may leave the capillary before sample application, whereas solutions of high viscosity may incompletely enter or leave the capillaries, high volatile solvents such as acetone, diethyl ether may undergo partial evaporation before application. Under such circumstances, the use of microsyringe is recommended if laboratory is not equipped with automatic application devices.

Usually application of 1–10 μl for TLC and 0.5–5 μl for HPTLC is recommended keeping the size of starting zone(s) down to minimum; 2-4 mm (TLC) and 0.5-1 mm (HPTLC) in the concentration range of 0.1–1 μg/μl for TLC/HPTLC. Substance zones which are too large from the beginning cause poor separation as during development spots do tend to become large and more diffused. This difficulty is more pronounced in case of substances with high Rf values. It is therefore recommended that solution should be applied in small increments with intermediate drying (use cold or hot air or nitrogen in case of labile compounds, asymmetric accelerated evaporation of the solvent from the point of application can lead to local changes in the concentration in spotted substances) particularly when the sample solution is predominantly aqueous.

Note: Application in small increments has disadvantage as well, since previously applied zones may get chromatographed on each subsequent application leading to formation of horseshoe-shaped developed spot.

Analytical results of any experiment are likely to be affected by chromatographer's state of mind on a day, avoid hand application for quantitative work.

For application, sample and reference solutions should possibly contain the same matrix, otherwise matrix present in the sample can cause change in Rf values.

However, volume and concentration primarily depend on the component under analysis and their sensitivity to various detection techniques. If too much sample is applied, it may not be absorbed uniformly throughout the layer leading to overloading, as a result tailing of zones and poor resolution is observed. Problem arising out of such overloading when unavoidable, can best be overcome by applying the sample as band, the only apparent disadvantage being that only fewer samples can be accommodated on a given plate.

Bands are formed at thin line, whereas spots cover a wide area above and below the origin, the separation resolution for less migration distance is sharp for bands as compared to spots. When the spot is applied even using low polarity solvents for sample preparation, the analytes are concentrated in the centre of the spot with much lower concentration on the perimeter. With development, the analytes get further diffused into the layer. Under these circumstances, for densitometric scanning of spots, large slit width shall be required to cover the entire area of the developed spot. In contrast, band appears uniform after development. Slit width equivalent 2/3rd of the band length is sufficient for densitometric scanning. Further, as migration of spot is not very precise, automated track adjustment shall be required for scanning whereas same is not required for band scanning.

Separation parameters: R_f and R_{st}

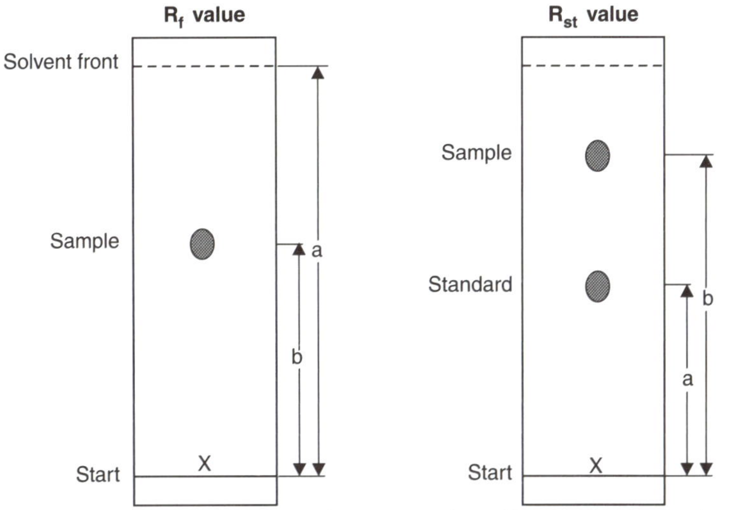

$$R_f = \frac{b}{a} = \frac{\text{Migration distance: sample}}{\text{Migration distance: solvent front}} \qquad R_{st} = \frac{b}{a} = \frac{\text{Migration distance: sample}}{\text{Migration distance: standard}}$$

R_f value is always ≤ 1, whereas R_{st} can be > 1.

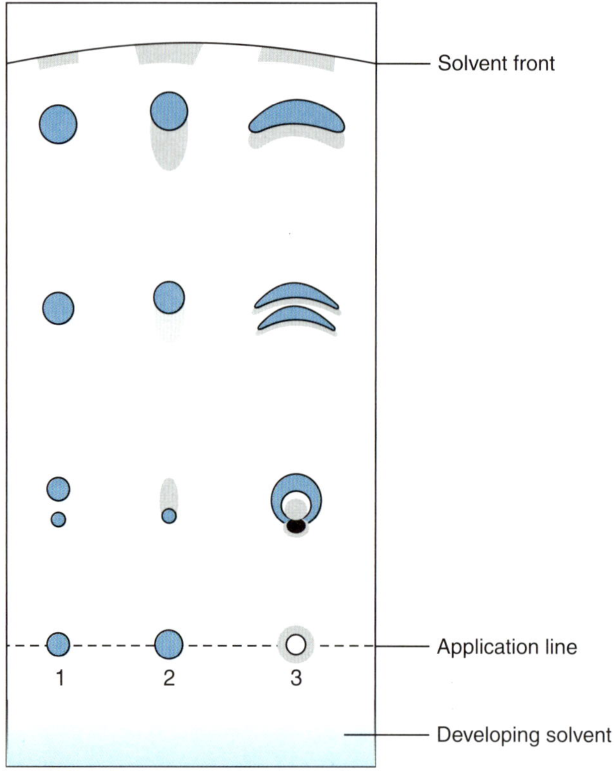

Sample application

1. Applied as compact round spot. 2. Layer overloaded with the sample leading to tailing, spots looking like tears. 3. Repeated application of sample in small increments without adequate intermittent drying of the solvent leading to local chromatography and also crescent type horseshoe bands or spots with tailing.

Although application of sample as spot does have few advantages such as less time, simplicity and less expensive but advantages of application of sample as band are more comprehensive.

Advantages of application of sample as band

- Even distribution of the sample.
- Better resolution.
- Greater accuracy i.e. lower standard deviation.
- More flexibility in sample application.
- Better separation because of rectangular area in which the compounds are present on the plate.
- Equal Rf values of the compounds from sample and reference solution.
- Matrix effect of extracted and applied excipients are significantly reduced as solution is distributed over a large area.

- Response of densitometer is higher than observed from an equal amount/ equal volume of the same solution applied as a spot. It appears that light may not gain access to all the sample material applied as a spot (point). This is supported by the observation that range of linearity is small for pointwise application than for bandwise application.
- Application of different volumes as bands from one solution gives same concentration-response curve as obtained by application of equal volumes of solution with different concentration. This correlation is absent when sample solution is applied as a spot. This is significant as while preparing the concentration-response curve, one need not prepare solution with different concentration while applying the sample as a band.
- Generally speaking, spot broadening in the direction of development is smaller in the case of bandwise application.
- Larger quantities of the sample can be handled for application, thus reducing the need for concentration step which may be quite damaging in case of labile substances.
- Position of plate for densitometric scanning is less critical as composition of the compounds is uniform in the entire area of band.

Note: It is recommended that samples should not be applied on outer (both) edges of the plate (leave at least 1–2 cm on each side) as the rate of solvent evaporation is usually greater at the edges than near the centre of the plate, Rf value is greater near the edges due to boundary/edge effect. Further, considering the method of manufacture of pre-coated layer, it is observed that usually layers at edges are thinner than the rest. Slight distortion in chromatogram and variation in Rf values are observed if the sample is applied near the edges, hence 1–2 mm is left in each side.

It is not only the size of the spot or length of the band, but the amount of sample loaded on TLC/HPTLC layers need special consideration. As the over-loaded spot or band migrates as result of development, diffusion into surrounding area of layer quickly occurs in the direction of migration. This leads to formation of streaks/tails, their length being dependant on the amount of overloading. In such cases, resolution is drastically affected. The amount of sample to be applied as spot or band depends on sample matrix, sorbent layer and its thickness, nature of sorbent, solvent used for sample preparation. Following guidelines may be useful.

In case of TLC, apply 0.1–2 µg/spot and 2–10 µg/band of 10 mm length, total volume in the range of 1–10 µl.

For HPTLC, we can apply 50–200 ng/spot and 1–4 µg/band of 10 mm length, total volume being 0.5–5 µl.

Samples can be applied manually with very simple equipments such as calibrated glass capillaries, microsyringe or micropipettes of set volumes. Several equipments are commercially available for semi-automatic or automatic application of sample, leading manufacturer being Camag (Switzerland), Desaga (Germany) and Baron (Germany).

Note: Manual application with pointed glass capillaries, or due to minisyringe prick can cause damage to the sorbent layer. Soft layer or repeated application of the sample at one spot are primarily responsible for layer damage. Polarity of the sample is also responsible for damage to the layer i.e. more polar he solvent, more easily the layer gets damaged. However, damage to the layer is not apparent until the development process is started. Damaged layer of sorbent shall give erroneous results as 100% application of the sample cannot be achieved. Other problems related with capillaries are:

(a) Surface tension and viscosity of the solvent leading to incomplete filling and delivery.

(b) Filling and emptying time varying.

(c) Inconsistent inner diameter of the capillary.

Role of humidity while applying sample

In general humidity is an important variable for optimizing chromatographic parameters. The moisture present in the sorbent layer affects the partitioning of analyte between stationary phase and mobile phase. However, problem relates to humidity around applied spot/band. After application of the sample, the volatile sample solvent evaporates from the surface of sorbent, the latent heat required for evaporation is taken from the surrounding atmosphere, thereby localized cooling is caused very close to the spot/band, thereby moisture is condensed onto the layer. So, if the area of application is not thoroughly dried at an elevated temperature, components of the sample shall move faster. However, care must be taken to ensure that while drying the application area temperature should not be very high to cause degradation of the analytes. It has been experienced that drying for 2–3 min at 75–80°C is adequate for complete removal of the sample solvent.

Drying of loaded plate before development

Following points need special consideration:

1. For volatile compounds such as essential oils, n-hexane or toluene is used as solvent. Do not use hair dryer or any other type of blower. Instead, after loading, allow the plate to dry for a few minutes at room temperature in horizontal position before keeping in chamber.

2. For thermally stable compounds in case of heavy loading for impurity testing uniform heating with hair dryer is usually not sufficient. Uniform heating such as in oven for 20 min is necessary to remove all the solvent. The temperature should be in the range of solvent boiling point.
3. If the plate is exposed to blower for a longer time, laboratory dirt is likely to be transferred to the plate making pre-washing step as suggested earlier ineffective.
4. For removal of solvent in case of oxidative prone or thermolabile sample laboratory experiment need to be performed to know the exact conditions.

Mobile phase (MP)

Thin layer chromatography is in variance with other chromatographic methods in that in addition to stationary phase and mobile phase, a gas phase is also present which influences the chromatographic results significantly.

Mixture of different components to make mobile phase should have appearance of a clear single phase without cloudiness and separation of any component. It performs the following functions:

1. Dissolves the analytes.
2. Moves analytes to be separated over sorbent layer.
3. Gives Rf values of medium range.
4. Provides reasonably good selectivity for the analytes mixture to get separated.

Requirements:

1. Must be of adequate purity.
2. Analytes must be stable.
3. Viscosity should be on lower side.
4. Should be least toxic (use of carcinogenic solvents such as benzene and pyridine should be avoided and look for suitable replacement such as toluene for benzene and use consistently).
5. Vapour pressure should be in medium range – not very low, not very high.

Note:

1. In case of solvent with similar elution power, the solvent with lower viscosity should be preferred as it gives shorter development time.

"No mobile phase can be most suitable for a given analytical problem unless proved by experiment."

2. It is important that solvent must wet the sorbent layer, otherwise no development shall take place as capillary force within sorbent layer would not be sufficient to overcome the repulsive forces between the stationary phase and solvent system. It is for this reason that in RP chromatography sodium chloride is one of the components of many mobile phases as it increases wetability of the layer.
3. Choose the mobile phase which gives better separation efficiency and shorter development time.

Developing solvent and mobile phase are considered synonyms. However, except neat solvent, in practical sense it is not correct. In fact, the liquid in the chamber is developing solvent, whereas the liquid moving through the sorbent layer constitutes the mobile phase. One is sure of the definite composition of the developing solvent when it is transferred to the chamber, while the composition of the liquid moving through the system shall be variable at a given time while it is moving till the equilibrium is established.

One of the most difficult problems is finding a most suitable mobile phase for separation of a given analyte mixture.

Poor grade of solvent used in preparing mobile phases have been found to decrease resolution, spot definition and Rf reproducibility. Mobile phase commonly called solvent system is traditionally selected by controlled process of trial and error and also based on one's own experience in the field. It is often possible that few layer-solvent combinations already reported in the literature for compounds of interest or similar compounds may be suitable in a given analytical problem with minor modifications. Nevertheless, it should not be forgotten that such conditions may have been chosen due to availability rather than suitability and often improvements are required. Manufacturers of sorbents and pre-coated plates usually supply bibliographies of separations that they have carried out in their application laboratories. However, mobile phase should be chosen taking into consideration chemical properties of analytes and the sorbent layer. Use of mobile phase containing more than three or four components should normally be avoided as it is often difficult to get reproducible ratios of different components.

- Solvent system composition is expressed by volumes (v/v) and usually sum of total volume is 100. This facilitates comparison of developed method in the laboratory with another method and for calculation of amount of each component in a given experimental situation.
- Various components of MP should be measured separately and then placed in the mixing vessel. This will not only prevent the contamination of solvent stock by evaporation from already partially filled mixing vessel but also any

possible volumetric error arising due to volumes expansion (dilation) or contraction on mixing.

- To minimize volumetric errors, MP should be prepared in a volume sufficient for one working day.
- Laboratories equipped with complete HPTLC system usually use smaller development chamber such as twin-trough chambers (10 × 10 cm) where comparatively smaller volumes of MP, usually 10-15 ml, is required. It is advisable that different components of the MP should be measured with volumetric pipettes.
- Different components of MP should be first mixed in mixing vessel with ground-glass stopper and then introduced into the developing chamber.
- Chambers usually containing multi-component mobile phase once used is not recommended for re-use for any future development work as composition of MP is likely to change during chromatographic development, due to differential evaporation and adsorption by the layer and also once the chamber is opened, each solvent component will evaporate disproportionately depending on their volatilities.
- Solvent components which are relatively volatile at room temperature and may play significant role in final MP such as pH of the solvent system. Solvents such as strong solution of ammonia, glacial acetic acid or diethylamine should not be used for long time once the original container is opened.
- Chemical reaction may occur between different components of MP such as acetic acid and ammonia or acetic acid and n-butanol or acetic acid and ethyl alcohol resulting in altered chromatographic results.
- Polar solvent portion of MP may get adsorbed by the layer during development.
- In bi-component MP, loss of more volatile minor component such as ammonia is worth considering. If the dissolved ammonia is lost, experimental results shall not be reproducible.
- Mobile phase should be as simple as possible and permissible by analytes and sample matrix.
- Some form of MP optimization is generally necessary.

Optimization of mobile phase (solvent optimization)

First level

Neat solvents from different selectivity area were tested. Within a selectivity area solvents may give similar separation. Usually ethanol, methanol, tetra-

"Selection of an appropriate mobile phase for a particular problem shall always remain a challenge for an analyst."

Relative humidity (%) of saturated salt solutions containing large quantity of undissolved salt

Saturated solutions	*Relative humidity (%) over the solution at 20°C*
di-Sodium hydrogen phosphate – $Na_2PO_4.12H_2O$	95
Sodium carbonate – $Na_2CO_3.10H_2O$	92
Zinc sulphate – $ZnSO_4.7H_2O$	90
Potassium chloride – KCl	86
Ammonium sulfate – $(NH_4)_2SO_4$	80
Ammonium chloride – NH_4Cl	79
Sodium chloride – NaCl	76
Sodium chlorate – $NaClO_3$	75
Sodium nitrite – $NaNO_2$	65
Ammonium nitrate – NH_4NO_3	63
Sodium bromide – NaBr	58
Calcium nitrate – $Ca(NO_3)_2.4H_2O$	55
Sodium dichromate – $Na_2Cr_2O_7.2H_2O$	52
Potassium carbonate – K_2CO_3	45
Zinc nitrate – $Zn(NO_3)_2.6H_2O$	42
Chromium trioxide – CrO_3	35
Calcium chloride – $CaCl_2.6H_2O$	32
Potassium acetate – $K(OOCCH_3)$	20
Lithium chloride – $LiCl.H_2O$	15

Note: Sulphuric acid (10–70% w/w in water) provides % RH ranging from 96% to 3%.

***Courtesy:* Merck Specialities Private Limited, India.**

Processes in the developing chamber

Thin-layer chromatography differs from all other chromatographic techniques in the fact that in addition to stationary and mobile phases, a gas phase is present. This gas phase can significantly influence the result of the separation.

The "classical" way of developing a chromatogram is to place the plate in a chamber which contains a sufficient amount of developing solvent. The lower end of the plate should be immersed several millimetres. Driven by capillary action the developing solvent moves up the layer until the desired running distance is reached and chromatography is stopped. The following

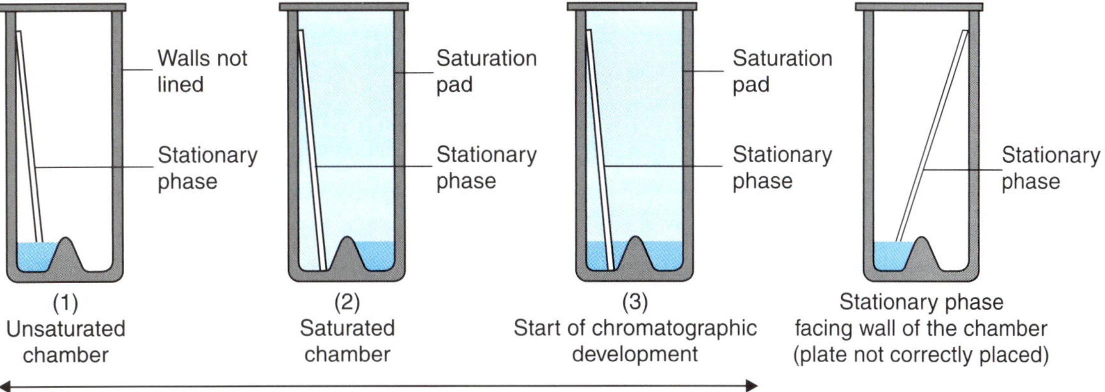

(1)

- Wall of chamber not lined with filter paper.
- Amount of solvent minimum.
- Plate placed immediately after chamber is loaded with solvent.
- The equilibrium between solvent and its vapours is partially established during chromatographic development.
- If chamber loaded with the solvent with tightly-closed lid is allowed to stand for some time before the plate is introduced (partially saturated chamber).

(2)

- Walls of the chamber are lined with filter paper soaked with developing solvent.
- Plate loaded with the sample is placed in empty trough opposite to the one containing solvent.
- Stationary phase is allowed to interact with gas phase prior to chromatographic development (pre-conditioning of layer).

OR

- Walls of the chamber lined with filter paper soaked with solvent.
- Developing solvent placed into the chamber.
- Wait for definite time before introducing plate loaded with sample into chamber to start chromatographic development (chamber saturation without pre-conditioning of layer).

(3)

- Development of plate when the solvent is introduced into trough with the plate.

"Habit of using mobile phase many times should be discouraged, each plate has the right for fresh mobile phase."

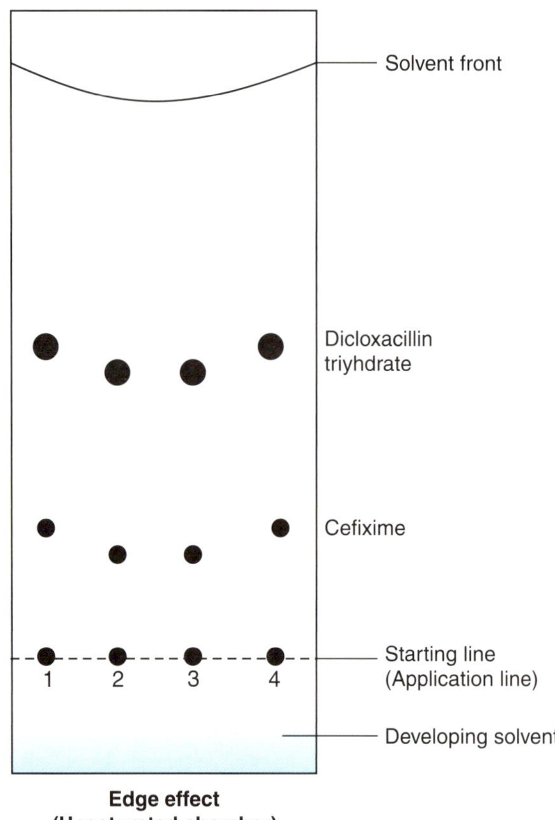

Edge effect
(Unsaturated chamber)

Four identical samples containing cefixime and dicloxacillin trihydrate developed in toluene–methanol–triethylamine (5 : 4 : 1 v/v) in an unsaturated chamber. Substances near the edge of the layer migrate faster than the same substances in the centre. The developing solvent evaporates more rapidly at the edges of the layer. Spots of each analyte have different Rf values with concave solvent front. Results not reproducible for identification and quantification. Rf values are higher on the edge.

considerations primarily concern silica gel as stationary phase and developments, which can be described as adsorption chromatography.

Provided the chamber is tightly closed, following competing processes occur:

1. Between the components of the developing solvent and their vapour, an equilibrium will be established eventually (1). This equilibrium is called chamber saturation. Depending on the vapour pressure of the individual components, the composition of the gas phase can differ significantly from that of the developing solvent.
2. While still dry, the stationary phase adsorbs molecules from the gas phase. This process, adsorptive saturation, is also approaching an equilibrium in which the polar components will be withdrawn from the gas phase and loaded onto the surface of the stationary phase (2).

3. Simultaneously the part of the layer which is already wetted with mobile phase interacts with the gas phase. Thereby especially the less polar components of the liquid are released into the gas phase (3). Unlike (1) this process is not as much governed by vapour pressure as by adsorption forces.

Note:

A. Except single component solvent (neat solvent), development solvent and mobile phase are not same. Their composition changes with progressing chromatography. Only the composition of the solvent at the time of placing into the chamber is positively known.
   (i) Developing solvent: The liquid placed in the chamber.
   (ii) Mobile phase: The liquid moving through the layer during chromatographic development.

B. Chromatographic results depend on the shape of the chamber. For reproducible results and comparative evaluation, type of chamber used and its saturation level need special attention.

C. Selection of chamber to be made during method development depending on availability, solvent consumption and economic aspect.

D. Rf values are lower in saturated chamber particularly on pre-conditioned layers as compared to unsaturated chamber.

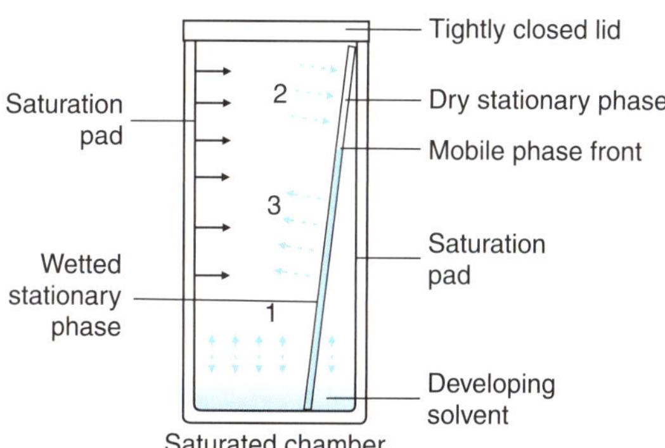

Saturated chamber

Development

One-dimensional (ascending, descending), two-dimensional, horizontal, multiple overrun (continuous), gradient, radial (circular), anti-radial (anti-circular), multimodal (multi-dimensional), forced flow planar chromatography are the most common modes of chromatographic development. Rectangular glass chambers, twin-trough chambers, V-shaped chambers, sandwich chambers, horizontal development chambers, KS-Vario chambers, circular and anti-circular, U chambers, forced flow development chamber, automated multiple development chambers and automatic development chamber are commonly used for carrying out different types of development.

General steps for development

- Place the chamber on smooth surface in diffused day light and a lid to give tight seal.
- Place suitable volume of developing solvent (DS), i.e., 10 ml for 10 × 10 cm TTS and 20 ml for 20 × 20 cm TTS.
- Open the chamber, place filter paper of suitable size in the rear trough.
- Pour 'DS' into the chamber so that filter paper is completely wetted and gets adhered to the walls of the chamber.
- Allow the chamber to saturate for 20 min.
- Tilt the chamber by 40–50° so that volume of the solvent is almost equal in both the troughs.
- Loaded plate is properly marked for the desired migration distance (usually 70 mm) on right edge of the plate with hard pencil.
- Slightly slide the lid of the chamber, insert the loaded plate in front trough, layer facing towards filter paper (keep the chamber open for minimum time for insertion of plate not to disturb the degree of saturation).
- Ensure that entire width of the plate dips into the mobile phase to same depth.
- Develop the plate to pre-marked distance.
- Open the lid and take out the plate.
- Dry the plate vertically in the direction of development with the aid of cold stream of air to remove excess of 'DS'.
- Proceed with detection and quantitative evaluation.

Note:

- After development, the 'DS' and filter paper are discarded.
- For next development, the chamber is cleaned and dried.
- 'DS' composed of solvents with widely varied polarities should be used only once.

Note: Under no circumstances, develop the chromatogram until and unless solvent of the applied sample is completely evaporated — it usually takes 5-10 minutes.

Since HPTLC is now a well accepted analytical technique for quantitative analysis, reagents often used for detection should no longer merely by visualized for identification only but should be expected to give reproducible and stoichiometric reactions suitable for quantitative analysis. It is therefore, important that once the chromatogram is developed, it should be handled with utmost care. Application of reagents, if required, has to be homogeneous ensuring uniform reaction and finally stabilizing of end reaction product.

Drying after development

After development the plate is removed from the chamber and MP is removed as completely and as quickly as possible to prevent any subsequent deterioration of chromatograms due to any diffusion or solvent having any adverse effect on detection procedure. This step should preferably be performed in fume cupboard to avoid contamination of laboratory atmosphere. The plates should always be laid horizontally so that while MP evaporates the separated substances will migrate evenly to the surface where they can be easily detected.

Usually analysts may employ hand dryer (hot or cold) to effect faster removal of the mobile phase; however, following need consideration:

- Volatile components such as essential oil components may evaporate, avoid use of high temperature.
- Compounds sensitive to oxygen may get destroyed due to rise in temperature while using hot air dryer.
- Particles of dust from laboratory may deposit on the chromatogram which may influence the ultimate densitometric scanning.
- Chemical vapours present in the laboratory are likely to be transported in the air stream onto the layer. This will positively interfere when post-chromatographic derivatization is resorted to.

If the MP contains derivatization reagent such as ninhydrin for amino acids, drying of the plate and reaction with reagent be completed by drying in oven or hot plate.

It is precisely for these reasons that drying of chromatogram should preferably be done in vacuum desiccator with protection from heat and light.

Note: If heating of the plate, after it is treated with the reagent, is not uniform, there always exists risk of reaction inhomogeneity on the plate. Usually, drying cupboard or hot plates are employed. Drying cupboard should have non-perforated shelf. Perforated shelf is not suitable as heat transfer is greater when there is contact with metal than with air. Therefore, holes in perforated shield will result in non-uniform heat transfer, thus inhomogeneity in heat dependent reactions adversely affecting the direct quantitative analysis. It is preferable to keep the TLC plate down vertically, edges touching walls of the cupboard. Hot plates with regulated range of temperature, i.e., 50–190°C ± 2°C are extensively being employed for heating the chromatogram. It has definite

Parameters affecting HPTLC performance

Separation	*Quantitative analysis*
• Sorbent quality • Type of sorbent (TLC/HPTLC) • Activity of stationary phase • Layer thickness and format • Binder in stationary phase • Different brands of sorbents • Pre-washing of pre-coated plates • Sample volume spotted (spot/band) • Purity of solvents • Composition of mobile phase • Quantity of mobile phase • Viscosity of mobile phase • Type and size of chamber • Chamber saturation time • Relative humidity • Temperature (Rf values usually increase with rise in temperature) • Mode of development • Distance between start zone and level of eluent in the chamber • Development distance • Solvent for sample preparation • Gradient formation • Pre-conditioning of layer	• Sample preparation, extraction time • Solubility of analyte (a) Stability of analyte during sample preparation (b) Stability of analyte in solution (c) Stability of analyte adsorbed on sorbent layer (d) Stability of analyte adsorbed on sorbent layer during development (e) Stability of analyse on sorbent layer after development • Post-chromatographic derivatization (a) Heating time (b) Heating temperature • Densitometry – scanning wavelength

Note: For reproducible results, various parameters and conditions under which results for specific analysis have been obtained must be kept constant and detailed method description be recorded.

advantage – reaction can be followed visually, can be terminated as soon as optimal colour is developed and reagent's vapours will escape directly.

Precautions:

- Solvent residue left in the chamber after development work is completed should be disposed of carefully. Special precaution is required to be taken while disposing of halogen containing (chloroform) solvents.
- Glass trough chamber should be dried by placing them on side. Chambers should never be turned upside down as it will damage flat ground glass tip of the chamber. This will adversely affect the quality of air-tight seal and further, due to hardly any air circulation, drying of the chamber may take longer time.

Detection and visualization

One of the most characteristic features of TLC/HPTLC is the possibility to utilize post-chromatographic off-line derivatization. With availability of many visualization reagents, findings can be confirmed which the HPLC is lacking. These visualization reactions are possible for identification even if the separation is not optimal (in such cases in-situ UV spectra gets disturbed due to closer HRf of related substances).

As soon as the development process is complete, the plate is removed from the chamber and dried to remove the mobile phase completely. The zones can be located by various physical, chemical, biological-physiological methods. There is apparently no difficulty in detecting coloured substances or colourless substances absorbing in shortwave ultraviolet (UV) region (254 nm) or with intrinsic fluorescence such as riboflavin, quinine sulphate. The substances which do not have above properties have to be transferred into detectable substances by means of chromogenic or fluorogenic reagents which are more expensive, time-consuming and complicated.

Detection sensitivity depends on the specificity for the reagent employed. Iodine is the universal detection reagent, the detection is usually non-destructive and reversible but certain substances may be altered through non-reversible derivatization such as ethambutol hydrochloride, a totally non-UV absorbing compound, which forms a UV-absorbing complex with iodine through charge transfer. Iodine is the least sensitive reagent. After the plates are exposed to iodine vapours, the compounds can be identified/located by slightly yellow-coloured iodine-containing spots. Best results are often obtained by dipping the plate in 0.10 to 0.25% solution of iodine in chloroform-methanol (1 : 1). After evaporation of excess iodine, the plate is covered with a glass sheet and four sides may be sealed with tape to prevent further evaporation of iodine from the spots/bands. This technique has been successfully employed by the author for quantitative estimation of certain non-UV absorbing compounds such as dicyclomine hydrochloride, ethambutol hydrochloride by densitometric scanning of the resultant spot/band at 440 nm (detection with iodine is not suitable for layers containing starch as binder). Although detection reagents to be used in gas phase, such as iodine, hydrochloric acid and ammonia vapours give uniform distribution, but dipping, as suggested above, is the method of choice for application of the reagent for reproducible results.

Detection under UV light is the first choice and is non-destructive in most of the cases and is commonly employed for densitometric scanning. However, certain drug substances such as steroids and vitamins (D_2, D_3) are highly sensitive and may undergo molecular rearrangement.

can conveniently be added to mobile phase without altering the chromatographic profile for converting peptides or amino acids to coloured derivatives. Whether spraying or dipping technique is used for application of the reagent, following points must be kept in mind about the detection reagent:

- Sensitivity of the reagent for detection of analytes.
- Whether the reagent is suitable for detection of analyte of interest.
- Stability of the reagent.
- Stability of the final chromatogram after application of the reagent.
- It should be easy and simple to prepare the reagent.
- The reagent should not be hazardous.
- It should not interfere in the scanning of the chromatogram.

When the analyst has to resort to post-chromatographic derivatization for detection or quantitative analysis, dipping technique for application of the reagent is preferred for following reasons:

- By using dipping techniques, the coating of the adsorbent layer with the reagent is more uniform.
- Distribution of the reagent is not influenced by viscosity of the reagent or drop size of spray mist.
- Distribution of the reagent on the layer does not depend on the manual skill of the user.
- Detection limits are appreciably lower than in case of chromatogram sprayed as dipping transfers more reagent to the layer than spraying.
- Reproducibility of results is improved due to homogeneity of reagent application.
- Consumption of reagent is very less.
- Reagent is less concentrated than used as spray.
- Contamination of the laboratory with the reagents particularly which are corrosive and hazardous/injurious to health such as sulphuric acid is less.
- Spray facilities such as fume cup board are not required.
- Results are more uniform, precise and reproducible.

Note: For derivatization, using dipping technique for application of the reagent, one is confronted with the risk that separated compounds or reaction products may dissolve in the solvent present in the reagent or sorbent layer may get disturbed if the reagent is aqueous or polar solvents of the reagent may have elution effect on the fractions of the sample. It is therefore desirable that time of immersion in the reagent should be as short as possible but not more than five seconds to avoid dissolving of substances out of stationary phase. It is therefore more than necessary that due care should be taken in the choice of solvent for preparation of reagent solution. The solvent thus chosen should neither dissolve the separated substances nor their reaction products nor it should lead to tainting effect, otherwise ultimate analysis (quantitative) will be adversely effected. Further, after post-chromatographic derivatization if the plate is visually inspected, colour intensity of the zone must be more intense at the top surface of the layer than when it is viewed from back of the plate. If this is not the case, reagent must be made less polar to avoid development across the thickness of the layer.

Automated time controlled dipping apparatuses are now commercially available and are free from ripple effect which is usually observed with manual dipping technique. Distribution of the reagent on the layer does not depend on the manual skill of the user.

Note: For derivatization, time of dipping in the dipping chamber should be determined experimentally and documented for every testing procedure.

Precautions:

1. Clean off back of the HPTLC plate which is wetted with the reagent before keeping it on hot plate, laboratory bench or scanning platform.
2. After dipping operation ends, the dipping chamber should be closed with the lid to avoid loss of solvent and contamination of the laboratory environment.
3. Spraying of the reagent is not recommended particularly when ultimate aim is quantitative analysis as densitometric scanning of such plates results in irregular baseline.
4. Propellant gases in ready to use spray guns contaminate the environment and well-ventilated fume cup board is essential to ensure effective removal of reagent clouds and toxic solvent vapours.
5. Most of the chemical reactions proceed more rapidly at elevated temperature, heating at 100–110°C for 5–10 minutes is usually adequate to ensure complete reaction (with heating at higher temperature or for longer time, entire background of the plate tends to get darkened as binder present in the layer often char). In such case, silica gel H (without binder) may be suitable.
6. For quantitative analysis after post-derivatization, it is desired that heating if used should be uniform. Use of non-perforated stainless steel trays is recommended as support while drying in oven for uniform heat distribution.
7. Although by spraying, uniform distribution of the reagent is difficult to achieve, however, in certain cases, it is unavoidable while using two or more reagents in sequence such as diazotization, followed by coupling with NED in case of sulphonamides or conversion of thiamine hydrochloride (vitamin B_1) to a fluorescent derivative.

Preparation of methanolic sulphuric acid: To 80–85 ml of ice-cold methanol while further cooling in freezing mixture, add cautiously and slowly 5–10 ml (as required) of sulphuric acid (already cooled in freezing mixture). Mix and make up the volume to 100 ml with ice-cooled methanol.

Almost every chemical reaction which can be performed in a test tube can be carried out on a TLC layer.

Note:

- Since reagent vapours are usually highly toxic, TLC plate heater must always be operated in fume cupboard. Further, because of loss of heat in fume cupboard, it is preferred that temperature of plate heater be set at 120°C instead of 100°C.
- The temperature and heating time be indicated in testing protocols.
- For quantitative work, exact time of heating and temperature need experimental verification for a given analytical problem.

Post-chromatographic derivatization by spraying

Since, for derivatization, application of reagent by spraying is most common, the chromatographers must keep in mind some of the most important practical aspects.

1. Spraying of the reagent on the plate must be done in TLC spray cabinet. These cabinets are designed in such a way that spray produced by spray reagent particularly that rebound from the plate are contained without losing the spray stream before it reaches the plate.
2. Since aerosol formed during spraying being toxic, in addition to efficient extraction system, use of goggles, gloves and mask is advised.
3. It must be noted that spraying produces less homogeneous coating, and volume of reagent sprayed is difficult to control.
4. Spray reagent should be freshly prepared. If stored longer, it should be tested for specific use before using.
5. Nozzles of the glass sprayer should neither be too narrow as it will take longer time for spraying process nor too wide as it will yield large drops of reagent thus damaging the layer making evaluation too difficult.
6. Spray head should be cleaned and dried after every use to avoid contamination of reagents to be sprayed at later date.
7. Reagents containing explosive solvents should never be used.
8. As it is difficult to spray on plates of smaller format (5 × 5 cm), it is advisable to keep the plate on used larger plate and then carry out the spraying.
9. When sequencing reagents are to be applied, the plate should be kept on hot plate for applied solution to evaporate quickly for spraying process to proceed further with different reagent.

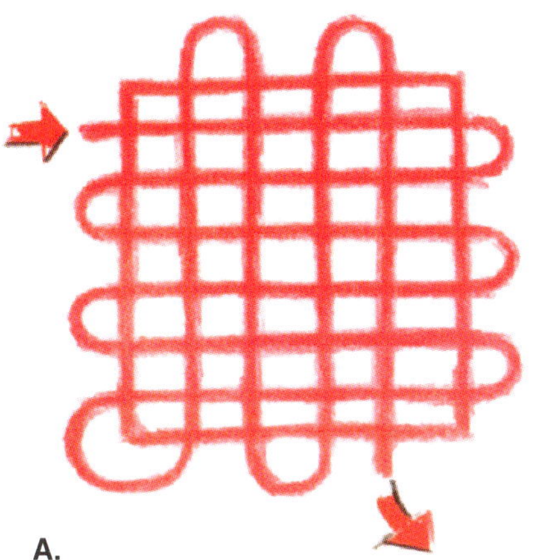

A.

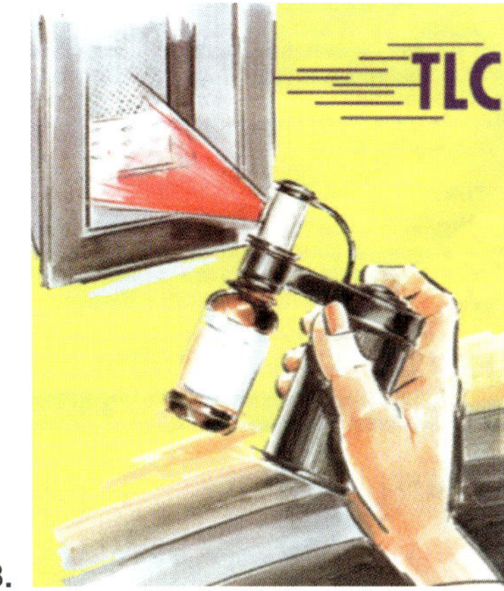

B.

A. Recommended spray scheme (meandering pattern). **B.** Spraying a TLC plate with the TLC sprayer.

Stabilization of developed zones

After treatment with the reagent as part of chromatographic derivatization, coloured or fluorescent chromatographic zones are used for quantitative evaluation. It is therefore desirable that the colour or fluorescence thus produced should be stable at least for 30 minutes for carrying out various steps involved in quantitative analysis. There is no general procedure laid down to stabilize the coloured chromatographic zones except to store in atmosphere of nitrogen and protected from light till they are evaluated. However, fluorescent chromatographs can not only be stabilized but often intensified. For extensive details on stabilization and augmentation of fluorescence intensity, one may refer to compilation by Jork et al., 1990 and 1994.

For this, the developed chromatogram is dipped in viscous lipophilic (hydrophobic) solvents such as 10–20% solution of liquid paraffin (mineral oil) in n-hexane. The stabilization is due to exclusion of oxygen responsible for oxidative degradation of the substance. Mixture of chloroform-liquid paraffin-triethanolamine (60 + 10 + 10) has been employed in stabilizing and augmentation of fluorescence in case of thiamine hydrochloride (vitamin B_1) and ethinylestradiol (fluorescence is stable up to 24 h and usually two-fold augmentation is observed). Mixture of 33% liquid paraffin in cyclohexane can be employed for stabilizing and augmenting fluorescence in case of amiloride.

A dipping solution containing 2% PEG in dichloromethane has been reported (*J. Pharm. Biomed. Analysis*, **39**, 581–586, 2005).

Mechanism: PEG causes excitation energy to be less dissipated during vibration/relaxation process. The last step enhances the fluorescent signals.

Precautions:

(a) For stabilizing the fluorescence, the plate may be immersed twice for 1 second each in the mixture of lipophilic solvent with brief intermediate drying.

(b) Quantitative evaluation should be resorted to at least 60 minutes after dipping as it takes longer time for fluorescent emission to stabilize.

Quantitation (Evaluation)

Requirements for various steps in TLC/HPTLC are more stringent for quantitative analysis. Accurate and precise application of samples is the most critical. Further, the chromatographic development should clearly and completely separate all the compounds of interest with no loss by decomposition, evaporation or irreversible adsorption during application or development. Sample and standard as a rule should be chromatographed on the same plate under similar conditions.

Earlier, a typical approach was scrapping the separated analyte zones from support material and extracting with a suitable solvent, compounds thus eluted could be analysed by any convenient analytical method; spectrophotometric, fluorometric or by suitable colour development method. To compensate for any interference from the sorbent, usually a blank area of the layer is also eluted simultaneously and used as a blank for final analysis. Such blank's values can be lowered by pre-washing of TLC layer with methanol, methanol-chloroform (1 : 1) or methylene chloride prior to chromatographic procedure. However, this method of separating and elution has limited application as the compounds under analysis may be irreversibly bound to the TLC/HPTLC support or elution/isolation steps may cause some chemical transformation or there is likelihood of analyte loss during extraction. In spite of these limitations, spot/band elution method is still widely used because it is simple and inexpensive. Layers containing gypsum as binder are considerably softer and especially suited for preparative chromatography involving scrapping from plate and subsequent elution and estimation.

The simplest method of in situ quantitative TLC is based on visual comparison of size and or intensity of coloured, fluorescent or UV (254 nm) absorbing compounds. The method is simple, quick and needs no elaborate instrumentation and laboratory facilities, however, the results are semi-quantitative (±10%). Accuracy can be improved when standard and sample concentrations are bracketed. Such visual comparisons are more meaningful on TLC plates than on HPTLC plates because of wider particle size of the sorbent in the former. The author has extensively made use of TLC for quick assessment of the quality of drugs during routine quality control of drug samples received for analysis. Basically, this technique involves bracketing the concentration of standard at 90 and 110% of the claim in respect of components present in the sample under analysis. Both samples (presumed to be 100%) and standards are chromatographed on the same plate under similar conditions. Comparison of the intensity and spot size is used for estimation. For such visual comparison of size of zones of sample and standard, it is important that Rf values are same. However, due to matrix effect, Rf values with the sample may not exactly compare with the standard, thus zone size may differ due to different diffusion pattern of the substance on the chromatogram. This procedure though semi-quantitative is extremely useful to establish whether analytical values so obtained are above or below preset limiting values.

In-situ densitometry

Densitometry is the in situ instrumental measurement of visible, UV absorbance, fluorescence or fluorescence quenching directly on the layer without resorting to scrapping and elution. Since chromatographic zones emit a lower light intensity than the environment around it, absorption spectra can be determined directly on the plate by comparison with substance free area of the sorbent layer. The measurements are usually made by reflection from the plate using single beam, double beam or single beam-dual wavelength operation of scanning instruments. The purpose of the scanner is to convert the spot/band on the layer into chromatogram consisting of peaks similar in appearance to HPLC. The position of the scanned peaks on the recorder chart are related to Rf values of the spots on the layer and peak height or area is related to the concentration of the substance on the spot. The signals which are measured represent the adsorption of transmitted or reflected light that passes through the band compared to blank portion of the sorbent layer.

To carry out a HPTLC densitometric analysis, three or four standard and purified samples are applied on the same plate. After development, detection (if necessary), the chromatogram is scanned. A calibration curve consisting of scan area of standard versus amount of analyte is constructed and amount of analyte in the sample represented by scan area is interpolated from the standard curve. Depending upon the analytical problem, one can resort to single-level or multi-level calibration. Single-level calibration is suitable when known target values are to be verified such as stability testing, dissolution profile. Single-level calibration utilizes simple proportion calculations. For multi-level calibration, select calibration functions (linear regression, non-linear regression, polynomial regression or Michaelis Menten regression) are best suited for method validation. Concentration of the analyte in the sample is calculated by considering the weight of the sample initially taken and dilution factors. Since contents of active ingredients in pharmaceutical formulations are usually well-defined, part of linearity curve falling in the range of 75–125% of the labelled/declared amount is adequate. It has been observed that a straight line fitting through 75–125% in a three point curve yields assay values with ±1% accuracy than those obtained with five point curve usually recommended in analysis, thus three levels of calibration curve usually serves the purpose for quantitative analysis. This advantage is significant in view of additional space available on the plate without sacrificing the quality of the analytical results. It may be emphasized that without reference compounds, identification is rather difficult and ultimate quantification is always questionable. Spot/band intensity on the developed chromatogram is likely to change as the time passes, particularly in case of sensitive substances. It is therefore, desirable that developed spots/bands should either be stabilized or scanned as early as possible, though it is the inherent advantage of HPTLC that all fractions remain stored on the plate. They can be scanned at different wavelengths consecutively.

Criteria for selection of most suitable wavelength for densitometric scanning of chromatogram

UV absorbing compounds such as paracetamol, caffeine, aspirin are determined by in-situ densitometric scanning after chromatographic development. The light intensity remitted by chromatographic zones is usually lower than the sorbent layer around it. Therefore absorption spectra of a compound can directly be determined on HPTLC plate itself in comparison to substance free portion of sorbent layer. It has usually been observed that spectra of the substance as recorded directly on the HPTLC plate (in-situ) is almost similar to the one recorded when the substance is in solution form, although modified layers such as silanol, amino, cyano, do cause bathochromic or hypsochromic shifts. For single component formulations, the quantification should be done by scanning at wavelength of maximum absorption (λ_{max}) in absorbance/reflectance mode.

The main reason for scanning at wavelength of maximum absorption is that difference between absorption by the chromatographic zone and the blank area of sorbent layer around it is the largest, background black being least. However, the analyst is often confronted with a problem while handling complex formulations containing several ingredients with variable concentration and having absorption maximum spread over a longer ultraviolet range. Under these circumstances, if the analyst resorts to scan the chromatogram at absorption maxima of each compound, then real purpose of using the HPTLC is forfeited and i.e. sample throughput, the main advantage of the method is adversely effected. It is therefore desirable that analyst should explore the possibility of selecting a single wavelength at which the entire chromatogram could be scanned without sacrificing vital information about different components. This single wavelength is usually referred to as "most suitable wavelength". It cannot be denied that limit of detection (LOD) and limit of quantitation (LOQ) will be substantially altered, we had frequently come across such instances during the course of laboratory evaluation of several multi-component pharmaceutical formulations. This problem is frequently encountered in formulations which contain different components at very different levels. A typical formulation frequently used as analgesic and anti-pyretic contains aspirin 300 mg, paracetamol 400 mg, caffeine 30 mg. If sample is diluted to an extent to bring aspirin and paracetamol within scanning range, then concentration of caffeine at that dilution will fall below detection or scanning limits. Analyst has therefore to take a judicious decision to select suitable dilution of the sample so that all the ingredients/components of a formulation can be simultaneously scanned. Whenever, the analyst has to take a decision for selecting a single most suitable wavelength, he may consider the following parameters before proceeding with selecting the required wave-length:

1. As already discussed, the absorption spectra of compound when recorded in solution or in situ from TLC plate is almost similar. Pre-recorded spectra of these compounds as available in literature may be considered for taking decision.
2. In-situ spectra of each component of the formulation may be simultaneously considered for selecting the most suitable wavelength for scanning.
3. Extinction coefficient (E 1% 1 cm) and actual concentration of a compound in the formulation has to be taken into consideration, particularly in respect of compounds with low extinction coefficient.
4. While selecting single wavelength, the interest of minor component in the formulation shall need special consideration such as caffeine in formulation containing aspirin and paracetamol. It is therefore obvious that single wavelength of choice in above formulation must be as close to absorption maxima of caffeine (λ_{max} 272 nm) as possible. In other words, if single wavelength near to absorption maxima of aspirin or paracetamol had been chosen for scanning, estimation of caffeine would not have been possible.
5. If absorption maxima of individual component of the formulation are quite apart, then the chromatogram must be scanned at individual absorption maxima for obtaining meaningful results.

Note: Overlaid UV-spectra of few formulations are provided to support above criteria for selection of suitable wavelength for densitometric scanning.

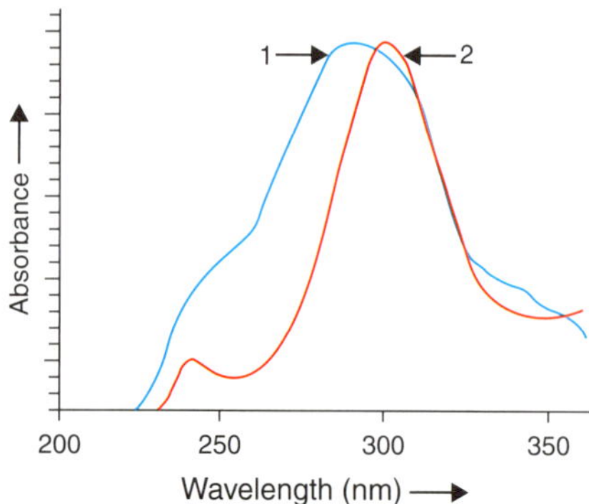

Overlaid UV-spectra of aspirin (1) and dipyridamole (2). UV-290 nm being the iso-absorption point of drugs (1) and (2) and close to λ_{max} of both the drugs was selected as most suitable wavelength for scanning densitogram of the formulation containing above two drugs for quantitative evaluation.

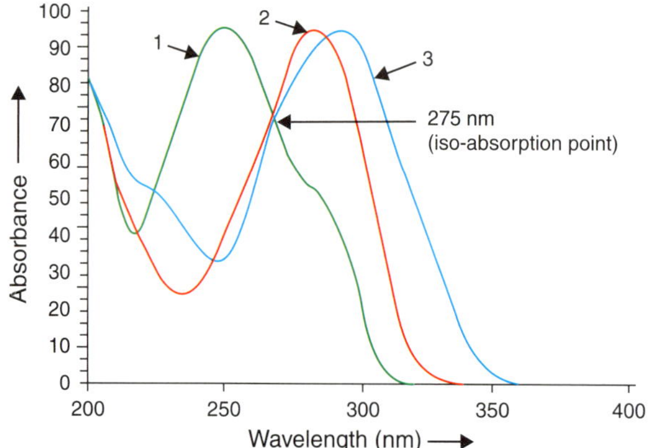

Overlaid UV-spectra of paracetamol (1), aceclofenac (2) and rabeprazole (3). UV-275 nm being iso-absorption point for all the three drugs was selected as most suitable wavelength for scanning densitogram of the formulation containing above three drugs for quantitative evaluation.

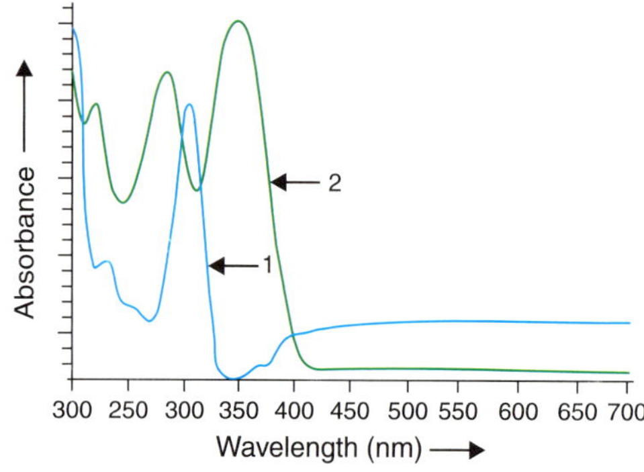

Overlaid UV-spectra of ethamsylate (1) and mefenamic acid (2). UV-300 nm being iso-absorption point was selected as most suitable wavelength for scanning densitogram of the formulation containing above two drugs for quantitative evaluation.

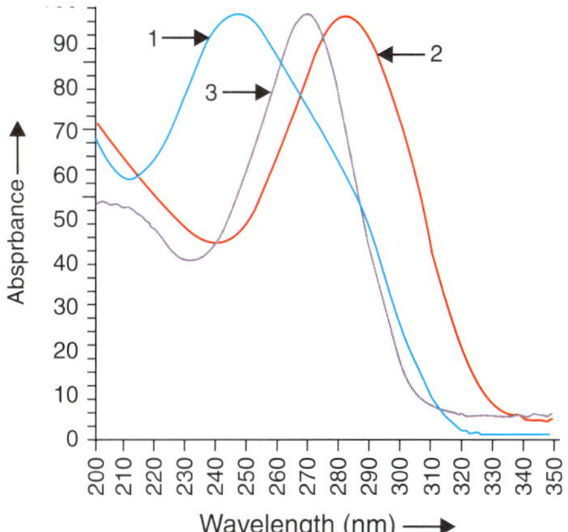

Overlaid UV-spectra of paracetamol (1), diclofenac sodium (2) and famotidine (3). UV-274 nm being iso-absorption point for (2) and (3), and (1) having significant absorption at 274 nm was selected as most suitable wavelength for densitometric scanning of the formulation containing above three drugs for quantitative evaluation.

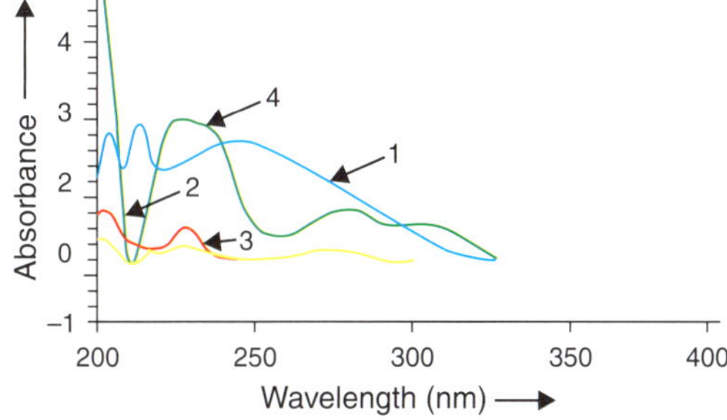

Overlaid UV-spectra of metoprolol succinate (1), ramipril (2), atorvastatin calcium (3) and aspirin (4). In the entire spectra (200–400 nm), no wavelength was found suitable for simultaneous quantitation of all the four drugs. UV-210 nm was selected for densitometric evaluation as at this wavelength all the four drugs exhibited absorption as is the case with all organic molecules.

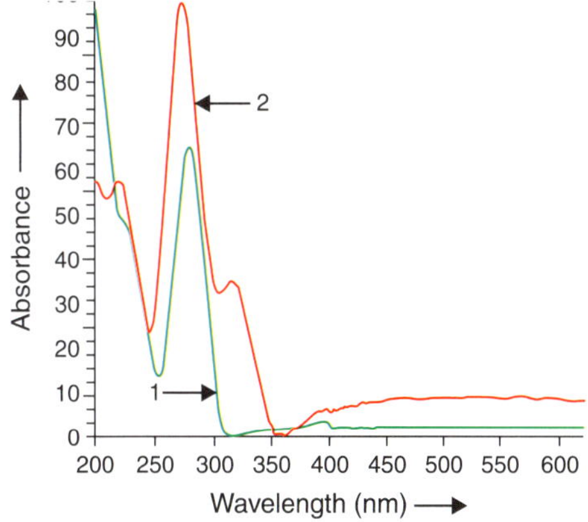

Overlaid UV-spectra of aliskiren (1) and hydrochlorothiazide (2). 280 nm, being very close to the absorption maxima of both the drugs, was selected as suitable wavelength for densitometric scanning.

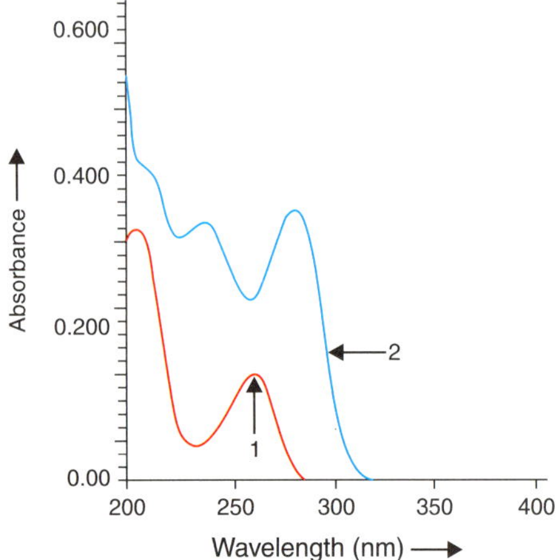

Overlaid UV-spectra of tenofovir (1) and emtricitabine (2). UV-265 nm was selected as suitable wavelength for densitometric scanning. Both the substances have reasonably good absorption at 265 nm.

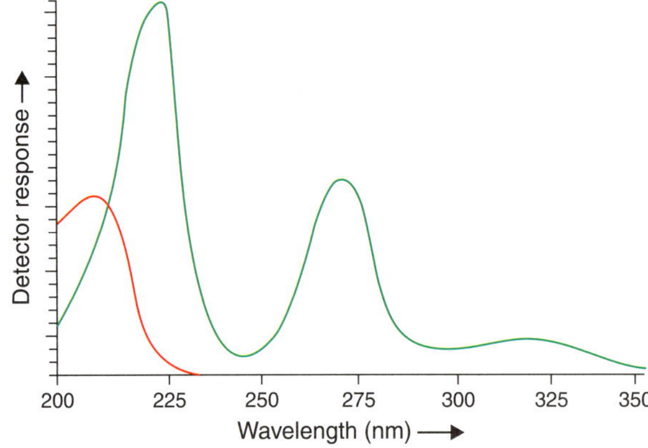

In-situ overlaid UV-spectra of hydrochlorothiazide (1) and lisinopril (2). Lisinopril being the minor component was scanned at 210 nm. Hydrochlorothiazide could not be scanned at 210 nm for accurate quantitation as its spectral curve was falling on slope. Hence, hydrochlorothiazide was scanned at its λ_{max} i.e. 275 nm.

REVERSED-PHASE TLC/HPTLC

Most separation by TLC is performed with unmodified silica gel pre-coated layers. However, due to complexity of certain separation problems and in response to the increasing demands and expectation of chromatographers to design mobile phases for HPLC without involving risk to costly columns, new layers with chemically modified silica gel have been introduced. Selectivity of adsorbent is continuously being increased by chemical modification of the layers, some of the most common modifications are amino, cyano, diol and silanization (commonly represented as RP_2, RP_8 and RP_{18}). The use of silanized (reversed-phase) plates provide quick and inexpensive previewed separation traits prior to HPLC (an estimated 80–90% of HPLC analysis is performed using reserved-phase columns). While using reversed-phase layers, it is relatively easier to find a good mobile phase as there are only a few volatile water miscible solvents available and most of them are generally found suitable such as methanol, acetonitrile, dioxane. It is increasingly being experienced that different components of a formulation which could not be resolved using normal-phase TLC could easily be resolved by reversed phase TLC often resulting in partial or complete reversal of retention order. Substances migrate in a general order of decreasing polarity (the most polar solute moves the fastest) and mobile phase strength increases with decreasing polarity (acetonitrile is a stronger solvent than water). On the other hand, wide variety of mobile phases available for use in normal-phase silica gel TLC increases separation potential. HPTLC silica gel 60 with a mean particle size of 6 nm and mean pore size of 60 Å is used for RP re-coated plates. Octadecyl chains are chemically bounded to the silanol groups on the surface of silica gel. These layers are designed to correlate to C_{18} bounded HPLC reversed-phase columns (usually 10–12% carbon loading). Chemically bound octadecyl chains are responsible for the reversed-phase character of the layer, remaining silanol groups which are not converted determine the hydrophilic properties of the sorbent, thus degree of wettability. Lower the modification, lesser the interaction between solute and sorbent, hence higher Rf value.

Note: Difference between Rf values with mobile phase of similar eluotropic strength are much lower than silica gel. Therefore, in identity testing by RPTLC, use of more than one mobile phase does not elicit much additional information.

Sample preparation

The samples spotted onto a RPHPTLC plate shall meet the same requirements as for normal-phase silica gel HPTLC. The samples that require extraction and clean-up prior to cellulose or silica gel TLC can sometime be applied directly to

RP plates, such as analysis of dyes in suspension and syrups and food products, the sample need only be diluted with methanol prior to RPTLC.

As RPTLC plates have high capacity and can accept large quantity of samples, clean-up of the sample or its concentration is often not necessary. Because of high capacity, less concentrated sample solution can be employed, thus reducing the need for plates with pre-adsorbent or pre-concentration layers.

Standards and samples should be dissolved in most polar solvent to avoid band spreading. By using weak solvent, purification of the complex samples is also achieved as highly non-polar impurities get eliminated being insoluble in weak solvents (selective solvation). Taking into consideration the stability of the compounds, wettability limitations, sample solutions should be prepared in predominantly organic solvent than in water. Methanol which is quickly evaporated and usually wets the layers adequately is suitable for substances capable of hydrogen bonding. For less polar compounds, methylene chloride and acetone are the suitable solvents.

Mobile phase selection

The greatest advantage of RPTLC is the simplicity of mobile phase. This is usually a two component mixture of water and a polar organic solvent miscible with water such as methanol, acetonitrile, acetone, dioxane. By adjusting the proportions of the components of the mobile phase, separation can be tuned. As a rule, more non-polar the sample, higher the proportion of organic components of the mobile phase. As polarity of the mobile phase increases, so does the contents of water in the mobile phase. While using water-alcohol mixtures as mobile phase, resolution may be improved by changing the alcohol to one of higher or lower chain lengths with constant concentration or by altering the alcohol-water ratio such as methanol « ethanol « propanol.

To start with chromatographic work with RPTLC, mixture of ethanol-water (80 : 20 v/v) is the most useful starting mobile phase. Selectivity may be improved by altering the ratio with water. Addition of 1–20% of tetrahydrofuran or dimethylformamide can prove useful in difficult separation problems. Mixtures of water with polar solvents often offer wettability problem. Separation of organic acid is facilitated by addition of weak acid such as formic acid or acetic acid to the mobile phase to give a pH value below the pH of the acid solutes.

Solvent mixtures containing more than 40% water may damage binding properties of the layer in addition to wettability problem, bad spot shape and irregular solvent front. This can be overcome by adding ion-pair salts or sodium chloride (0.1 to 0.5 M) instead of water. The addition of salt usually does not affect the separation, rather increases the migration rate of the mobile phase.

Addition of 0.5 M sodium chloride to acetonitrile-water mixture containing less than 25% of water, usually demixing of phase is observed, then ammonium acetate (0.5 M) may be employed instead of sodium chloride)

- RP plates normally do not require activation.
- Adjustment of water content is not critical as with silica gel because virtually all accessible silanol groups are de-activated by chemical bonding with hydrocarbons.
- Solvent demixing is less of a problem.
- Independent of humidity.
- Non-chlorinated solvents.
- Higher the percentage of carbon loading of the layer, more the developing time, usually carbon loading of about 12% gives good results.
- Rate of development decreases with increasing water contents of mobile phase.
- Chemically bonded RP layers offer advantage over otherwise impregnated layer (with paraffin oil) of non-contamination of solute with impregnating liquid.

Note:

(a) If with use of polar solvents, diffuse spots with high Rf values are obtained, use of polar silica gel layer might be advantageous because spot sequence will change.

(b) While using neutral solvents (methanol-water) if the coated surface is damaged, use of 0.5 M sodium chloride can prevent the damage to some extent.

(c) The bonded layers can be washed with methanol, methylene chloride or acetone and re-used up to 4–5 times with no apparent change in chromatographic separation profile. Washing is usually continued till previously chromatographed solvents are visually undetected under UV.

(d) Reduction of 10 ml of methanol per 100 ml of mobile phase reduces HRf value by 10–20.

Detection on RPHPTLC

Sensitivity of detection depends on the absorptivity (extinction coefficient) of each compound. The problem of water instability and wettability of RP layers usually limits the use of totally aqueous or water rich detection reagents; reagents in methanol or acetone are usually employed. Use of aggressive (charring) reagents such as sulphuric acid is limited on chemically bonded plates as presence of organic phase leads to discoloration of background.

Correlation of HPTLC to HPLC (silica gel)

Most of the versatile and efficient mobile phase used in normal-phase TLC/HPTLC using silica gel as sorbent containing toluene, acetone, ethylacetate cannot be used in silica gel HPLC because of their UV absorbing property. Only solvents such as hexane or dichloromethane mixed with methanol, isopropyl alcohol or tetrahydrofuran can be employed. Such mobile phases are relatively inefficient in TLC/HPTLC and their versatility is limited. Therefore use of silica gel TLC/HPTLC as a pilot technique for silica gel HPLC has limited application.

Correlation of RP-HPTLC to RP-HPLC

C_{18} HPLC columns from different suppliers have different selectivities and same is true for different makes of RP-HPTLC plates as well. The work carried out by Robert et al., 1984, on neutral substances establishes excellent relation between RP-HPTLC and RP-HPLC. The capacity factor (K′) in column HPLC is related to Rf value of a HPTLC spot by the equation:

$$K' = \frac{1 - Rf}{Rf}$$

Optimum K′ range for HPLC is 2–6 which corresponds to Rf values of 0.1–0.3. It is therefore obvious that mobile phase that gives HRf values between 10 and 30 may be the proper strength for use as a solvent in RP-HPLC. As an empirical rule for practical work using methanol-water mixture, decreasing methanol concentration by 10 ml per 100 ml of solvent mixture roughly doubles the K′ values in RPHPLC and reduces HRf values in RP-HPTLC by 10–20.

It is often claimed that TLC on C_{18} layers can be used to scout solvent systems for transfer to column RPHPLC. The speed, ease of operation and low cost of TLC renders it ideal for determining the conditions for RP-HPLC. Uncharacterized samples may be preliminarily evaluated without risking expensive HPLC columns having limited life can thus be spared from experimental runs required to establish the separation conditions. However, such correlation is not possible in each and every case. Major problem in obtaining correlation is the lack of complete equilibration with the mobile phase in TLC/HPTLC compared to column HPLC because of fundamental differences in experimental procedures used for the two techniques. However, it is possible to obtain order of elution of solutes which will help the analyst to fine tune this solvent on column HPLC before actual analytical run. Generally 3–5% more polar mobile phase is required for equivalent results in RP-HPLC compared to RP-HPTLC.

Determination of purity profile by RPTLC and RP-HPLC

In HPLC, low level of substances or impurities with relatively high retention time are poorly resolved and detected owing to peak broadening. On the other hand, in RPTLC, substances with low Rf values form tight and sharp zones, hence have better detection sensitivity. In contrast, the substances with low retention time may appear as unresolved in HPLC but in RPTLC, they will usually appear between HRf value of 50–90 and can easily be detected. In RPTLC, the impurities either at starting line or near the solvent front can be detected provided the plates have been properly cleaned by pre-washing prior to development. Large quantities of slowly eluting substances would completely spoil the HPLC column after injections and may show memory effect, whereas slowly eluting substances in RPTLC will be retained near the origin.

Precautions:

- TLC plates to be used for purity profile should not be dried at elevated temperature in order to avoid any decomposition, oxidation and hydrolysis during chromatography.
- The solvents to be used for preparation of sample or as component of mobile phase should be first checked by running a blank TLC plate in the solvent. The plate should not show any spot visible under UV light or with the reagent likely to be used for detection of the impurity/impurities. This is absolutely essential because any impurity present in the solvent can give erroneous results, in that the additional spot/spots can be mistaken to have been contributed by the substance under examination.

PREPARATIVE THIN LAYER CHROMATOGRAPHY (PLC)

This technique is used when significant quantities of sample components are to be isolated and purified for subsequent analysis (IR, GC-MS, NMR).

- To achieve higher loading capacity, sample may be applied by streaking across the full width of the plate instead of spotting.
- Pre-coated plates of 20 cm height (20 × 20 cm) with a thickness up to 2000 mm are commercially available for preparative TLC. Preparative TLC plates (20 × 40 cm), 1000 mm thick have also been introduced by Whatman.
- Laboratories having facilities for coating their own plates, can prepare plates of any height and thickness as required.
- Preparative plates having both pre-adsorbent and analytical layers are most suited for the purpose. Pre-adsorbent edge of the plate is dipped in the sample solution allowed to cover the pre-adsorbent area but before it reaches the interface with analytical area. The plate is taken out, dried and the process repeated. The plate is finally dried and subjected to development process as usual.

- Since sole purpose of preparative thin layer chromatography is to recover pure sample components, reversed-phase TLC plates give higher sample recovery, hence recommended particularly while dealing with valuable samples.
- After development, the plates should be dried in vacuum desiccator and never heated.
- No destructive detection technique should be used, most common technique being fluorescent quenching.
- Exposure to iodine vapours – the reaction with most of the compounds is reversible, but care should be taken to avoid oxidation.
- Spraying plates with water locates lipophilic and other water insoluble compounds.
- For eluting the detected zones, the entire plate should be sprayed to dampness with absolute alcohol, area marked and scrapped off with sharp blade, about 10% additional area than marked may preferably be scrapped to compensate for 3-dimensional development of the band in the layer.
- Minimum volume of the solvent should be used for eluting the components from scrapped material, usually mobile phase is recommended for the purpose. Volume of solvent required can be calculated as follows:

  Volume of solvent required = Volume of scrapped material × 10 × (1 – Rf)

  For eluting 0.5 ml of scrapped material of sample with Rf value of 0.2, we require 0.4 ml of the solvent.

  Volume of solvent required = 0.5 × 10 × (1 – 0.2) = 0.4 ml.
- Scrapped material and solvent is homogenised in vortex mixture to ensure complete elution, centrifuged, supernatant collected for evaporation.
- Solvent mixtures containing 20–30% methanol are preferred.

One may also encounter the following problems in preparative chromatography:

1. Sample may be lost through irreversible absorption – can be minimised by using reversed-phase chromatography.
2. Contamination from other sources.
   (a) Solvent: Use chromatographic grade solvent.
   (b) TLC plates: Pre-wash the plate before use and always store in vacuum desiccator.

Dual-phase TLC plates (layers)

Two-dimensional chromatography first described by Kirchner in 1951 made use of the same plate but either one or two different mobile phases for both the dimensions were used; the first to resolve polar constituents and second for non-polar components. By this procedure diverse species could be separated. However samples usually leads to streak in second dimension if difference in composition is too significant, thus leading to poor reproducibility. In 1979, Whatman introduced TLC plates having both normal and reversed-phase layers side by side on the same TLC plate (3 cm band of reversed-phase layer, the remaining being normal phase layer). Development in the first direction usually occurs on reversed phase strip, followed by second development on the normal phase region. This technique allows separation of complex, crude and samples of diverse polarity without any sample loss due to prior clean-up.

Application of dual-phase plates

1. While using reversed-phase area of the plate, and dealing with crude and complex samples (liquid formulations of vitamins and expectorants), the polar mass will migrate to the solvent front, lipophilic substances will be strongly bound and will remain near or at the point of application thus leading to cleaner separation in the second direction.
2. Complex samples are likely to contain components which are either too different or too similar to be separated by single phase TLC. One of the approaches may be to use two different plates, extracting the unseparated components from first plate and re-chromatographing them on second plate. However for separation of such complex mixture, use of dual phase TLC plate is the right answer.
3. Preparing finger printing of complex samples and mirror image.
4. Identification of sample: By subjecting the sample and standard to both the phases on a dual phase TLC plate, one can confirm the identity of the unknown, the combination of two very different separation mechanisms is a very reliable source of confirming the identity of an unknown sample.

Most important application of this technique is in the area of obtaining “finger printing” such as analysis of herbal formulation containing mixture of several plant extracts. To obtain mirror image, spot the sample at either end of reversed phase strip, develop towards centre line (scored before development) in the first mobile phase. It may be ensured that first direction development is carried out to exactly the same distance for both samples. Sample and standard chromatographed side by side and mirror image/finger prints obtained. Use of certain sulphonamides is restricted by law due to their suspected carcinogenicity in animal field, these can be detected by mirror image technique.

With the reversed-phase band along the bottom, this region of the layer can serve as pre-adsorbent clean-up area for removal of lipophylic impurities from samples in which polar compounds are to be analysed by one-dimensional TLC.

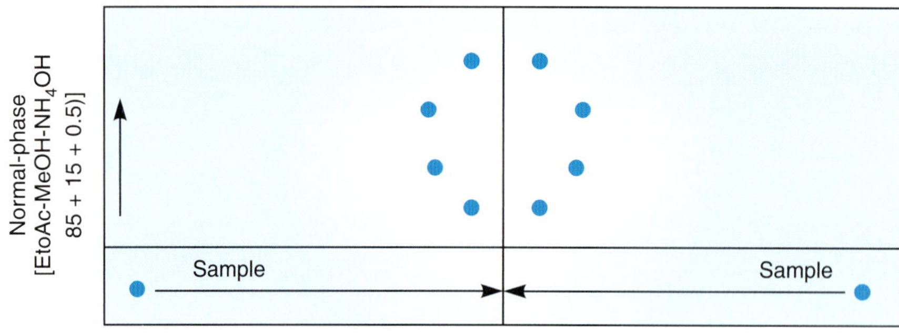

Sample application scheme for obtaining fingerprint/mirror image.

To obtain even solvent front on the first direction on reversed-phase region, the reversed-phase region may be first covered, silica gel area sprayed with 95% ethanol, the object being to neutralize silica completely to ensure uniform migration of solvent on reversed-phase layer. Alternatively, about 0.5 cm strip of the silica gel layer is scrapped off so that normal phase region is not immersed in first mobile phase used for reversed-phase TLC.

Aqueous contents of mobile phase for reversed-phase TLC should not be more than 40%. Use of 0.5 M sodium chloride in place of water is recommended to increase wettability. Ammonium acetate can also be used (it volatilises completely to ammonia and acetic acid on drying the plate at 110°C).

If chromatography in the first direction is on reversed-phase layer, it will be necessary to reactivate the plate at 110°C prior to second dimensional chromatography on normal phase layer. If compounds of interest are heat labile, removal of mobile phase used for reversed phase chromatography should be carried out is a vacuum oven or desiccator at room temperature.

HPTLC plates with pre-adsorbent layers (concentrating zones)

Such plates consist of 2–3 cm strip of non-adsorbing inert material such as kieselguhr (inert to large number of compounds) along with lower edge of a standard silica gel layer or RP layer (analytical layer). This strip serves as quick application zone. Even if the sample has been applied with unsteady hand (careful sample application is time-consuming and requires special equipment such as Linomat V), quantitative evaluation of the chromatogram is possible. Irrespective of shape, size or position of the spot, analyte will form a sharp narrow band at the junction of two layers (kieselguhr and silica).

Separation proceeds on analytical layer. Resolution and sensitivity is superior as compared to use of conventional silica gel layer due to vertical compactness of the initial zones. This inactive strip is also known as staging area for application of samples.

Plate preparation

Depending on the length and condition of storage, pre-washing may be necessary, use of chloroform or methylene chloride-methanol (1 + 1) or mobile phase is recommended, followed by heating in oven at 70–80°C for 30 min to ensure removal of traces of wash solvent (pre-washing improves sensitivity, accuracy and precision of densitometric scanning by increasing the contrast between the zones and background, and reducing the baseline noise). Pre-washing is essential while using bioautography or extracting zones for identification by HPLC, GC, MS, NMR.

Sample preparation

As sample clean-up takes place on the pre-adsorbent layers, minimal sample preparation is required, thus dilute samples can be directly applied. Prime steps involved in sample purification (extraction, separation of phases, evaporation and reconstitution of analyte) are eliminated resulting in saving of time and avoidance of loss of analyte due to these steps. Crude samples such as biological fluids, herbal extracts can be directly applied to the pre-adsorbent layer.

Sample application

Maximum realization of the pre-adsorbent effect is obtained by application of sample across the entire layer. Samples should be more dilute (4–10 times) than for application in conventional HPTLC plates. To avoid partitioning mechanism, moisture left in the applied sample must be removed by hot air, in a desiccator over P_2O_5 (for unstable compounds). Spraying of plate with alcohol near the end of drying operation and subsequent heating will remove the water as azeoptropic mixture. In case of directly applied samples (biological fluids), it is preferable to use stronger solvent such as methanol or methanol-ethyl acetate (1 + 1) and carry out the development up to layer junction for 2–3 times with intermittent drying. This pre-development gives compact and uniform band for further chromatography on analytical layer.

Advantages

- Rapid application of high volumes and dilute solutions.
- Improved resolution.
- Improved sensitivity of detection.
- Improved precision of resolution.
- Improved precision of quantitation by scanning.
- Less sample clean-up required.
- If very dilute solutions or large volumes are to be applied, one can immerse the pre-adsorbed strip of the plate in sample solution.

Applications

1. Separation of fatty acid esters.
2. Aflatoxin.
3. Alkaloids.
4. Aquarium microbial agents.
5. Food dyes.
6. Penicillins.
7. Phenothiazines.
8. Purines.
9. PTH-amino acids.
10. Steroids.

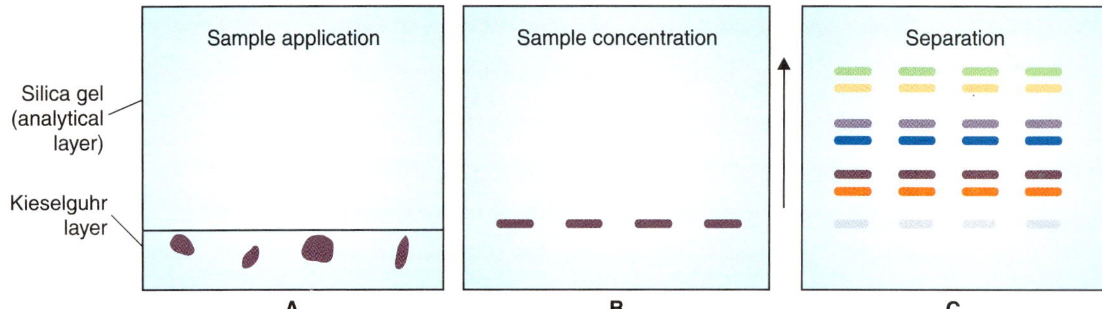

(A) A strip coated with kieselguhr serving as concentration zone for application of samples in any shape, size and position. **(B)** Sharp bands at the interface of two adsorbents (kieselguhr and silica gel). **(C)** Silica gel layer for development and separation of complex mixture of fatty acid esters.

Stability studies

Analyte should not decompose during development of the chromatogram and should be stable in solution and on the sorbent for at least 30 and 15 minutes respectively. The intensity of the spot on the chromatogram should be constant for at least 60 min. While optimizing the extraction/purification procedure, one must keep in mind the chemical properties and purity of the extraction solvent. Chemical reaction of the solvents and their impurities can form artifact, which may produce extra spot/peak, thus leading to false assay values. Other important factor is pH of the aqueous phase for extraction/purification which may lead to hydrolysis, oxidation, isomerization. Evap oration of organic solvent to dryness may also lead to formation of artifact, complete removal of organic solvent to dryness may also lead to formation of artifact, complete removal of organic solvent should be avoided.

(a) *Stability in sample solution:* Many solutes may decompose in sample solution prepared prior to TLC/HPTLC investigation. Solutions of same concentration are prepared from stock sample solution and stored at room temperature for 240, 120, 60, 30 and 10 min. and then applied on the same chromatoplate, after development the chromatogram is evaluated for additional spots if any. The chromatogram should not contain any spot absent in the initial chromatogram (zero time) and any spot present in the initial chromatogram should not be absent from the final chromatogram.

(b) *Stability of the analyte adsorbed on the sorbent layer prior to development (spot stability):* Further possible source of error is the decomposition of the analyte due to active sites of the stationary phase. Sample application (spotting technique, size and shape of spot, temperature of air stream used for drying the spot, chemical effect of light, air and the time the sample is left to stand on the sorbent prior to chromatographic development are some of significant factors which can influence the stability of separated spots and are required to be investigated for validation. Usually, it is recommended that spot should be stable for at least 15 minutes on sorbent layer. Two-dimensional chromatography using same solvent system should enable to find out any decomposition occurring during spotting and development. General procedure of validation as described under stability in solution may be followed.

(c) *Stability of analyte during development:* Many compounds are very sensitive to the conditions used for chromatographic development, most important are oxidative or hydrolytic decomposition primarily due to dissolved oxygen (O_2), light and temperature. This problem is related to method development or mobile phase optimization. To evaluate any detrimental effect of temperature and exposure to light, one may design the experiments separately at room temperature, cool place, both in reflected light and protected light.

Oxidative decomposition can be reduced by use of protective gas (nitrogen or argon) both in chamber and to remove any dissolved oxygen from eluent by flushing or use of stabilizers (antioxidants) such as use of BHT in TLC of vitamin D_2 and danazole – this will protect the sample from oxidative decomposition.

Evidence of analyte decomposing during spotting and chromatographic development can be confirmed by resorting to two-dimensional chromatography using same solvent system in both directions. If decomposition occurs during spotting and spot drying only, the chromatogram obtained in the second direction of the eluent flow will be free from any impurity peak (single peak chromatogram shall be obtained). If decomposition occurs during development, peak(s) of decomposition product(s) shall be obtained for the analyte both in the first and second direction of the run. The shape of peak of decomposition product usually shows significant tailing compared with that of analyte, peak area of decomposition product in both the directions being similar to each other.

Alternatively the decomposition may occur both during spotting/spot drying and chromatographic development. The situation is similar to one encountered above, but the peak(s) of decomposition products in the first direction exhibit less tailing than that obtained in the second direction and area of peak in first direction is significantly higher than that obtained with second direction.

(d) *Stability of analyte after chromatographic development:* When sensitive substances are subjected to TLC/HPTLC, intensity of the spot sometime may change on the developed chromatogram as the time passes. This difficulty is often encountered when eluent cannot be easily evaporated from the sorbent layer. Constant spot signals during densitometric evaluation can indicate the stability of the spot(s) after chromatographic development. Usually spot(s) showing constant signals up to 30 minutes are adequate for quantitative densitometric evaluation.

Note: For proper understanding whether the sample has decomposed during spotting and spot drying or during chromatographic development as described under (c) above, refer to chromatogram (A) and (B) on page 78.

(e) *Purity of reagents and solvents:* During most stages of chromatographic procedures, the substances are in dissolved form. It is therefore essential to know the quality of the solvents employed and types of additives present to stabilize the solvents. When large quantities of solvents are required for extraction and subsequent concentration to a small volume, the solvent must be free from residual water, non-volatile or not readily volatile impurities as these impurities if present become enriched on concentration and can cause serious contamination problems. Most of the commonly used organic solvents contain stabilizers which can influence the polarity of the solvents.

Note:

- These stabilizers may have a positive or a negative effect on separation.
- Purity of reagents and solvents must be specified, preferably guaranteed by two independent analysis method.

- To further satisfy the purity of solvents particularly for detection of impurities, one may follow the procedure described under "Purity profile for HPTLC and HPLC.
- In case any degradation of sample or reference material occurs during sample preparation or different chromatographic steps, change of solvents or sorbents may be required. Use of antioxidants, N_2/CO_2 atmosphere may also be considered to evaluate the stability of analyte.

	Solvent	*Stabilizer*
Chloroform	Ethanol	0.5–2%
	Amylene	0.01–0.02%
Dichloromethane	Cyclohexane	100–350 ppm
	Amylene	20–25 ppm
Diethyl ether	Ethanol	2%
	BHT	5–7 ppm
Dioxane	BHT	15–25 ppm
Tetrahydrofuran	BHT	0.02–0.03%

Take recourse to your own experience or that of others or literature search to find solution to many separation problems – do not experiment in the dark.

Stability profile by 2-dimensional chromatography

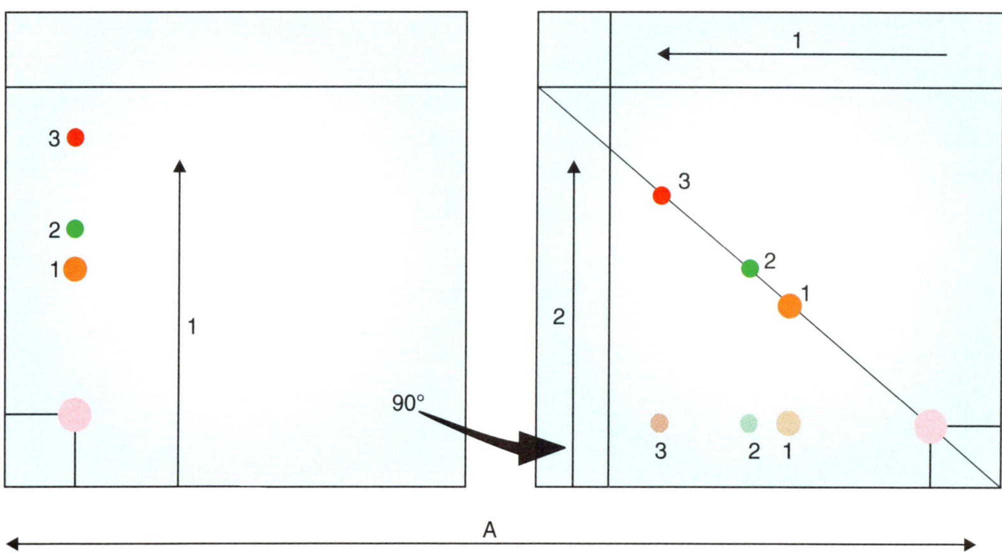

Diagrammatic representation of chromatogram (A) of 2-component analyte mixture. Spot 2 was suspected to be decomposition product. On two-dimensional chromatography (second direction) in same mobile phase, both analytes (1 and 3) gave single spot indicating that the spot 2 obtained in first direction was the result of decomposition of one of the analytes during **spotting and spot drying** and not during development.

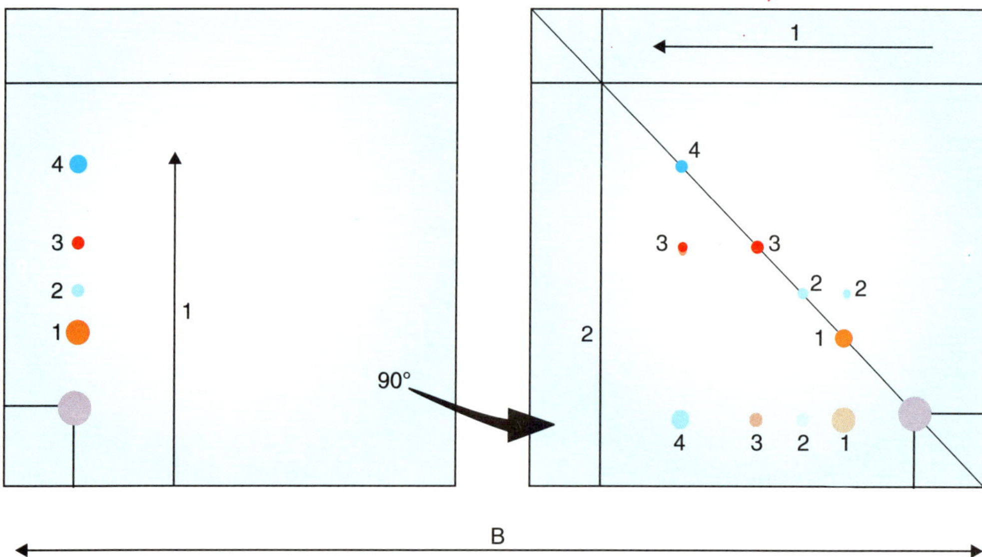

Diagrammatic representation of chromatogram (B) of 2-component analyte mixture. Spots 1 and 4 correspond to analytes whereas spots 2 and 3 were suspected to be decomposition products. As both the analytes (1 and 4) showed secondary spots during two-dimensional chromatography (second direction) similar to the one shown in first development, it confirmed that sample **decomposed during development** and not during spotting and spot drying.

Comparative evaluation of HPTLC and HPLC techniques

	HPTLC	*HPLC*
1.	Simultaneous processing of sample and standard under similar conditions leads to better analytical precision and accuracy; less need for internal standard (I.S.); instability problem, if any, can be detected immediately.	Simultaneous processing of sample and standard not possible; I.S. is frequently required for precision and accuracy of the analysis.
2.	Extreme flexibility for various steps (stationary phase, mobile phase, developing technique, detection, pre- and post-chromatographic derivatization).	Limited flexibility.
3.	Co-chromatography (co-TLC) possible and often practised.	Co-chromatography (co-HPLC) usually not practised.
4.	Several analysts either of the same laboratory or of different laboratories can simultaneously work on the system.	Only one analyst can work at a given time.
5.	Technically, it is simple to learn and operate.	Skilled and well-trained personnel are essential.
6.	High sample throughput of similar or different nature of samples, hence lower analysis time and less cost per analysis.	Even with total automation, HPLC cannot compete with HPTLC in terms of sample output in a given time.
7.	Low cost pre-coated HPTLC plates/rolls are available.	HPLC columns are very expensive.
8.	Pre-coated plates are disposable and for single use only.	Columns require washing and regeneration at the end of each experiment.
9.	Not applicable.	For longer life of the column, use of guard column is recommended.
10.	Entire spectrum can be seen at a glance.	Closed system.
11.	Negligible wear and tear, hence low maintenance cost i.e. less spares and consumable.	High maintenance cost, cost of the spares and consumables significantly adds to the cost of system.
12.	Cannot be fully automated.	Can be fully automated.
13.	Sample preparation is simple.	Sample preparation is the most critical step, is laborious and time-consuming, filtration through membrane filters is mostly needed.

(*Contd.*)

	HPTLC	*HPLC*
14.	Choice of solvent for dissolving sample is not very critical as it is to be removed completely before developing the chromatogram.	Solvent to dissolve the sample must be compatible with HPLC column and mobile phase.
15.	Samples rarely require clean-up; dirty or turbid samples can be directly applied. Strongly adsorbed impurities or presence of solid particles do not interfere as plates are not re-usable.	Samples require purification/clean-up before being introduced into the column. Strongly adsorbed impurities and solid particles if present in the sample can damage the HPLC column, hence exhaustive clean-up required, column being re-useable.
16.	In-situ derivatization possible and routinely employed.	In-situ derivatization not practical.
17.	Solvents need no prior treatment like filtration and degassing.	Degassing/filtration of solvent is absolutely essential.
18.	Solvents of analytical grades are suitable.	Solvents of only HPLC grade are recommended.
19.	Mobile phase consumption per sample is extremely low, thus reducing the acquisition and disposal cost.	Mobile phase consumption is very high, increased acquisition and disposal cost, an economic impediment.
20.	Sample application (a) Variable volumes can be applied. (b) Spot or band. (c) Manual or automatic.	Sample application (a) Normally fixed volume is selected. (b) Injected/introduced. (c) Manual as well as automatic.
21.	Chromatographic development (a) Vertical, horizontal, single or multiple, two-dimensional, continuous, circular, anti-circular, etc. (b) Variety of stationary phases including modified layers are commercially available. (c) Wide combination of stationary-mobile phase is possible.	Chromatographic development (a) Tubular elution by pressure. (b) Limited number of stationary phases are possible. (c) Limited combination of stationary-mobile phase exists.
22.	There is no possibility of interference from previous analysis as fresh stationary and mobile phases are used for each analysis (**no memory effect**).	HPLC columns are reused, hence possibility of interference from previous analysis always exists (**memory effect**).
23.	No carry over, hence no contamination.	Possibility of carry over, hence chances of contamination exist.

(*Contd.*)

	HPTLC	HPLC
24.	Formation of artifact not possible provided various steps are carried out under due care.	Formation of artifacts possible.
25.	Corrosive and UV absorbing mobile phases can be used.	Not possible.
26.	Mobile phases having pH 8 and above can be employed.	Not recommended as stationary phase is unstable in highly alkaline media.
27.	System equilibrium time is small.	Equilibrium time is usually much larger.
28.	Quantity of solvent required on absolute basis and on per sample basis is quite low, hence reduced disposal problem.	Quantity of mobile phase required is comparatively large, hence disposal problem.
29.	Detection	Detection (limited by mobile phase used)
	(a) Visual detection possible, being open system.	(a) Visual detection not possible, being closed system.
	(b) Derivatization is simple and routinely used (sequential application of series of compatible reagents can be employed on each layer such as in case of sulphonamides, thiamine hydrochloride and hydrochlorothiazide.	(b) Difficult, rarely used.
	(c) Non-UV absorbing compounds can easily be detected by post-chromatographic derivatization.	(c) Difficult to detect.
	(d) Chromatographic results can be photographed for documentation.	(d) Not feasible.
30.	Quantitative measurement	Quantitative measurement
	(a) UV, visible, fluorescence, MS.	(a) UV, visible, RI, fluorescence, EC, MS.
	(b) Multiple repeated scanning of the same developed chromatogram at different wavelengths possible.	(b) Only one time scanning is possible.
	(c) Each fraction can be quantified at wavelength of its maximum absorption.	(c) Usually not possible.
	(d) Spectra of each separated compound can be taken.	(d) Routinely not feasible.
	(e) Identification by Rf, UV spectrum and derivatization possible.	(e) Identification by retention time.

(Contd.)

HPTLC	HPLC
(f) Fractions of interest only may be scanned.	(f) All the separated fractions are scanned and measured.
(g) Rf values are not always reproducible.	(g) Capacity factor (K') is reproducible.
(h) Multiple development after each scanning possible to separate certain slow moving solutes.	(h) Not possible.
31. Stationary phase is usually not susceptible to sample poisoning.	HPLC columns are susceptible to sample poisoning.
32. Irreversible absorption of samples on sorbent rarely observed.	Problem of irreversible adsorption may be encountered which can cause potential problems in subsequent separation.
33. Resolution is inferior to HPLC.	Resolution is superior.
34. Substances sensitive to light and oxygen can create problem, being open system.	Substances sensitive to light and oxygen give least problem as it is a closed system.
35. Quality of separation can be continuously monitored as whole chromatogram can be seen at a glance.	Not feasible.
36. Sorbent requires no regeneration as TLC/HPTLC plates are disposable.	HPLC columns require regeneration after each chromatographic run which is a time-consuming process.
37. From starting line to solvent front, almost everything is detectable.	It is difficult to ascertain whether all components of an unknown sample have been eluted out or not.
38. Low analytical requirement.	High analytical requirement.

Note:

- HPTLC technique is most suited for impurity profile of drug substances and content uniformity test as per compendial specifications.
- Large number of development tanks containing different solvent systems may be maintained to optimize the solvent system for TLC/HPTLC.
- HPTLC is unrivalled in rapid and matrix robust-screening of many samples in parallel.
- TLC/HPTLC is the fastest chromatographic technique. It is a time machine that can speed up your work and allows you to do many things, usually not possible with other techniques.
- TLC/HPTLC gives more information about the sample.

Take recourse to your own experience or that of others or literature search to find solution to many separation problems – do not experiment in the dark.

PROCUREMENT OF ANALYTICAL INSTRUMENTS

The need for a particular laboratory instrument usually depends on the analytical functions to be performed. The analysts are usually aware which instrument is required to accomplish the job but are not aware which particular specifications are required to match their requirement and also often lack the expertise to use the system effectively. Before planning purchase of an instrument, one should have sound rationale for purchasing the instrument and should justify the expenses involved.

The purpose of acquiring an instrument may be:

(a) Increasing productivity
(b) To meet specific needs as per protocols
(c) To meet regulatory requirements
(d) To enhance the capability of the laboratory

Procedure for purchasing the laboratory instrument(s)

Buying laboratory instruments is one of the most expensive exercises. Adequate homework is required for finding the right instrument with required specifications and reliable vendor.

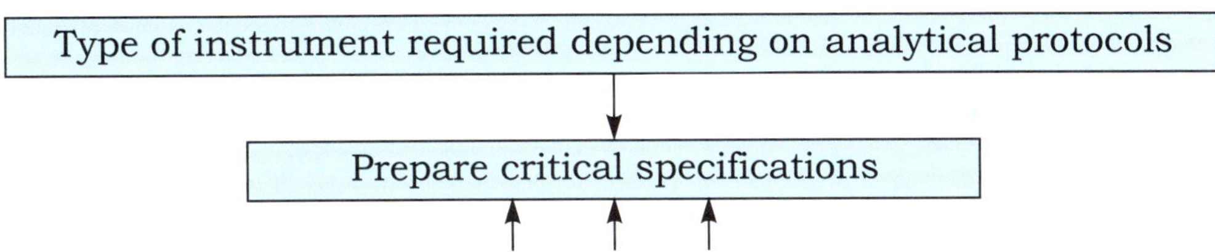

- Consider present and future requirements depending on different functions of the laboratory.
- Consider different applications of the laboratory (flexibility).
- Consult sale brochure/literature.
- Consult knowledgeable experts in the field.
- Consult your colleagues (senior technicians, analysts actually using the instruments).
- Consult colleagues in other laboratories handling similar jobs.
- Consider installation, after-sales service, training, application support and spare parts required.
- Contact vendors, manufacturers' sale representatives.

For any wrong decision/selection, you will be reminded of it almost every day.

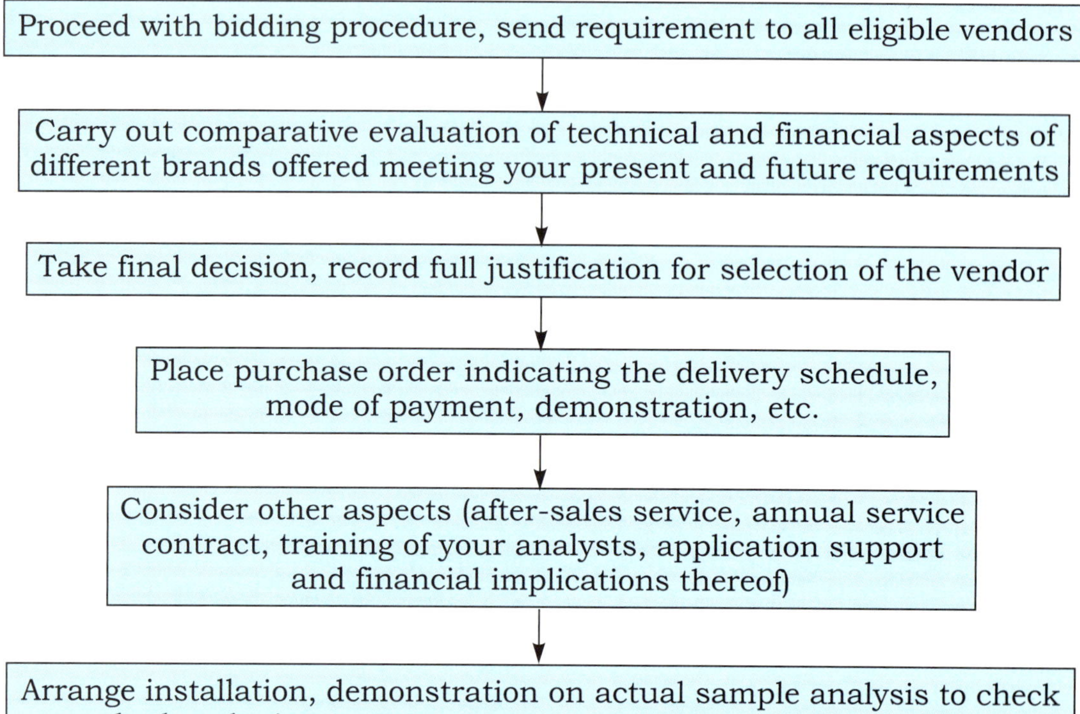

Note:

1. Write down simplified operating protocols of the instrument.
2. Maintain log book for use of the instrument.
3. Assign responsibility to one of the analysts for overall maintenance of the instrument.
4. Arrange training of technicians/analysts for proper and effective use of the instrument.

Preparing Specifications and Configurations of Analytical Instruments

1. Nature of analytical work (quality control, R&D, in-process control).
2. Is the analysis required qualitative, semi-quantitative or quantitative?
3. Are the reference standards available for comparison?
4. What is the degree of analytical precision and accuracy required?
5. What is the expected range of analyte concentration?
6. What is the quantity of sample usually available for each analysis?
7. What is the probable sample matrix and which component of the matrix is likely to interfere in the analysis?

8. Are you required to follow only compendial (USP/BP/IP/EP/JP) methods or alternative methods of analysis can also be employed?
9. Pre-installation requirements.
10. What safety practices are required?
11. Number of samples to be analysed per day (throughput per day).
12. How quickly the results are required?
13. Is automation required? If so, to what extent?
14. Do you plan to upgrade the instrument at later date to meet future requirements? (Flexibility)
15. What type of instruments are being used in other laboratories engaged in similar analytical work?
16. Spares and consumables.
17. Are there any economic constraints?
18. Academic qualifications and training level of the personnel who will handle the instruments.

Note:

1. Some degree of compromise may sometimes be necessary. One must assign priorities to various factors considering the ultimate objective of analysis and future planning.
2. All the users (analysts, technicians) may not have expertise due to lack of professional competency; they may need specific training for useful operation of a particular instrument.
3. The specifications for routine analytical work, such as identification, assay of main active ingredients in dosage form for product release, may be different. However, if the laboratory is involved in stability testing, impurity profiling, instruments with very specific specifications may be required.
4. Do not hesitate to consult a colleague who has considerable expertise in selection and use of such instruments for his/her investigations. This will help you in taking final decision.

Rule of thumb: The more complex the specifications are, the more it will cost and more things can go wrong as they often do. The instrument may run unattended but if any error creeps in, it will rapidly generate large quantities of useless analytical data.

The person who understands the laboratory ultimate goal can make intelligent decision on which type of instrument fits into laboratory's needs.

SELECTION OF VENDORS (SCIENTIFIC EQUIPMENT SUPPLIERS)

"Certification and qualification of vendors/suppliers of raw material, instruments and other inventories should be the responsibility of quality control department and be part of pre-approval programme of all potential vendors/ suppliers."

One of the most difficult tasks in choosing an instrument is selecting a vendor because human interaction, personalities and emotions come into the picture. It is advisable to make several contacts with one or more vendors' representatives before selecting an instrument as people will be your main source of information about the product and the manufacturer. You should feel comfortable while speaking with them, asking them questions and hearing their advice. Try calling the technical support line and see how quickly and accurately they answer your questions. The best measure of a vendor is the satisfaction of the current users of the product you are planning to purchase.

Most vendors will supply you the names, addresses and telephone numbers of only selected users, who are almost always happy with the product and after-sale service. To get less biased evaluation of a vendor, it is preferable if you can find users through other channels such as professional societies, scientific seminars/conferences and other professional contacts. However, it is preferable that the vendor should have greater expertise than the customer on the technique and the instrument being offered.

It is suggested that except common laboratory apparatus such as heaters, centrifuges, mixers, ovens, stirrers, etc. one should get major analytical instruments from major manufacturers as they offer complete package of hardware, service support, and their representatives are more knowledgeable for the instrument. Further, warranty services are quite prompt in keeping the instrument running and fixing them if anything goes wrong as it often can. They provide training in their application laboratory and often provide support in solving difficult analytical problems.

To help the analysts to select the vendors and in procurement of instrument with required specifications, some important guidelines have been elaborated. These are:

1. Is the vendor specialized in the analytical field or is just a trader?
2. Is the vendor dedicated to selling analytical instruments only or is just a small part of a big organisation?
3. What is the financial status of the vendor?

4. For how long the vendor has been in the field of selling analytical instruments (vendor's previous experience)?
5. Vendor's familiarity with CGMP and CGLP?
6. Does the vendor have the list of customers particularly in your region to whom he has supplied the instruments during the last two years.
7. Can the vendor establish that the instruments under consideration are proven to operate satisfactorily in Indian conditions?
8. Will the vendor carry out after-sales service of the instrument? Has he the facilities for annual service contract? If so, what will be the charges? Find out from the current users.
9. Before finalising the purchase, can the vendor arrange practical demonstration of the instrument with actual sample analysis of your field?
10. Is the vendor equipped with application laboratory and trained technical personnel?
11. Will the vendor provide necessary help and guidance in developing and validating methods of analysis?
12. Does the vendor support the customer for training including the level of training in his application laboratory? If so, are there any financial effects?
13. Does the vendor usually stock substantial amount of consumables required for maintenance and after-sales service of the instrument?
14. Does the vendor have the facilities for updating the knowledge of your analysts from time to time with application notes?
15. Will the vendor be arranging workshop/seminars from time to time? If so, what shall be the charges for participating in them?
16. Has he informed you the additional facilities required in your laboratory for installation and operation of the said instrument and has your laboratory been adequately equipped as suggested?
17. Have you any previous experience with the vendor either directly or through knowledge gained from other laboratories? If so, how do you assess his general performance particularly in respect of after-sales service and your own confidence in vendor's ability?
18. Have you prepared the detailed specifications of the instrument you are looking for, considering the requirements of your laboratory before making trade enquiries.
19. Have you consulted your fellow analysts in the field known to you before making final choice of the instrument?

If you are not happy with your decision of selecting the vendor, you will probably be reminded of it almost every day.

20. Are you satisfied that the instrument to be procured shall meet your present requirements and can be updated to meet future requirements?
21. If you are duplicating the instrument, take into consideration the past performance of the existing one.
22. While making budgetary provisions for the purchase of an instrument, consider procurement of consumable spares for at least two years.
23. Carry out comparative evaluation of technical and financial aspects of various marketed brands of the instrument meeting your specifications before making the final choice.
24. Has any of your technical personnel been trained in the operation and maintenance of different analytical instruments including the one under consideration for purchase?

Note:

1. Although technical and economic factors have significant bearing on the selection of vendor, however, final decision should be made after properly assessing each prospective vendor's capabilities in respect of above factors. This will help you in short-listing the vendors.
2. Strong relationship with fewer but better suppliers is mutually beneficial to facilitate improvement in quality, cost and overall responsiveness.
3. Once the vendor is chosen, he should be considered important player of your team. The vendor should provide all the possible assistance in establishing the equipment validation. The vendor will carry out normal operations checks for its pre-qualification acceptability criteria.
4. Once the vendor has demonstrated the equipment validation, optimal limitation of the instrument should clearly be understood by the analytical chemist.

Some manufacturers or their exclusive distributors have well-established application laboratory primarily for training of analysts of prospective buyers or those already have their instruments. These laboratories often have very good collection of general methods that have been validated and they make it available to their customers on request free of charge. However, such methods may still need optimization to fit into individual laboratory's needs. The trained laboratory specialist can help the customers in solving difficult analytical problem or in developing a specific method.

If you buy a good instrument from a reliable vendor, it will free you to spend your time in generating useful analytical data.

TLC / HPTLC INSTRUMENTATION

As an author and pharmaceutical analyst, I have been interested in application of TLC/HPTLC in the field of pharmaceutical analysis for the last 35 years. In view of my interest in the field, I am regularly scanning literature related to application of TLC/HPTLC in pharmaceutical analysis appearing in important national and international journals since 1990. To the best of my information, only two companies i.e. Camag, Switzerland and Sarstedt AG & Co (Desaga), Germany, are manufacturing complete HPTLC system. From the information available in published work and also in respect of applications compiled in this manuscript, it was observed that almost all the institutions carrying out research on application of this technique and publishing their work are using Camag HPTLC system. It is quite possible that laboratories equipped with Desaga HPTLC system may not be publishing their work. For practical reasons, it was not possible to include detailed description of both the commercially available instruments. Based on information available from published literature as included in three volumes of this book, it will be appropriate to provide brief description of different equipments comprising **Camag HPTLC System**. This should help the chromatographers in choosing the correct configuration depending on the requirement of their laboratories and the type of analytical work involved. It is interesting to note that a basic configuration for TLC work can be upgraded to a concise system for quantitative work by adding instruments at any time i.e. transition from conventional TLC to HPTLC is simple and straightforward – just add the appropriate instrument as and when required. The upgrading of basic configuration is also possible with Desaga HPTLC system as well.

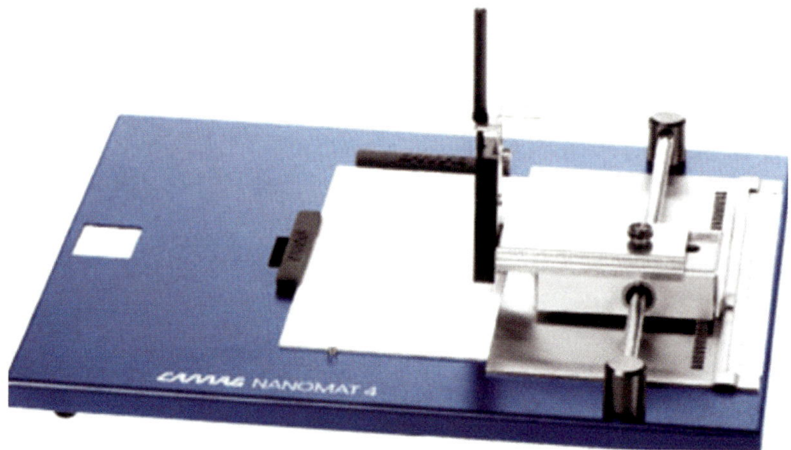

Camag Nanomat

For easy manual but instrumental application of precise volume of sample in the form of spots on TLC/ HPTLC plates by contact without damage to the layers. Sample is filled in disposable graduated glass capillaries precisely guided by a capillary holder onto the layer. Capillaries have no carry over.

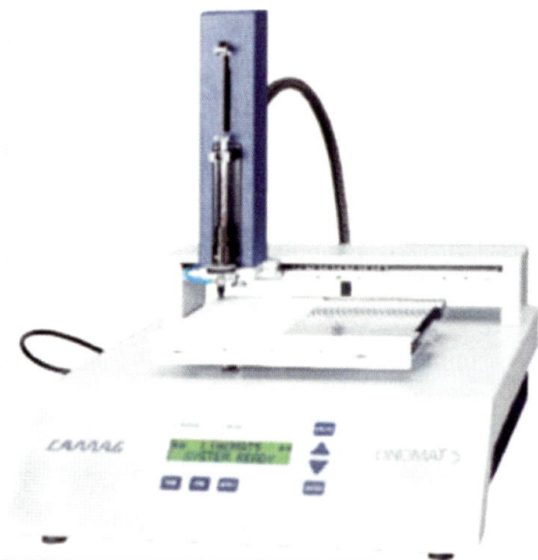

Camag Linomat

Linomat offers semi-automatic application of samples as bands or lines for qualitative, quantitative analysis as well as for micro-preparative separation . The samples are sprayed on chromatographic layers in the form of narrow bands allowing larger volumes to be applied than by contact transfer (spotting). By spraying, solvent for sample gets evaporated leading to concentration of sample as narrow band leading to higher resolution and better quantification.

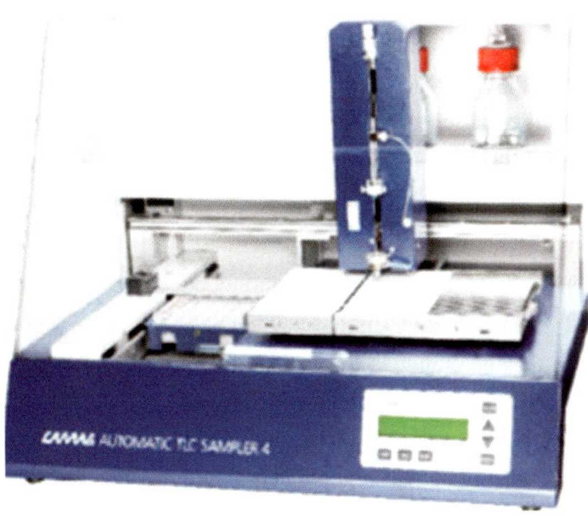

Camag Automatic TLC Sampler-4 (ATS)

ATS-4 offers fully automatic sample application for quantitative, qualitative analysis as well as for micro-preparative separation. Sample can be applied as a spot through contact transfer or as a band by spray-on technique. The system allows over-spraying i.e. sequential application on the same position, useful for pre-chromatographic derivatisation or spiking of sample. Optional heated nozzle and rectangular application is ideal for aqueous samples.

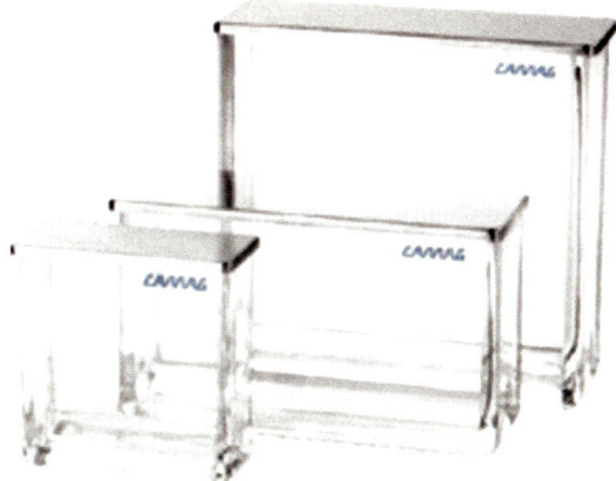

Camag Twin-Trough Chamber (TTC)

The bottom of twin trough chamber is divided into two troughs allowing control over gas phase saturation, humidity and pH. They are economical, requiring minimum solvent consumption (10–20 ml), thus less disposal problems. Development is possible without disturbing equilibrium status i.e. without opening the chamber lid. Different sizes are available for analysis such as for 20 × 20 cm, 20 × 10, 10 × 10 TLC plates.

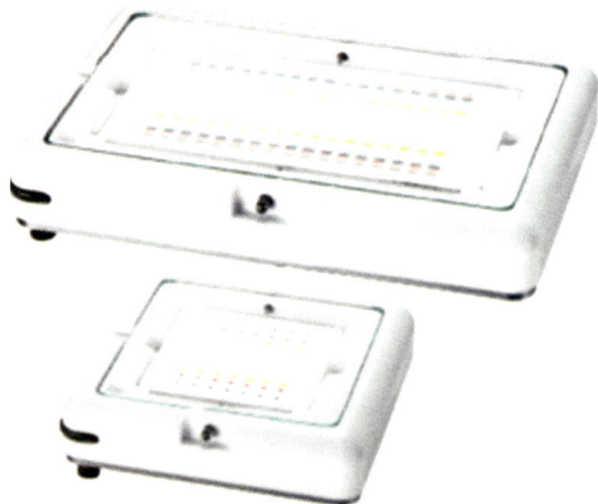

Camag Horizontal Development Chamber

Horizontal development chamber is designed for chromatogram development from both sides of a glass plate. As many as 72 samples and standards can be run in parallel simultaneously, with or without layer saturation. Very rapid and cost effective, provided the development distance of about 40 mm is enough.

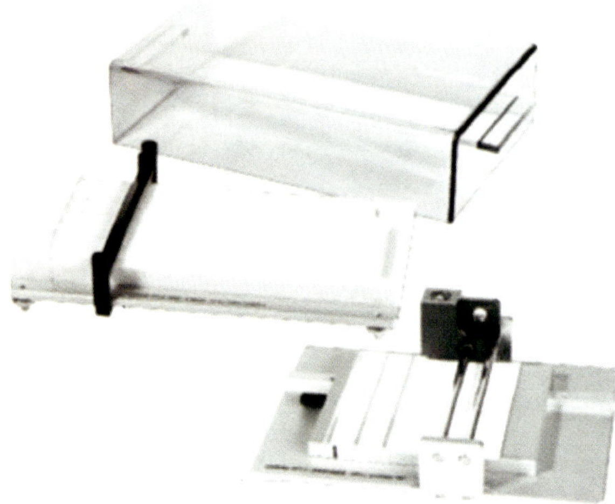

Camag Vario Chamber

The vario system helps in method development. Six solvents with different elusion strength can be tested side by side. The system allows six different conditions of pre-equilibration and also a horizontal development mode. Useful for development and optimization of new methods.

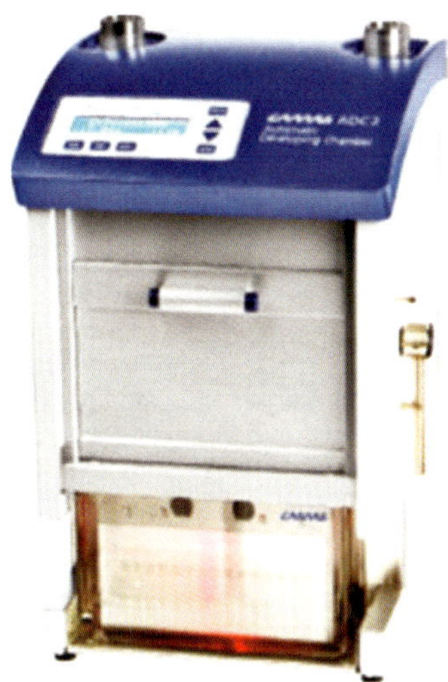

Camag Automatic Development Chamber (ADC)

Automatic Development Chamber (ADC-2) offers convenience and reproducibility for isocratic development of TLC/HPTLC plates. It performs development steps fully automatically independent of environmental effects. Preconditioning of layer, chamber saturation, development distance and final drying can be preset and automatically monitored. An accessory helps to achieve desired humidity level during development.

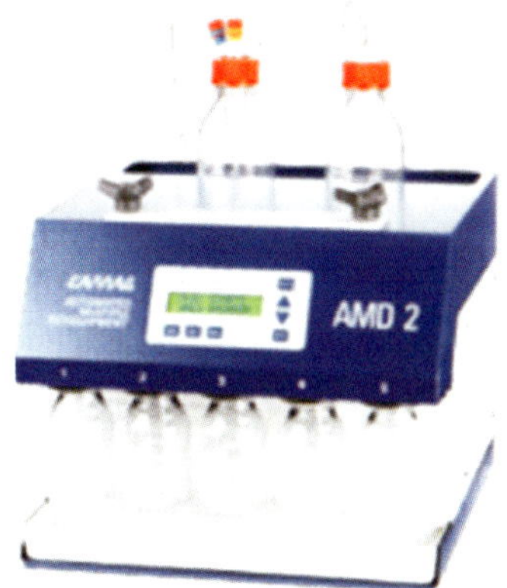

Camag Automatic Multiple Development System (AMD)

The AMD-2 system allows reproducible gradient elution on silica gel pre-coated plates. Gradient elution with up to 5 solvents with different elution strength leads to high resolution. The plates are repeatedly developed in same direction, each successive run extended over a longer migration distance than the one before. After every run the solvent is completely removed from chamber and the layer is dried under vacuum. The system is controlled through System Manager Software – Samples that are complex or have different polarity fractions or a large number of fractions are best resolved by AMD-2.

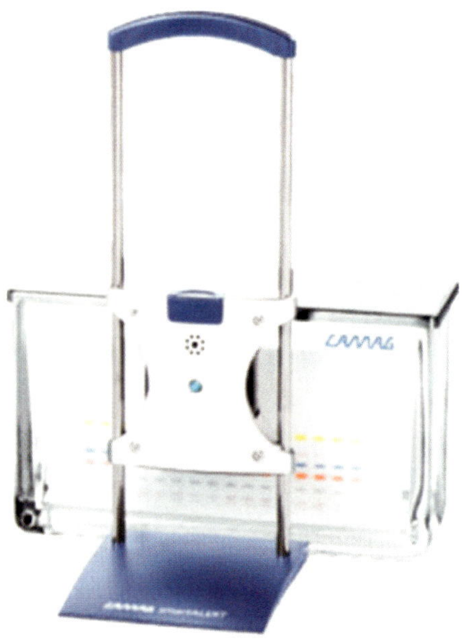

Camag Solvent Front Monitor (smartALERT)

smartALERT provides acoustic and visual notice when mobile phase reaches the desired developing distance. It runs on batteries and replaces the stop watch. A must for every laboratory as its eliminates human monitoring.

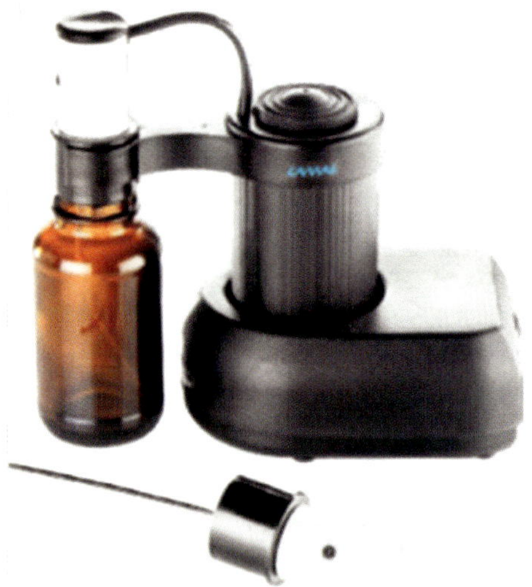

Camag Auto Reagent Sprayer

The Auto Reagent Sprayer gives out a uniform and consistent fine spray using a small pump and rechargeable batteries. If spraying has to be used (when reagents are unsuitable for dipping), this uniform sprayer proves to be far superior to the glass sprayer with bellow. It is provided with spray heads for spraying solutions of both normal as well as high viscosity.

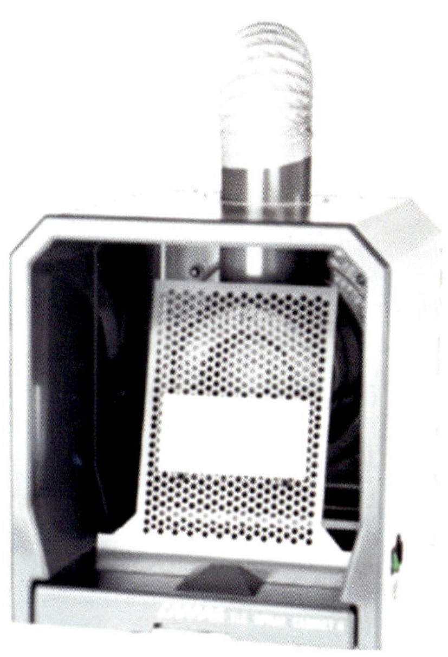

Camag TLC Spray Cabinet

The TLC spray cabinet ensures complete removal of reagent mist without deflection of spray mist before it reaches the chromatogram. The cabinet is made of reagent resistant PVC and is equipped with exhaust system for the analysts' safety. The bottom of the cabinet has a built-in removable tray for easy cleaning.

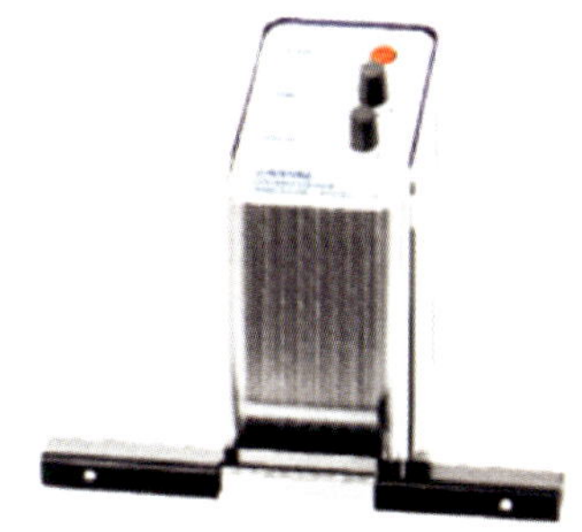

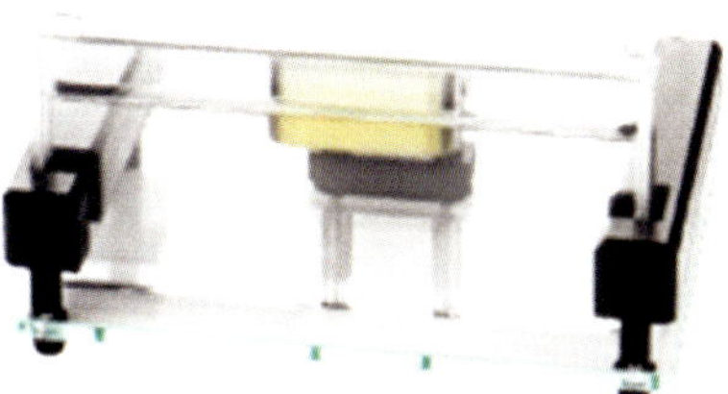

Camag Immersion Device

The device used for immersion of plates into a derivatising reagent to provide uniform and quick spreading of the reagent on the plate leading to improved detection. There is no pollution, no tide marks, gives better results than spraying.

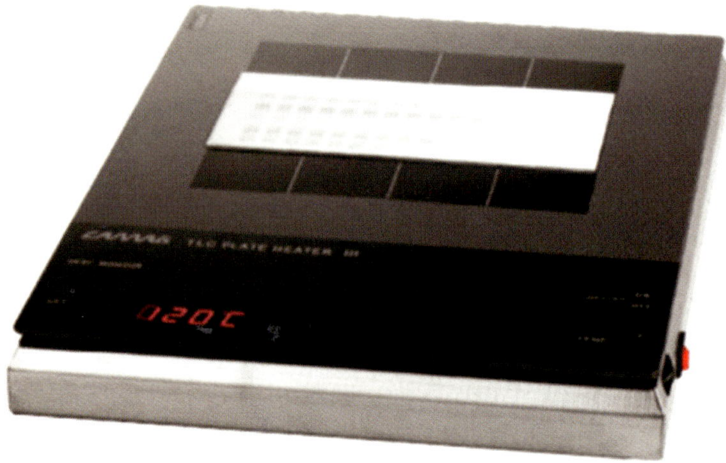

Camag Plate Heater

Plate heater is designed for uniformly heating of TLC pre-coated plate to a set temperature. Ceramic heating surface is resistant to chemical corrosion and easily cleaned. The heating surface has a grid to facilitate correct positioning of the plate . It is most useful for in-situ derivatisation or for plate activation. Programmed and actual temperature is digitally displayed and is selectable between 25–200°C. The plate heater is protected from overheating.

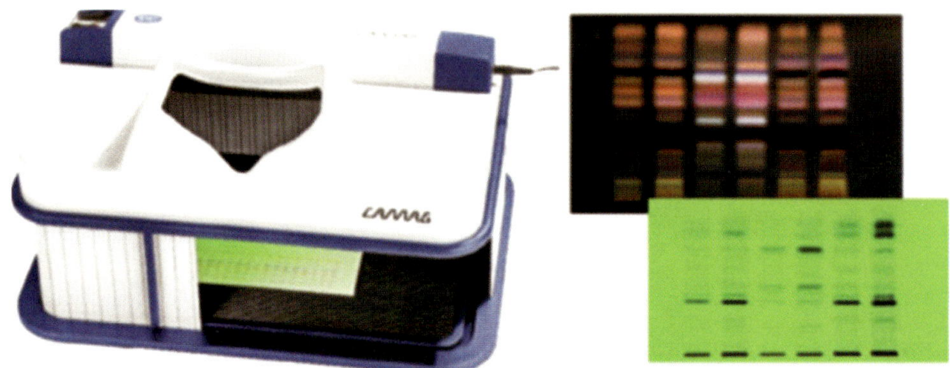

Camag Smart Digi: UV Modified Cabinet with Camera

Inspection of the plate is done at every step of HPTLC using UV (254 nm) or fluorescence (366 nm) in a non-destructive manner inside the UV cabinet. The Camag modified UV cabinet has provision for attaching consumer digital camera for recording images. Useful for non-GLP or R&D documentation.

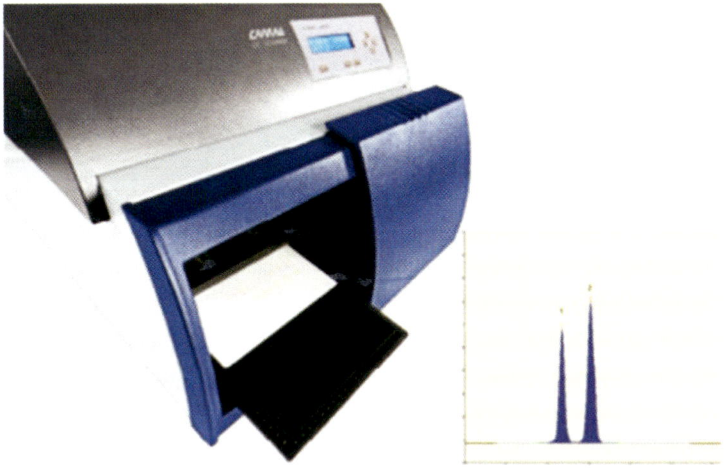

Camag TLC Scanner-4

The most advanced fully automatic densitometric evaluation of TLC/HPTLC plates by scanning in UV, visible and fluorescence modes for quantitative analysis, suitable for densitometric measurement of other planar objects, equipped with different lamps i.e. deuterium, halogen-tungsten and high-pressure mercury lamp. It can record in-situ UV-visible spectra with range of 190 to 900 nm for identification and purity check. Only high quality chromatograms with well resolved sharp bands should be scanned.

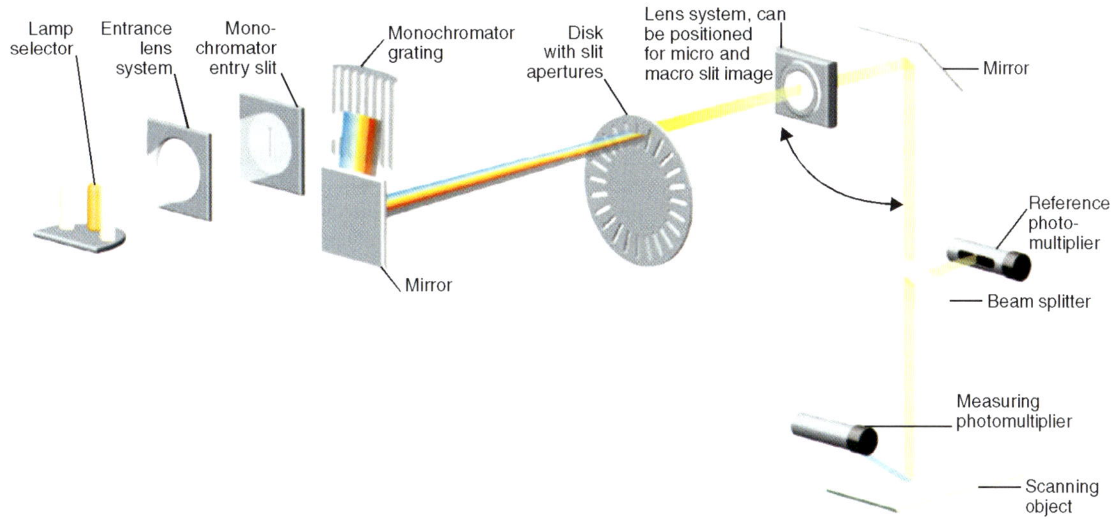

Optical System of TLC Scanner-4

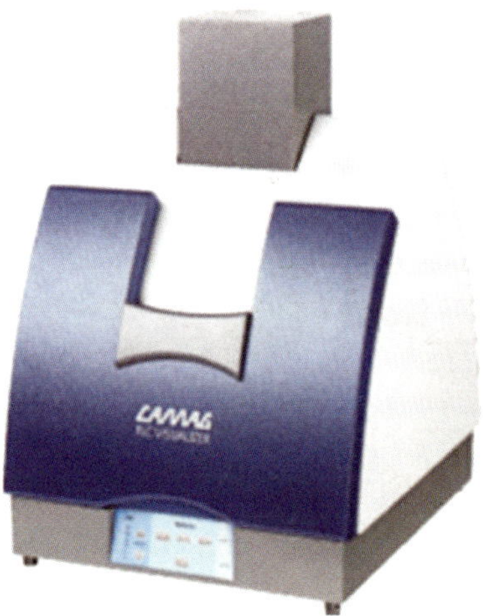

Camag TLC Visualiser

The "Visualiser" captures thin layer chromatogram's images of best quality with the use of 12-bit industrial camera. The system provides illumination with direct, and/or transmitted white light as well as direct UV 254 nm and UV 366 nm light. It is most useful for herbal finger-printing and correct identification as well as to detect adulteration.

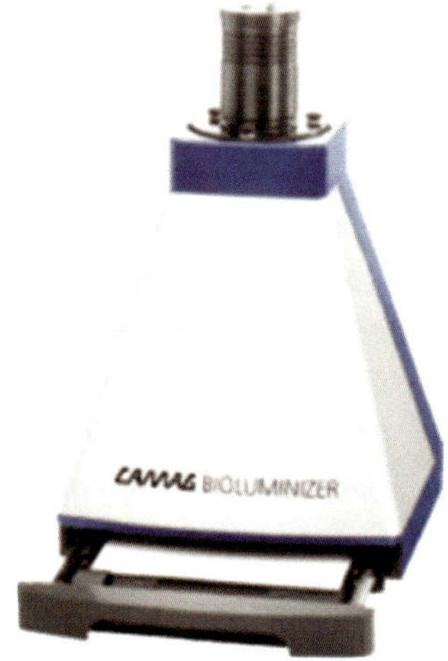

Camag Bioluminizer

A system to document bioluminescence on HPTLC plates. The samples are first separated on HPTLC plates and immersed in the bioluminescent Vibrio Fischeri bacterial suspension. Any toxic substance present kills the bacteria (i.e. the bioluminescence) while some substances may cause increase in bioluminescence. A 16-bit cooled CCD camera ensures that even the faintest variation in bioluminescence is recorded.

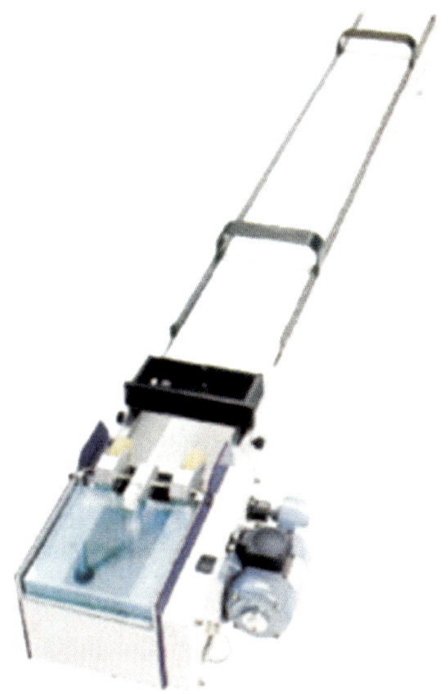

Camag Automatic Plate Coater

The coater provides economical source of glass coated plates of 20 × 20 cm or 20 × 10 cm size. Layer of adsorbent is very uniform. Most useful in large laboratories or laboratories consuming their own coated plates.

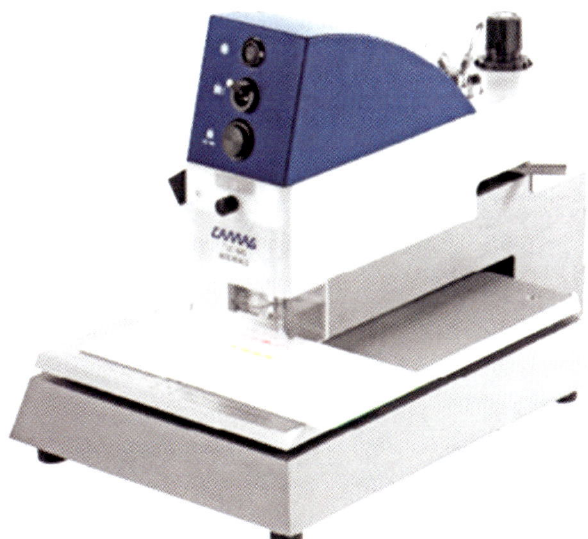

TLC-MS

Definitely a major tool for mass spectroscopist. The TLC-MS interface allows direct elution of separated fractions on a plate, direct into any LC-MS or LC MS-MS.

GLOSSARY OF TERMS USED IN TLC/HPTLC

Activity: Surface properties of a sorbent: the activity of a sorbent is affected by its water content which can be adjusted by relative humidity. Silica gel and aluminium oxide layers are activated at 105–110°C to desorb the physically bonded water. Aluminium oxide according to Brockmann is classified according to activity grades (I to V) depending on the residual moisture, grade V being the least active.

Adsorption chromatography: Chromatographic separation in a solid-liquid phase by competitive interaction between adsorption at the sorbent surface and dissolution in the moving mobile phase, resulting in separation of mixture according to the polarity of the individual components.

Anti-circular chromatography: The substances are applied around the outer circle and mobile phase is applied around the peripheral arc and migrates towards the centre. The substances with large Rf values are well separated as compared to linear chromatography.

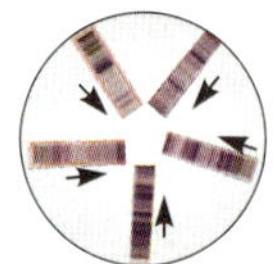

Chamber saturation: Before and during development, the components of the mobile phase are in equilibrium with the entire space in developing chamber. For uniform equilibrium, inside of the chamber is lined with filter paper on three sides. Usually Whatman filter No. 1 or of 3 mm thickness is used.

Chromatogram: Developed TLC plates (result of chromatographic separation), one may obtain photocopy, photograph or densitometric scan.

Chromatographic system: It comprises sample under analysis, sorbent (stationary phase) and eluent (mobile phase).

Circular chromatography: The layer is in a horizontal orientation. The substances are applied on a circle around a central point and the mobile phase is applied to the mid-point of this circle. The components migrate outwards with the mobile phase in the form of segments located on concentric rings and are separated in the process. The substances with small Rf values are separated particularly well in comparison to linear development.

Clean-up: Process for removal of interfering matrix (excipients) from the sample for purification before subjecting to chromatographic analysis.

Densitometer: Chromatogram scanning spectrophotometer, usually called scanner, used for quantitative evaluation by recording absorbance or fluorescence in reflectance or transmission mode. The substance to be measured must either absorb light, stimulated to fluorescence or may be subject to post-chromatographic derivatization prior to evaluation.

Detection: Visualisation of separated substances after chromatographic development in order to assess their separation. Detection is based on specific colour of the substance, intrinsic fluorescence at 366 nm, property of fluorescence, quenching or post-chromatographic treatment of the plate with suitable reagent.

Development chamber: Glass trough chamber commercially available are commonly used for ascending chromatography. Chambers for horizontal or automatic development are available. Twin-trough chambers are suitable when equilibrating the layer is required.

Dyeing reagents: To detect colourless compounds which neither absorb in UV region nor have intrinsic fluorescent property. Dyeing reagents can be sprayed on the plate or the plate is dipped into them. 5% sulphuric acid in methanol, vanillin in sulphuric acid are the most common nonspecific dyeing reagents. One can use specific reagent such as ninhydrin for amino acid.

Edge effect: In an unsaturated chamber, the substance spotted near the edge of the sorbent layer migrates faster than the same substance in the centre. This is due to faster evaporation of developing solvent at the edges in order to saturate the chamber. Evaporation from the edges of the plate causes Rf values of the substance spotted on the outer side of the plate to be higher than the same substance spotted in the middle. This effect is obtained normally when mixture of solvent differs considerably in polarity, vapour density and density and can be prevented by equilibrating the chamber by lining with filter paper.

Caution: For reproducible Rf values, one may avoid spotting of the substance very close to the outer edges of the plate.

Eluent: Usually known as mobile phase.

Fingerprint: Sequence of peaks or zones appearing on chromatography which are specific for a sample.

Fluorescence: Molecules with rigid structures and π electron systems can be stimulated by radiation of suitable wavelength usually in UV region and emit radiation of lower energy, i.e., longer wavelength, mostly in visible region of the spectrum.

Fluorescence indicator: Such indicators are usually incorporated into the layers and make colourless substances visible by fluorescence quenching. Commonly used indicators are:

- F_{254}: Manganese-activated zinc silicate which when stimulated by short wavelength UV (254 nm) gives green fluorescence.
- F_{254s}: Acid stable indicators (magnesium wolframate) usually useful in RPTLC when stimulated by short UV (254 nm) give pale blue fluorescence.
- F_{366}: When stimulated by long UV (366 nm), intense blue fluorescence results. Optical brightners are commonly employed.

Fluorescence quenching/inhibition: When the layers containing fluorescence indicators are stimulated by UV radiation (254 nm), colourless substances absorbing UV light appear as dark chromatographic zones by fluorescence quenching on a green or pale blue fluorescent background-fluorescence indicator.

Forced flow technique: Movement of mobile phase under pressure or by centrifugal force in addition to the capillary forces present in the sorbent.

Gas phase: Vapour phase in the chromatographic chamber. It is one of the important factors affecting separation.

Gradient technique: Changing composition of the mobile phase during development (gradient elution or AMD technique).

HPTLC: High Performance Thin Layer Chromatography. In this case, the sorbent has finer particle size and the narrower distribution than conventional sorbents used for TLC. HPTLC layers are more homogeneous and thinner resulting in improved resolution, shorter analysis time, suitable for in situ quantitation.

Impregnation: Depending on the type of analysis, layers are treated with liquid paraffin, buffers, acids, either by spraying or dipping for impregnation prior to development.

Horizontal development: Special development tanks which allow linear development from both sides of the TLC plates. This has advantage of high sample throughput.

Mobile phase: Solvent or mixture of solvents that move through the porous sorbent layers because of capillary action resulting in separation of substances under chromatographic analysis. Its composition is not known.

Multiple development: Development of chromatogram several times with intermediate drying of layer using the same mobile phase or different mobile phase. This brings about improvement in separation of complex mixtures such as that of amino acids (intermediate drying even at room temperature causes broadening of spots, resulting in diffusion).

Particle size: Smaller the particle size, narrower the distribution, better the separation efficiency. HPTLC plates have mean particle size of 4–6 μm whereas TLC plates have 10–12 μm.

Partition chromatography: Chromatographic development separation is based on solubility differences of individual components of a mixtures in mobile and stationary phases [layer of liquid (water) on the sorbent layer].

Preparative layer chromatograph (PLC): This technique is primarily used for purification and isolation of substances required for other chemical studies such as IR, GC, MS, NMR, etc. In this case, preparative plates with layer thickness of up to 2 mm are employed. The samples are applied as bands. The substance can be isolated by extracting the scrapped layer with suitable solvent.

Post-chromatographic: For detection of substances after development, the chromatogram is treated with suitable reagent, either by spraying or dipping. This is commonly known as post-chromatographic derivatization.

Pre-chromatographic: Subjecting substances to chemical derivatization prior to chromatographic separation.

Pre-coated layers/plates: When sorbent is coated as a thin layer on a suitable plate (glass, aluminium or plastic). The sorbent may contain suitable binder and fluorescent indicator. Layer thickness is usually 0.25 mm (TLC), 0.2 mm (HPTLC), or 0.5–2 mm (PLC).

Pre-conditioning: Adjustment of properties of the stationary phase by exposing to the gas phase prior to chromatographic development.

Relative humidity: Degree of saturation of atmosphere with water at a particular temperature. It is possible to control the relative humidity with sulphuric acid solution of particular concentration or with saturated salt solution in contact with excess salt such as 25% sulphuric acid gives relative humidity of 65%, saturated solution of potassium chloride 85%, and saturated solution of sodium chloride 75%.

Resolution: This is also called separation efficiency. This is judged by differences in Rf values of separated substances and conciseness of separated bands/ spots. Band broadening, spot diffusion should be least for better resolution.

Retention factor (Rf): It is a parameter for qualitative analysis. It only serves as guide for sequence of elution of different compounds in a chromatogram and are approximate.

$$\text{Rf} = \frac{\text{Distance from starting line} - \text{middle of spot}}{\text{Distance from starting line} - \text{solvent front}}$$

Rf values are between 0–1, best between 0.1 to 0.8 or 10–80 for HRf. Owing to the numerous factors influencing the migration of a substance, which are rather difficult to control all the times, Rf (HRf) should therefore be regarded as an approximate value. It is therefore, desirable that a standard substance should be chromatographed on the same plate and under identical conditions, R_x or R_{st} value can be calculated as follows:

$$R_x \text{ or } R_{st} = \frac{\text{D stance (starting zone} - \text{substance zone)}}{\text{Distance (starting zone} - \text{zone of reference substance)}}$$

Rf value is always ≤ 1. R_{st} value can be >1.0.

Reversed phases: Stationary phases (sorbent layers) are modified either by impregnating the normal layers with hydrophobic substances such as liquid paraffin or chemically modifying the layers by treatment with hydrocarbons such as alkyl chlorosilanes of different chain length. Common reversed phase plates (RP_2, RP_8, RP_{12} and RP_{18}) are available. Hydrophobic character increases as the hydrocarbon chain increases. For such plates the mobile phases are predominantly polar aqueous.

Sample application: After proper clean-up, the samples are applied to the starting line of a TLC plate. The samples may be applied either with the help of a syringe or capillary. However, for the quantitative TLC, the use of automated sample applicators are recommended for reproducible results.

Silica gel: Most commonly used sorbent; more than 80% chromatographic analyses are done using silica gel as stationary phase. It involves separation by adsorption and partition chromatography. Usually available in pore size of 40-60 Å (4 to 6 nm).

Sorbents: These can be inorganic such as SiO, Al_2O_3 or organic such as cellulose.

Surface area: Surface area of the sorbent expressed as m^2/g, includes both internal (surface area of pores) and external (surface area of particles), larger the surface area, stronger will be the interaction between sample and stationary phase. Surface area in respect of silica gel 60 is 550 m^2/g and pore volume is 0.65 ml/g.

Stationary phase: Sorbent including any other molecule retained on its surface as a result of impregnation.

Stepwise development: Multiple development with mobile phase of graded polarity. Useful for separation of substances varying in their chromatographic behaviour (this is commonly referred as AMD technique). Each development step cover longer development distance than the previous one.

Two-dimensional development: After first development, the chromatogram is dried and rotated through 90° and again subjected to ascending chromatographic development. One may use same or different mobile phases in two directions. This method is employed to improve separation of complex mixture or in validation of chromatographic conditions in respect of stability during spotting or development of a chromatogram.

A new approach for multi-dimensional planar chromatography has been suggested by V.G. Berezkin & S.S. Khrevotova (2011) in their paper presented at International Symposium on HPTLC (Abstract No. 0.1C). After development the plate was cut into 4 narrow strips after grouping the separated zones on the basis of their Rf values. Then each sub-plate was again developed at right angle to the first direction. For each sub-plate, most appropriate mobile phase was used. The proposed new variant in multi-development chromatography was suitable for separation of complex multi-component analyte mixtures.

Varo-KS chamber: These chambers are suitable for horizontal chromatography. For optimising the chromatographic conditions, several mobile phases alongside each other can be employed.

SOME GENERAL REFERENCES

1. H. Jork, W. Funk, W. Fischer & H. Wimmer. Thin Layer Chromatography, Reagents and Detection Methods, Volumes 1a & 1b, 1990, 1994.
2. Peter E. Wall. Thin Layer Chromatography, A Modern Practical Approach, RSC Chromatography Series, 2005.
3. Elke Hahn Deinstrop. Applied Thin Layer Chromatography (Practices and Avoidance of Mistakes), 2nd ed., 2007, Wiley-VCH Verlag GmbH & Co., KGaA.
4. Merck Chrombook, 2nd ed.
5. Journal of Planar Chromatography – Modern TLC.
6. Camag TLC Catalog.
7. Stahl, E. Thin Layer Chromatography, 2nd English ed., 1967.
8. Thin Layer Chromatography, Application Manual, Macherey-Nagel (M&N), Germany.

Important Practical Tips

Read carefully. It will provide valuable support to novice analyst to be sound chromatographer.

HAND-MADE LAYERS (SELF-MADE LAYERS)

Although in-house preparation of TLC layers is no more a good option but in certain special cases analyst may be required to prepare the plate. Hence, the analyst ought to keep in mind the general practical aspect while preparing such plates, if so required.

- Amount of water required for preparation of sorbent slurry shall vary on the layer thickness required.
- Layer thickness obtained after coating and drying shall be slightly less than one fixed on the coater.
- Coating should be performed rapidly owing to fast hardening process because of gypsum being used as binder, otherwise layer shall not be uniform.
- Coating should be carried out at constant speed to ensure reasonable uniformity of layer.
- During drying process all draught must be avoided, otherwise cracks will appear in the layer.
- Allow the coated plate to remain on the plate holder till the sorbent layer is transluscent.
- While drying in the oven, keep the plate in the vertical position as in horizontal position water vapours may condense and fall on the coated layer, thus damaging the layer.
- Heating oven with air circulation system is preferable.
- Glass plates should be of uniform thickness and dimensions, free from dirt, grease and scratches.
- Final layer thickness is slightly less on edges, remove 1–2 cm of layer on both edges with the help of thumb and index finger; this will ensure uniform Rf value in the remaining width of the plate.
- Do not change the sorbent's brand frequently.

- Use of starch and carboxymethyl cellulose as binder is not suitable for post-chromatographic charring reactions.
- Use of starch as binder does not allow use of iodine as universal detector because of adduct formation between iodine and starch.
- Quality and reproducibility of hand-made layers is generally inferior to those of pre-coated plates because of poor adherence and less constant layer thickness.

PRE-COATED LAYERS

Before proceeding further examine the plate under 254 nm and 366 nm. The plate should be free from scratches.

- Polyester-backed plates, though rarely used, cannot be heated above 120°C as they tend to lose shape.
- Mineral acids or strong ammonia solution cannot be used with aluminium-backed plates as they chemically attack aluminium (Al^{+++}).
- Aluminium-backed plates are compatible with organic acids such as acetic acid and formic acid.
- TLC/HPTLC plates coated with silica gel 60 with or without fluorescent indicators manufactured by different manufacturers vary in particle size, pore size distribution, and amount of binders used.
- Smaller the particles, narrower the particle size distribution, better the separation efficiency.
- Larger the surface area, more intense interaction between the sample and the stationary phase, hence greater the adsorption or stronger the retention.
- Do not frequently change the brand of pre-coated layers.
- During method validation, never change the brand of pre-coated plates.
- For repeating a reported validated method, use the same brand of pre-coated plates as given in the method.
- Never store more than one box of a product in the laboratory to avoid contamination.
- Pre-coated layers are reactive and because of large surface area are likely to take up moisture and contaminants from the laboratory which can affect chromatographic results. Hence, both opened and unopened packages should preferably be stored in storage cabinet or desiccator.
- If you are using more than one type of plates in the laboratory, mark the item number on the top right hand side as soon as the plate is taken out of the box as it will be difficult to identify the type of plate once the plate is taken out as all the TLC/HPTLC plates are white.
- For rarely used plates, do not remove the original packing and labelling.
- While storing the opened package, sorbent layer should face down to avoid contamination with laboratory atmosphere.

- Touch the plate with fingers on the outer cut edge only.
- Fingerprints should not be left on the layers as they can become visible particularly after derivatisation with certain reagents such as anisaldehyde-sulphuric acid or ninhydrin reagent.
- Before loading the plate with sample, observe the plate under short and long wavelengths to ensure that layer is free from scratches and foreign particles.

PLATE FORMAT

- Keep the format constant for a particular separation for comparability and reproducibility.
- Before cutting a plate to required format, look for abrasion marks as produced during production. Development of chromatogram has to be carried out in the same direction only irrespective of the size of the plate employed.
- For cutting aluminium- or plastic-backed plates angle of the scissors should be inclined to right by 35–40°.
- The blades of a scissors should be sharp and long to give fine and fewer cuts.
- Cut edges should be gently wiped off with spatula to remove loose sorbent, if any. This will provide constant Rf values over the entire width of the plate.

Note:

1. Different formats such as 20 × 10, 10 × 10, 5 × 10 cm are commercially available.
2. Unlimited choice of plate formats can be cut as required from 20 × 20 cm plates.
3. Ensure that each cut plate is marked with direction of abrasion marks to determine the direction of development.

PRE-WASHING OF PRE-COATED PLATES AND ACTIVATION

- Pre-washing should be done 1–2 cm longer than the desired development distance.
- Pre-washing should be done in the direction in which the layer of the sorbent has been applied; for direction look for abrasion marks on the back of the plate.
- Ascending blank chromatography provides the most efficient cleaning but it takes longer time.
- During pre-washing, active dirt gets accumulated at the solvent front which may interfere in identifying analytes with Rf values of ≥ 0.75.
- Cut off about 1–2 cm of the portion where dirt has accumulated to identify even fast moving substances.
- Methanol is the most commonly used solvent for pre-washing, but may not provide efficient cleaning in case of non-polar contaminants.

- Pre-washing with the proposed mobile phase can lead to formation of secondary front where impurities get collected.
- After pre-washing, direction of washing and washing front be marked as further chromatographic development has to be carried out in that direction only and not beyond the washing front.
- Since the plastic packing of TLC/HPTLC plates is not impermeable to gases, it will not completely protect the plates from environmental contamination, hence pre-washing/cleaning of plates is required.
- Activity of the layer is inversely proportional to the relative humidity.
- Best way to control RH and the temperature is to actually record the same during actual development.
- Select a mobile phase which is least prone to small changes in humidity and temperature.
- After washing, drying the plate at 110°C for 10–15 min is quite adequate to activate the plate.
- Time required for constant activity depends on layer thickness and increases therewith.
- Higher the activity, lower the Rf values.
- Drying for too short a time and at too low temperature may result in incomplete removal of pre-washing solvent.
- Heating at higher temperature and for longer time leads to very active layers thus risk of sample decomposition and formation of artifacts. In such an eventuality, use of modified layers is recommended.
- High activity is not a pre-condition for high separation performance.
- Activation of layer is particularly important in tropical countries for reproducible separation.
- In general, catalytic activity of the layer increases with increasing activity.
- Air-conditioned room with air locks maintains the effects of activity at an essentially constant rate.

SAMPLE PREPARATION

- Many clean-up steps have to be worked out and optimized empirically.
- Sufficient quantity of sample should be cleaned to permit replicate determination.
- After clean-up the sample should be chromatographed as quickly as possible.
- Any error in clean-up process will persist all the way through to the evaluation of final densitogram.
- Solvent should be safe, stable and non-reactive with the layer and the sample.
- Use reasonably pure solvent particularly when large sample volumes are to be applied as impurities present in the solvent shall get accumulated on the layer.

- The solvent should have optimal volatility requiring minimum time for application and to ensure appropriate drying of application zone.
- Use of benzene, because of its carcinogenic effect, is banned for laboratory use; can be easily substituted with toluene.
- Halogenated hydrocarbons such as chloroform are hazardous solvents, their use should be avoided as far as possible.
- Use dichloromethane instead of chloroform.
- Use of polar solvents such as water, dimethylformamide, dimethylsulphoxide, n-butanol should be avoided as they take longer time to be removed from the layer after sample application.
- Use of acetone should be avoided as on active layer of silica gel, it is likely to form condensation product acetylacetone which shall interfere in detection of analytes after chromatographic development.
- Avoid use of low boiling solvents such as acetone, diethylether as they will quickly evaporate from the capillary after it is filled and before sample is applied to the layer, thus transferring <100% of the sample to the layer.
- In case of solution of analyte in high density solvent such as chloroform, solution leaves the capillary in an uncontrolled manner.
- Standard and sample solutions should be prepared in the same solvent and should preferably contain similar matrix.
- The sample should be correct representative of the batch under analysis.
- Order smallest packing of concentrated ammonia solution (250 ml) and once the bottle is opened, it should always be stored in refrigerator.
- When small volume of ammonia (25–50 ml) is left, do not use for TLC/HPTLC separation as amount of dissolved ammonia is extremely critical for chromatographic separation.

SAMPLE APPLICATION

- Samples of high density are likely to leave the capillary before sample application.
- Solutions of high viscosity may reluctantly or incompletely enter or leave the capillary.
- High volatile solvents undergo partial evaporation before application from the capillaries.
- Concentration should be selected in such a way that single emptying of capillary should provide adequate sample to the layer as multiple application is likely to lead to spot deformation.
- Disposable capillary can be re-used after multiple filling after emptying on filter paper.
- All samples to be applied on the plate must be correctly positioned for comparative Rf values.

- The position from right and left edges and from sample to sample must be controlled to avoid edge effect.
- Apply samples about 10–15 mm away from edges for reproducible Rf values.
- Overloading the plate with sample leads to poor separation and excessive tailing.
- The bands should be as thin as possible for good resolution.
- For repeated application of sample ensure intermittent removal of sample solvent to avoid local chromatography.
- Local chromatography due to repeated application of sample can produce dog bone shape of spots in finished chromatogram.
- To speed up removal of sample solvent after application, excessive use of hair dryer should be avoided as it can contaminate the layer and there is possibility of loss of volatile constituents of the sample.
- While applying sample, keep a clean glass plate above the application zone to retain activity of the layer for longer time.
- Starting line of application should not be very close to the bottom edge of the plate to avoid risk of extending application line to the solvent; preferable application line should be 1–1.5 cm above the bottom edge.
- While using capillaries for sample application, the beginners should practice the sample application on upper portion of the plate to know filling and emptying time of the capillary and should have feel of pressure required for releasing the sample onto the layer.
- Rf values of the sample applied very near to the edges is always higher and not reproducible than the samples spotted in the middle of the plate.

DRYING THE PLATES BEFORE DEVELOPMENT

- Ensure that the solvent used for sample preparation is completely removed after application before starting development, i.e., start zone must be completely dried.
- For volatile samples such as essential oils, do not dry with hair dryer to avoid loss of constituents – just keep the loaded plate at ambient temperature for few minutes in horizontal position facing layer upward.
- Do not expose the plate to blower as laboratory contaminants can get deposited on plate, thus defeating the purpose of pre-washing the plate.
- For thermolabile samples or samples prone to oxidation, laboratory experiments need to be carried out for suitable drying conditions (temperature and time) to ensure integrity of the sample.

MOBILE PHASE (SOLVENT SYSTEM)

- Mobile phase (MP) should have apparently appearance of a single phase with no cloudiness.

- Should give Rf values in the medium range.
- Should be selective.
- Vapour pressure not very low and not very high.
- Consult literature or seek help from an experienced chromatographer for selection of suitable MP.
- Sorbent layer should be so chosen that it is adequately wettable with MP, otherwise development shall not occur satisfactorily.
- Out of two solvent systems with similar elution strength, use the one with lower viscosity.
- Separation on RP-HPTLC is not possible with MP containing high water content.
- Use of solvents such as pyridine, benzene being carcinogenic should be avoided; look for alternative.
- Mobile phase should be freshly prepared. If at all to be stored, store in a dark bottle at cool place.
- To minimize volumetric errors, developing solvent can be prepared in a volume sufficient for one working day.
- Each component of the mobile phase should be measured separately and then mixed to avoid any problem due to volume contraction or dilation.
- Storing solvent system containing alcohol and acids leads to esterification, thus change in chromatographic conditions.
- Use of diethylether (ether), a solvent with very low boiling point and flash point, should be avoided. Further, presence of peroxides in ether can cause oxidative decomposition of analytes and also there is disposal problem.
- Use of halogenated hydrocarbons (chloroform) should be avoided.
- Mobile phase containing mixture of solvents with widely varied polarities should be used only once.

DEVELOPMENT DISTANCE

- Mark the required development distance of mobile phase (MP) on one edge of the plate – few mm in length with pencil.
- Whole breadth of the plate should dip into mobile phase to the same depth.
- Do not mark along the entire width of the plate as if by chance the MP exceeds the marked line, MP shall stagnate at the marked line causing diffusion of analytes.

Note:

1. Development time required for marked distance will depend on the viscosity and surface tension of the solvent system, i.e., greater the viscosity and smaller the surface tension, longer the development time.
2. Slight fluctuations in room temperature do not have significant effect on Rf values.

- Dipping technique requires large volumes of the reagent, though the reagent is less concentrated.
- The plate should be dipped absolutely vertically, otherwise risk of broadening of separated zones.
- The solvent to prepare the reagent should not be very polar, otherwise there is risk of diffusion of the zones or dissolution of the analytes in the solvent.
- After immersion clean the back of the plate before keeping on heating surface.

HEATING THE PLATE AFTER DERIVATIZATION

- Heating surface must be very smooth for uniform transfer of heat to the plate, use of non-perforated metal tray is recommended to support the plate for uniform heat distribution.
- While heating in an oven, risk of contamination due to aggressive fumes is there.
- While heating in an oven, it is difficult to terminate heating process as it cannot be observed.
- To achieve smooth surface in a heating oven, keep the derivatized plate between two thick blank glass plates. This will allow uniform transfer of heat and also avoid curling of the plate and contamination of the layer. Curling of the plate shall make densitometric scanning impossible.
- The plate should not come in direct contact with the heating surface, instead keep the derivatized plate over blank glass plate. This shall prevent lifting of outer edges of the aluminium plate.
- Commercially available plate heater should be operated in fume cupboard to remove the toxic vapours of the reagent.

DENSITOMETRIC SCANNING, SELECTION OF SUITABLE WAVELENGTH

- While selecting suitable wavelength for scanning, do not sacrifice analytical information about any of the sample compounds.
- The analytical information about the minor compound is most important.
- For selecting suitable wavelength, analysts are advised to read relevant portion of the text in this monograph.

STABILITY STUDIES

- 30–50% decomposition of the substance should be taken as reasonable for different stress conditions.
- If no decomposition occurs, stress conditions to be reviewed.
- If 100% decomposition occurs, reduce the stress level.

Validation of HPTLC Method

Dr. Nitin Dubey, Dr. Nidhi Dubey, Dr. D.K. Jain

- Introduction
- International regulatory requirements for method validation
- Validation plan: Strategies for HPTLC method validation
- Method validation parameters (accuracy, precision, repeatability, specificity and selectivity, LOD, LOQ, linearity, range, robustness, ruggedness, system suitability, filter retention studies, extraction efficiency, forced degradation studies)
- Glossary of terms related to HPTLC method validation
- Practical examples for developing and validating HPTLC method
- Bibliography

Dr. Nitin Dubey, M.Pharm. (Q.A.), Ph.D.
Head of the Department (Pharm.Chem.) & Associate Professor,
College of Pharmacy, IPS Academy, Indore
nitindubeympharm@yahoo.com

Dr. Nidhi Dubey, M.Pharm. (Q.A.), Ph.D.
Reader, School of Pharmacy, Devi Ahilya University, Indore

Dr. D.K. Jain, M.Pharm., Ph.D.
Professor & Principal, College of Pharmacy, IPS Academy, Indore

DEFINITIONS

AOAC: *The planned and documented procedure to establish the method's performance characteristics. The performance characteristics or the validation parameters of the method determine the suitability for its intended use. They define what the method can do under optimized conditions of matrix solution, analyte isolation, instrumental settings and other experimental features. The inclusion of particular validation parameters in a validation protocol depends on the application, the test samples, the goal of the method and domestic or international guidelines or regulations, as applicable.*

CITAC: *Validation of a method established by systematic laboratory studies that the method is fit-for-purpose, i.e. its performance characteristics are capable of producing results in line with the needs of the analytical problem.*

EU guideline: *Action of proving, in accordance with GMP principles, that any procedure, process, equipment, material, activity or system actually leads to the expected results.*

EURACHEM: *Analytical method validation is the process of defining an analytical requirement, and confirming that the method under consideration has performance capabilities consistent with what the application requires.*

Irish National Accreditation Board: *Confirmation via the provision of objective evidence that the requirements for specifically intended use or application have been met.*

ISO 8402:1994: *Validation is confirmation by examination and provision of objective evidence that the particular requirements for a specified intended use are fulfilled.*

NATA: *Method validation provides objective evidence that a method is fit for purpose, meaning that the particular requirements for a specific intended use are fulfilled.*

USFDA: *Methods validation is the process of demonstrating that analytical procedures are suitable for their intended use.*

INTRODUCTION

'Valids' a word of Latin origin means 'strong'. Method validation is a critical component of a comprehensive quality assurance system (Fig. 2.1). Method validation is not about a method, it is about a complete analytical system. When we validate a method, indirectly we are demonstrating that a complete system is in control, it includes a defined procedure, specific analyte, concentration, analyte matrix, and chromatographic peculiarities. It requires that the data is useful, accurate, acceptable, and true. It is all about identifying, documenting and demonstrating performance characteristics (fitness-for-

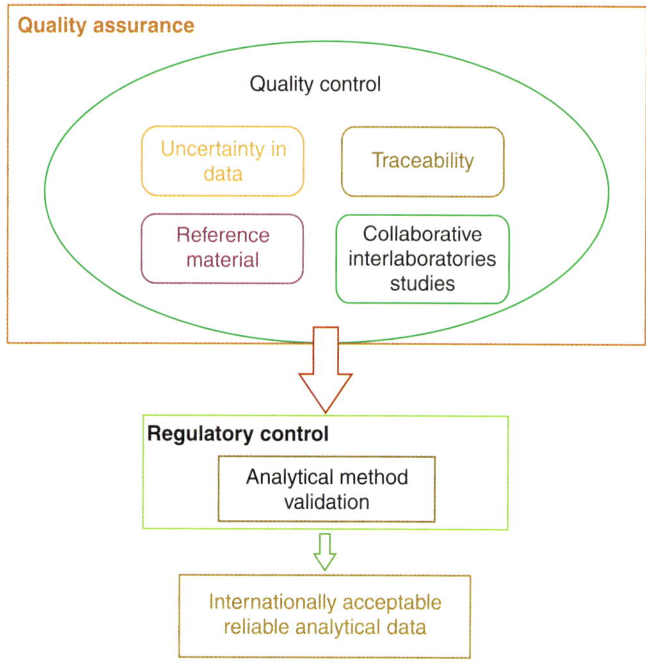

Fig. 2.1: Quality Assurance of Analytical Method.

purpose), measurement uncertainty, effect of matrix variation and limitations of an analytical method on the basis of a set of official or recommended parameters.

IUPAC defines *fitness for purpose* as the degree to which data produced by a measurement process enables a user to make technically and administratively correct decisions for a stated purpose. It involves identification of factors affecting the method performance and their acceptable extent so that reliable and internationally acceptable data may be generated.

Measurement uncertainty is a critical indicator of 'fitness for purpose' and reliability of results. It is a statistical non-negative parameter, which describes the possible fluctuations of the results. As per the ISO definition, it is a parameter associated with the result of a measurement that characterises the dispersion of the values that could reasonably be attributed to the measurand. It is generally denoted as standard deviation or the width of a confidence interval. Measurement error should not be confused with measurement uncertainty. Measurement error indicates the difference between determined value and its true value. While measurement uncertainty should be treated as an interval or region of routine result in which real unknown true value falls with certain probability.

The sources of uncertainty may be inappropriate sampling, inappropriate extraction of analyte, inappropriate methodology, insufficient resolution or lack of calibration of instrument, environmental conditions, inadequate signals, etc. (Table 2.1). Matrix variation is an important source of variation as composition of matrix may seriously affect the performance of method. Method suitable for one type of analytical matrix may not be suitable for the other type.

Table 2.1: Major sources of uncertainties in measurements as per ISO 17025/AOAC guidelines

1. Weights	Within ±10% (but use actual weight for calculations)
2. Volumes	Volumetric flasks, graduated beakers, and transfer pipettes (stated capacity with negligible uncertainty)
3. Burettes	Stated capacity except in titrations
4. Graduated pipettes	Use volumes >10% of capacity
5. Temperatures	±2° of specified temperature
6. pH	Within ±0.05 unit
7. Time	Within ±5%

The drive is to develop simple and economical validated methods. This requires comprehensive quality management of laboratories involving accreditation of laboratories, internal quality control, quality audits and external proficiency exercises to generate confidence in performance of the quality control unit.

Validation may include single laboratory validation or development of '*fully validated*' methods. It may be achieved through interlaboratory method performance study or collaborative study including test material and minimum numbers of laboratories (Table 2.2). Full interlaboratory validation requires a study of minimum of five matrices using eight laboratories, which is an expensive and time consuming exercise. Relatively cheaper but reliable alternatives includes minicollaborative studies that reduces the required number of matrices and laboratories, single laboratory validation protocol by IUPAC, the *Peer-Verified Methods Programme* and *Performance Tested Methods* for test kits. The *Peer-Verified Methods Programme* merely requires verification of the analytical parameters by a second laboratory, It is not always required to conduct '*full validation*' and single laboratory method validation may be acceptable.

This chapter deals with analytical method validation strategies with special reference to High performance thin layer chromatography (HPTLC). Chromatography is a technique in which the components in a sample, carried by the liquid or gaseous phase, are resolved by sorption-desorption steps on the

Table 2.2: Conditions requiring full/single/cross validation

Full validation

1. Method development for the first time.
2. Method development for new chemical entity, new formulation, etc.
3. New analyte addition in formulation.
4. New metabolite in matrix.

Single laboratory validation

1. Any change in analytical methodology such as detector, sample holder, etc.
2. Analytical method transfers between laboratories or analysts.
3. Any change in anticoagulant used in biological fluid analysis.
4. Any change in analytical matrix, within species (e.g., rat plasma to rat urine), amongst species (rat plasma to human plasma) or dosage form (tablet to syrup, oil), etc.
5. Change in sample processing procedures.
6. Change in target concentration range.
7. Changes in instruments and/or software platforms.
8. Use of restricted sample volume such as used in paediatric studies.
9. Use of rare analytical matrices such as phospholipids, triglycerol, etc.
10. Selectivity estimation of an analyte in multicomponent system.
11. Selectivity estimation of an analyte in the presence of specific degradation product or metabolites.
12. Analysis for specific purposes like dope test, cleaning validation, etc.

Cross validation

1. Sample analyses performed at different laboratories within a single study.
2. Sample analyses performed at same laboratory but different sites within a single study.
3. Sample analyses using spiked matrix at different laboratories to check interlaboratory reliability.
4. Sample analyses using different analytical techniques (i.e., Gel electrophoresis vs. Capillary electrophoresis vs. ELISA, HPLC vs. HPTLC).
5. When revised method is being tested against original validated method across the same or different studies.

stationary phase. Thin layer chromatography is a manually performed chromatography where separation occurs on a stationary phase (layer thickness: 250 μm, particle size 10–15 μm) that consists of a thin layer applied to a solid substrate as a support material (glass, aluminium foil or plastic). It is also known as planar chromatography. If the plate (particle size of stationary phase is 3–4 μm, thickness of the layer is 100–200 μm) is scanned through the densitometer, the separation technique is known as high performance thin layer chromatography. HPTLC may be used for identity (qualitative) test, semi-quantitative test (limit test) and quantitative estimation of impurity or active moiety (assay) (Table 2.3).

Table 2.3: Purpose of HPTLC analysis

1. To establish identity of the product or components.
2. To check purity of the product.
3. To check efficacy and safety of the product.
4. To demonstrate that the product meets desired specifications.
5. To check the presence of specific analyte such as contaminant, pesticide, etc.
6. To demonstrate that the product is acceptable to the regulatory authority.

Qualitative methods confirm the presence or absence of a particular analyte in the sample. If a particular analyte is absent, it means that the analyte is below the detection limit of the instrument or is absent. *Identity testing* is the most common qualitative application of HPTLC to ensure the identity of an analyte in a sample. It requires comparison of a property of the sample with a standard. In TLC/HPTLC, R_f value and colour of the spot after derivatization and UV absorbance spectrum (190– 400 nm) is used for qualitative evaluation. R_f value (retardation factor) is defined as the ratio of distance travelled by the spot from the start to the distance travelled by the mobile phase from the start. If an internal standard (IS) is used, the parameter 'R_f' will be replaced by 'RR_f'. It is the ratio of R_f of the analyte's spot to the R_f of internal standard. The analyte's spot can also be visualized using UV at 254 nm (if the compounds have UV absorbing functional group) or at 366 nm if the compounds are fluorescent. If the R_f values and/or the colours of two spots are different, it suggests that spots consists of two different compounds. Even if the R_f values and colours of two spots (sample and standard) are identical, it does not mean that the spots consist of same compounds. Even appearance of single spot of the sample (after development) does not mean that the spot contains only one compound. Using a scanning densitometry, the HPTLC/TLC chromatograms can be converted into densitograms, in which all spots will be observed as peaks. Identity of the spot/peak can be evaluated by overlain UV/VIS spectrum of sample and reference standard (Fig. 2.2). Fig. 2.2 compares the example of acceptable and poor quality of overlain spectrum. If the value of the correlation coefficient of up slope to apex ($r_{s,m}$) and apex to down slope ($r_{m,e}$) are more than 0.999, it may be concluded that the spot/peak is pure. Confirmation of the identity of an analyte's spot can also be determined by two-dimensional TLC with full UV/VIS spectrum scan and co-chromatography.

HPTLC method is widely used for qualitative analysis of herbal drugs or medicinal plants. In this case, a Botanical Reference Material (BRM) is required, instead of a reference standard compound. The HPTLC finger-print of the sample will be compared to its BRM finger-print for sequence (such as number of spots, colour, intensity, and position) in a densitogram. The quality of medicinal

3. When 'full' validation is required for compendial purposes. Verification of precision, linearity, ruggedness, matrix variation and bias studies are required.
4. When 'fully validated' method is being used but with different matrix. Verification of precision, linearity, ruggedness and bias studies are required in new matrix.
5. When method is available in scientific literature with exhaustive details. Verification of matrix specific precision, linearity, ruggedness and bias studies are required.
6. When method is published in scientific literature without much details. Verification of matrix variation, precision, linearity, ruggedness and bias studies are required.
7. When quantitative estimation is based on specified procedure (i.e. empirical method) and reference material is unavailable. Verification of laboratory bias, data related to interlaboratory precision using Horwitz function are required.
8. When method does not require establishment of general range of a value (*ad hoc* analysis), data related to interlaboratory precision, laboratory bias, ruggedness, recovery are required.
9. When revalidation is required specially due to change of equipment, premise, variable reagent, etc. may require specific parameters study that are most likely to be affected with general verification of already established parameters.
10. When assay, identification or limit test of new drug or pharmaceutical formulation alone or in combination with other drug, in same or different analytical matrix is required for marketing authorization or product registration, recommended parameters as per concerned regulatory authority should be developed.
11. When impurity determination, stability indicating method or cleaning validation studies are required then recommended parameters as per concerned regulatory authority should be developed.
12. When different performance characteristics are required for a validated method, then specific parameters are required to be re-established. Data related to interlaboratory precision, limit of quantitation and detection, laboratory bias, ruggedness and recovery are required.

Validation is required regardless of whether analytical method is used for release, stability, acceptance or pharmacokinetic study. The method may include qualitative or quantitative estimation for in-process quality control testing, shelf life evaluation, raw material validation or finished product testing. Methods related to active pharmaceutical ingredients, finished dosage forms, botanicals, polyherbal formulations in complicated analytical matrix, dietary supplements, veterinary drugs, alternative and complementary medicines, impurities, metabolites and degradation products, analytes in biological fluids, pesticide residues and industrial contaminants.

INTERNATIONAL REGULATORY REQUIREMENTS FOR ANALYTICAL METHOD VALIDATION

Method validation is a mandatory requirement for pharmaceutical product registration and accreditation by all pharmaceutical regulatory authorities including ISO 17025. A literature survey of the current regulatory control over analytical method validation revealed that many regulatory authorities have described different parameters to develop a validated method. This is sometimes challenging for an analyst to derive useful conclusion out of so many different requirements, and even the terminologies used for the parameters differ from agency to agency. The field is continuously changing and requires an analyst to remain updated. Regulatory enforcement has always been a major driving force for development.

This chapter provides an understanding of topic including, but not restricted to, the current recommendations of International Conference of Harmonization (ICH), United States Pharmacopoeia, United States Food and Drug Administration (USFDA), National Association of Testing Authorities (NATA), Australia, International Union of Pure and Applied Chemistry (IUPAC), Irish National Accreditation Board, Association of Official Analytical Chemists (AOAC), Eurachem, American Society for Testing and Material (ASTM), World Health Organization (WHO), International Organization for Standardization (ISO), Cooperation on International Traceability in Analytical Chemistry (CITAC), Codex Committee on Methods of Analysis and Sampling (CCMAS), International Laboratory Accreditation Cooperation (ILAC), European Committee for Normalization (CEN), Food and Agricultural Organization (FAO), British Pharmacopoeia, European Cooperation for Accreditation (EA), Analytical Methods Committee, UK, etc. (Table 2.4).

ISO/IEC 17025 is related to the general requirements related to analytical laboratories like testing, method development, sampling, calibration, etc. It specifically addresses the establishment of traceability for measurement. It has replaced EN 45001 and ISO guide 25 guidelines and serves as a basis of laboratory accreditation. However, ISO/IEC 17025 accreditation is not mandatory by USFDA. In accordance with article 12 of European Council Regulation 882/2004, laboratories designated for official control of pesticide residues must be accredited to ISO/IEC 17025. ISO 5725 covers quantitative estimation methodology and statistical models for analytical methods especially

Table 2.4: Method validation parameters as per recommendations of various regulatory bodies

No.	Parameters	ICH	IUPAC	USP	AOAC	ISO 17025	Eurachem	NATA	EU
1.	Accuracy	√	√$^{\Psi}$	√	√	√	√	√	√
2.	Trueness	√$^{\Psi}$	√				√	√	
3.	Selectivity		√		√	√	√	√	
4.	Specificity	√		√			√		√
5.	Precision	√	√	√	√		√	√	√
	Repeatability	√		√	√	√	√	√	√
	Intermediate Precision	√		√	√				
	Reproducibility	√		√$^{\Psi}$		√	√	√	√
6.	Linearity	√	√	√	√	√	√	√	√$^{\Psi}$
7.	Range	√	√	√	√		√	√	√$^{\Psi}$
8.	Sensitivity		√				√	√	
9.	Recovery		√	√	√		√		√
10.	Limit of Detection	√$^{£}$	√	√	√	√	√	√	
11.	Limit of Quantitation	√$^{£}$	√	√	√	√	√	√	
12.	Stability		√	√					
13.	System suitability test	√		√	√				
14.	Measurement uncertainty		√				√	√	
15.	Robustness	√$^{\Psi}$		√	√	√	√		
16.	Ruggedness	√$^{\Psi}$	√	√	√		√	√	√
17.	Decision limit								√
18.	Detection capability								√
19.	Filter retention studies			√					
20.	Extraction efficiency studies			√	√				

√$^{\Psi}$, Parameter exists with different name.
√$^{£}$, Parameter not required for assay.

for food analysis. It shares its terminologies and definitions from ISO 3534 Parts I and II. ISO 22971 assists in implementing ISO 5725-2 protocols. Fundamentals of linear and square regression are also given in ISO 11843. ISO 16140 is used for validation of microbiological methods. The Codex Alimentarius Commission (*Latin* for book of food) was framed in 1963 by FAO and WHO to develop internationally recognized food standards, guidelines and codes of practices under the Joint FAO/WHO Food Standards Programme. It follows the AOAC/FAO/IAEA and SANCO guidelines 10684/2009.

Codex Alimentarius has notably three committees which are working for validation of residue analytical methods: the Codex Alimentarius Committee on Analytical Methods and Sampling (CCMAS), the Codex Alimentarius Committee on Residue of Veterinary Drugs (CCVDF), and the Codex Alimentarius Committee on Pesticide Residues (CCPR). CCMAS is concerned with food monitoring while CCVDF and CCPR are involved with residual estimations.

AOAC (Association of Analytical Communities) has had official observer status in Codex Alimentarius. AOAC "Official Methods of Analysis" have been defined as "official" by regulations promulgated for enforcement of the Food, Drug, and Cosmetic Act (21 CFR 2.19). It prepares validated methods and guidance documents for method validation for single laboratory methods and collaborative trials.

European Commission (EC) directives 2002/657/EC provide basis for the analytical methods to be used in the testing of official samples and specifies common criteria for the interpretation of analytical results of official control laboratories. In 2011 guideline on bioanalytical method validation (EMEA/CHMP/EWP/192217/2009) was issued by European Medicine Agency (EMA). Q2(R1) Validation of Analytical Procedures: Text and Methodology (CPMP/ICH/381/95 - ICH Q2 (R1)) is adopted as reference for analytical method validation for characteristics applicable to identification, control of impurities and assay procedures by EC.

Eurachem is a network of organisations in Europe having the objective of establishing a system for the international traceability of chemical measurements and the promotion of good quality practices. It has issued guidelines such as Traceability in Chemical Measurement (2003) and The Fitness for Purpose of Analytical Methods: A Laboratory Guide to Method Validation and Related Topics (1998) covering various aspects of analytical method development and validation.

The International Union of Pure and Applied Chemistry (IUPAC) issued a technical report in 2002 as 'Harmonized guidelines for single-laboratory validation of methods of analysis'. In the past, ISO, IUPAC, and AOAC

International have developed common guidelines on the design, conduct and interpretation of method performance studies, proficiency testing of (chemical) analytical laboratories, internal quality control in analytical chemistry laboratories and the use of recovery information in analytical measurement.

Cooperation on International Traceability in Analytical Chemistry (CITAC) has also provided guidance with an aim to provide laboratories with guidance on best practice for the analytical operations.

ILAC – the International Laboratory Accreditation Cooperation – has also issued relevant guidance and rules.

USFDA has harmonized its requirements with ICH, but guidance documents including bioanalytical methods for the industry are helpful to achieve method validation. The US cGMPs mandates the requirements for validation in sections 211.165 (e), 211.194, Bioavailability and Bioequivalence Requirements 21 CFR 320 and USFDA GLP regulation 21 CFR Part 58. United States Pharmacopoeia has chapter 1224 on transfer of analytical procedures, chapter 1225 on validation of compendial procedures, chapter 1226 on verification of compendial procedures and chapter 621 on chromatography itself.

The International Conference on Harmonisation (ICH) of Technical Requirements for Registration of Pharmaceuticals for Human Use is unique in bringing together the regulatory authorities and pharmaceutical industry of Europe, Japan and the US. Under the set of quality guidelines, it has provided Q2(R1) guideline issued in 1996. Earlier, it was available as a set of two guidelines which were merged later into single guideline. It comprises of previously coded as Q2A guideline which includes validation parameters needed for a variety of analytical methods. It also discusses the characteristics that must be considered during the validation of the analytical procedures as a part of registration applications. Guideline on methodology (Q2B) included the actual experimental data required, along with the statistical interpretation, for the validation of analytical procedures.

National Association of Testing Authorities, Australia (NATA) is the authority responsible for the accreditation of laboratories, inspection bodies, calibration services, producers of certified reference materials and proficiency testing scheme providers throughout Australia. It is also Australia's compliance monitoring authority for the OECD Principles of GLP. It has issued many technical notes including (notes no. 17) guidelines for the validation and verification of chemical test methods.

American Society for Testing and Material (ASTM) has published many relevant standards including ASTM D6299-10e1 for 'standard practice for applying statistical quality assurance and control charting techniques to evaluate analytical measurement system performance', cleaning validation, etc.

Table 2.5: Method validation parameters as per ICH Q2(R1)

Parameters	*Assay*	*Identification*	*Test for impurity*	
			Quantitation	*Limit test*
1. Accuracy	√	×	√	×
2. Precision	√	×	√	×
3. Repeatability	√	×	√	×
4. Intermediate precision	√	×	√	×
5. Specificity	√	√	√	√
6. Limit of Detection	×	×	×	√
7. Limit of Quantitation	×	×	√	×
8. Linearity	√	×	√	×
9. Range	√	×	√	×

VALIDATION PLAN: STRATEGIES FOR HPTLC METHOD VALIDATION

An old proverb says, '*Analysts don't plan to fail but they fail to plan*'. An analyst should, first, determine the purpose of the method. It should include the requirements and specification limits to be identified and controlled. Further steps to a complete method validation includes development of a validation protocol or a validation plan, execution of the plan, documentation of validation experiments, results in validation report and designing change control procedure.

Validation plan should cover all the steps of the analytical procedure. It includes details of chromatographic system, all standard substances such as certified reference standard, working standards, reagents, solvents, samples, equipment used, sample preparation steps, preparation of reference standards, stability aspects and calculation of the final results. It should include detailed description of the method and defined personnel responsibilities of the validation team.

Prerequisite of validation

Certified reference standard

The reference standard should be dried (preferably) before use to eliminate residual solvent(s), unbound and bound moisture present in it. The drying is compulsory for hygroscopic compounds. However, drying may result in the loss of a hydrate or degradation of thermolabile compounds. Thus, care should be taken to prevent degradation or the loss of a hydrate compound. Quality of reference material is a critical parameter and is discussed in detail elsewhere (section 5, accuracy).

Sample preparation

Sample preparation should be optimized to ensure that complete extraction of active principle may be ensured without affecting the quality of the analyte. Stability of the analyte during sample preparation steps should be checked to optimize sample preparation steps. Filter retention studies and extraction efficiency determination is discussed in detail under section of validation parameter (section 13, 14).

Stability aspects

Stability of analyte during method development in an open system such as used in HPTLC is a critical aspect that must be carefully investigated prior to validation. There are high chances that substance sensitive to humidity or oxygen may undergo hydrolytic or oxidative degradation during pre-treatment, sample preparation, application on the surface of the sorbent layer and development.

- Stability of the analyte during sample preparation steps should be confirmed, especially when extraction involves series of solvent and long extraction time. This can be part of the optimisation of the sample preparation procedure.
- Stability of the analyte in solution may be checked by evaluation of plate at appropriate intervals from 10 min to 24 hrs after the application of analyte and reference solutions over same plate side by side following development and assessment. The acceptance criterion is that the peak area of both standard(s) and sample(s) solutions should be stable within ±2% RSD for 24 h.
- Stability of analyte adsorbed in stationary phase from 10 min to 4 hrs should be evaluated before development.
- Stability of analyte during development may be evaluated using two-dimensional separations in both directions at right angles to each other. When all the spots are situated on the diagonal of the chromatogram, it indicates no degradation, while spots originating from degradation in the first run will be observed out of the diagonal on the chromatographic plate.
- Stability of the analyte spot on the sorbent layer after development and before and after visualisation by densitometry or post-chromatographic derivatization can be done by scanning the spots of analyte periodically and recording peak areas or peak heights. In case of degradation, secondary spots are not observed but fading or change in light-absorption/emission occurs.

- An aged mobile phase should also give the same values of R_f, tailing factor (T), and number of theoretical plates (N) when compared to a freshly prepared mobile phase, and in addition, the results of analyses should be within ±2% RSD.

If degradation of the analyte or reference material is observed, different strategies like changing the method, changing the solvents, or sorbents, use of antioxidants, protection from light or providing nitrogen or carbon dioxide atmosphere during development may also be applied until the stability of the analyte is found suitable.

Instrument verification

Software and hardware of instrument must be "qualified' before use. Instrument should produce reliable and acceptable system suitability data. The "qualification" (formerly called validation) of the instrument (instrument qualification) is divided into design qualification (DQ), installation qualification (IQ), operation qualification (OQ), and performance qualification (PQ).

In HPTLC, the solution of standard and sample are applied using a precision gas-tight syringe of sample band applicator, which must be checked for volume accuracy. This is done by gravimetric method, where weight of volume delivered by the syringe is determined using thermostated low volatile liquid like water and bromoform. Performance of the applicator is to be checked for reproducibly delivering same volume of solutions. It may be tested by applying at least eight times the same (sample) solution of a standard substance over a chromatographic plate. The plate is scanned to record the peak area of the sample. The % RSD of peak area should not be more than 1%.

Detection at 254 nm and 366 nm requires a UV cabinet. The UV lamps used must be qualified on regular basis. Sodium salicylate is applied over fluorescent silica gel plate in various concentrations. The spot should be detected equally at 254 and 366 nm wavelengths. This indicates sensitivity of lamp. Visible difference should be observed for sample applied in decreasing concentration to confirm homogeneity. Scanner should be checked if it can reproducibly read the same spot ten times with same output having % RSD of less than 1. In HPTLC methods, analysts should apply one band over the plate and the same band should be analyzed six or nine times. This is used to verify instrument precision. The relative standard deviation obtained should not be more than 0.4% (preferably 0.2%). Now, the same may be studied using six bands of same solution (same concentration and volume) and analyzed six or nine times. The relative standard deviation obtained should not be more than 0.8–1.5%.

System suitability determination is discussed under the section of validation parameters (Section 12).

Handling and development of plate

One should be aware that, only precoated plates should be used for reproducible results. Amongst others, precoated TLC plates and precoated HPTLC plates are available in market which differ on the basis of particle size. Precoated TLC plates are widely used and are cheaper as compared to the precoated HPTLC plates. Precoated HPTLC plate may be used if results obtained through precoated TLC plate are not acceptable. Precoated plates of silica gel $60F_{254}$ of 20 × 20 cm or 10 × 10 cm should be cut appropriately and used without pre-treatment. Plate should be visually examined for irregularity in plate material, scratches or other deformities. Development may be carried out using 20 × 10 cm or 10 × 10 cm twin trough chamber. For reproducibility studies, plates may be prewashed using 20 ml methanol in each trough. Prewashing may help in removing any dirt or impurity over the plate due to accidental contamination or storage. Plates may be dried at 120°C for 20 mins. Plate should be carefully handled and should not be touched over the developing area. Side edges or top edges may be used for proper handling. The bands/spots on the plate may be applied using contact spotting or spray-on application. The diameter of spot should not be more than 1.5 mm for HPTLC plate or 2–4 mm for TLC plates for better resolution. Thus, 0.5–5 μL solution may be applied as band/spot on pre-coated TLC plate, while HPTLC plate allows 0.1–1 μL volume.

8 mm bands should be applied at minimum 4 mm apart using automatic sample applicators. Linomat-5 and Automatic TLC Sampler (ATS4) of CAMAG® use spray-on technique. The centres of spots are usually applied 5 mm (HPTLC) or 10 mm (TLC) apart. Spray-on technique ensures homogenous distribution of sample over entire length of the band. The concentration of stock solution should be adjusted such that the appropriate volume of spots correspond the appropriate concentration. If the solvent volume occupies up to 5 mm in twin though chamber (HPTLC plate) or 10 mm (TLC plate) height from the lower edge of the plate, the bands should be applied at minimum of 8 mm (HPTLC plate) or 15 mm (TLC plate) above the lower edge of the plate and minimum 15 mm (HPTLC plate) or 25 mm (TLC plate) from right or left edge of plate (Fig. 2.3). This may compensate any irregularity of plate material at edges. The volume of the mobile phase should be 10 ml for 10 × 10 cm chamber and 20 ml for 20 × 10 cm chamber, equally distributed by tilting the chamber at 45°. Filter paper soaked in mobile phase kept at rear trough may be used to check the chamber equilibrium. 20 minutes may be sufficient for chamber saturation. Plate may be dried vertically, in the direction of development using a clean stream of cold air. Hot air dryers may influence the band and may deteriorate the sample.

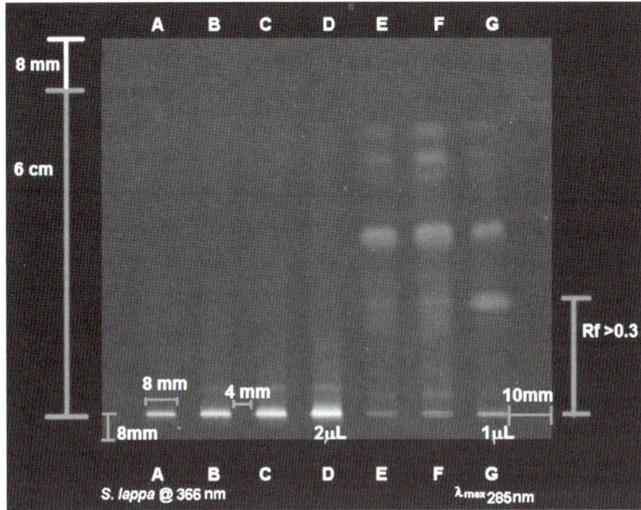

Fig. 2.3: Development of HPTLC plates.

Scanning densitometry

Scanning densitometry is very sensitive in the range of 190 nm–900 nm. Analyte present at nanogram level may be detected using absorbance mode and λ_{max} of the compound may be identified using UV spectrum. Scanning densitometry sequentially scans all the samples and standard on a plate. Multiwavelength scan also helps in sequential scanning of each track with up to 31 wavelengths in single chromatogram, so that each analyte may be quantitated at optimum wavelength. Detector at fluorescence mode may detect analyte at picogram levels. A micro-slit of 0.3–0.4 mm height with 20 mm/sec scanning speed may be used to optimally utilize light and resolution. Derivatization is performed in cases where compound is not detectable and chromophoric groups require chemical alteration for the same. It is also useful in cases where specific detection of any one compound is required; detectability may be increased by inducing fluorescence. Some common derivatization agents are Dragendorff's reagent, iodine vapour, anisaldehyde-sulphuric acid, etc.

Documentation of plates

Identification of sample requires documentation of number, colour, intensity, position and sequence of zones. Chromatogram may be photographed using three types of light sources. The use of a particular source depends on the visibility of band for proper documentation. Chemical derivatization may be used to increase the details of the bands on the plate. Bands, and thus analytes, present therein may absorb at 254 nm, 366 nm or white light. Short wave (254 nm) emitted by UV lamp excites the analyte and band may be illuminated in different shades such as blue or green. Long wave (366 nm) UV, also emitted by UV lamp, excites molecule to fluoresce. The details may be further enhanced using cut-off filter for better photograph using camera. White light may be used for coloured bands in three different modes: reflectance, transmission, and combination of reflectance and transmission. This increases the details that may be observed by an unaided eye. Pictures should be of uniform resolution (i.e. 640 × 480 or 1024 × 768) with constant camera parameters for comparative analyses. The details of resolution, zoom, white balance, etc. parameters should be documented for GLP compliance. A system manager software is now essential to control the HPTLC system and manage the data ('visionCATS' and 'winCATS – Planar Chromatography Manager' supplied by CAMAG).

ANALYTICAL METHOD VALIDATION PARAMETERS

Validation helps in proving the suitability of method for the intended purpose. Method may be used for identification, limit test, semi-quantitative purity test, assay, in-process or finished product quality control test, etc. A validation characteristic of a particular analytical method varies with its objectives. As per USP, the assay procedures differ from highly particular analytical determinations to subjective attributes analysis. These assay procedures may be divided into four categories depending on specific scheme of validation required.

Class I: For quantitative determination of bulk drug and active component in finished dosage form (including preservative).

Class II: Includes quantitative assays and limit tests. For impurity determination in bulk drug and degradation products in active component in finished dosage form.

Class III: For determination of particular performance characteristics such as dissolution test and drug release studies.

Class IV: For identification tests.

Apart from four-class classification by USP, a six-category classification given by AOAC and ISO 17025 also exists.

1. Confirmation of Identity.
2. Quantifying an analyte at a low concentration.
3. Limit test at low concentration.
4. Quantifying an analyte at a high concentration.
5. Limit test at high concentration.
6. Qualitative test.

However, whether it is a four-class or six-class classification, HPTLC can be used for identity (qualitative) testing, semi-quantitative test or quantitative estimation.

Validation of identity tests

The validation parameter evaluated for acceptance of an identity test is the specificity of the test. Matrix components which are expected to interfere and disturb the spot shape and R_f value of the analyte are developed simultaneously side-by-side to the analyte on the same chromatographic plate. No other spots or peaks should be observed at similar R_f value of the analyte and the peak should not be distorted. The identity of botanicals involves comparison of fingerprint chromatograms which are indicative for the composition and the ratio of the different components. Thus, in case of botanicals along with the prevalidation and the specificity test, the precision of the method at three concentration levels is also tested. The observed standard deviation of the R_f values of the separated zones is determined and controlled.

Validation of semi-quantitative HPTLC procedures

Semi-quantitative results are generally based on visual comparison of spot sizes and intensities, as in limit tests. Limit tests are used to check limits for the sum of ordinary impurities in a product as per chapter 466 of USP. No interfering peak should be present on the same R_f. Purity of the peak may be further confirmed comparing its UV spectrum recorded at three different positions. Derivatization may be opted, if required. The validation of a limit test consists of a specificity test and a check of the detection limit (LOD), the smallest quantity of the analyte that can be detected. As visual estimation is quite subjective, at least three analysts should perform this evaluation and the mean value is regarded as LOD. Precision of method is established at three concentration levels with % RSD of less than 2. The Eurachem Guideline recommends 10 determinations. In addition, it should be checked using different concentrations of the analyte, whether a difference of approximately 20% or 50% of the specification limit can be judged reliably.

Detailed investigation may be required in some cases. The spot of the impurity is compared to spots of either the main component or one particular known and isolated impurity applied in appropriate concentration. If appropriate, instead of the main component, a more suited, characterised impurity may be used as reference substance. The quantities of the individual impurities are then estimated by visually comparing the sizes and intensities of the spots to that of calibration spots.

Validation of quantitative TLC procedures

Quantitative TLC estimations involve evaluation of the chromatograms by scanning densitometry, video densitometry or using MS-detection techniques. According to ICH Guideline, the validation characteristics to be determined in case of a quantitative impurity testing are as follows: specificity, detection and quantitation limit (LOD/LOQ), accuracy, precision, linearity and range. For an assay procedure in pharmaceutical application with an expected label claim of the analyte, all the parameters except LOD/LOQ are determined.

It is evident from above discussion, that every analytical method based on the purpose requires different types of parameters to be validated and specifications to be set (Tables 2.5 and 2.6). There is no official sequence in which the validation parameters should be determined, but many of the method performance parameters are determined at the time of method development. There is no demarking line, where method development finishes and method validation starts. Method validation is very closely associated with method development.

Table 2.6: Performance characteristics required for method validation

Parameters	Qualitative estimation	Identification estimation	Limit test		Quantitative estimation	
			Analyte at low conc.	Analyte at high conc.	Analyte at low conc.	Analyte at high conc.
Linearity	×	×	×	×	√	√
Range	×	×	√	√	×	√
Accuracy	×	×	×	√	√	√
Precision	×	×	×	√	√	√
Specificity	√	√	√	√	√	√
Ruggedness	×	×	×	×	√	√
LOD	×	×	√	×	√	√/×
LOQ	×	×	√	×	√	√/×

The objective of the topic is to offer clear understanding of essential scientific parameters so that an internationally accepted, robust, reliable and valid HPTLC method may be developed. Typical validation characteristics, which should be considered, are listed below:

A. Accuracy
B. Precision
   - Repeatability
   - Intermediate Precision (Ruggedness)
   - Reproducibility
C. Specificity & sensitivity
D. Limit of Detection
E. Limit of Quantitation
F. Linearity

G. Range
H. Robustness

Other validation parameters:

I. System suitability determination
J. Filter retention studies
K. Extraction efficiency studies
L. Forced degradation studies

ACCURACY / TRUENESS

AOAC: *The closeness of agreement between the measured value and the accepted, "true," or reference value.*

EURACHEM: *'Accuracy' expresses the closeness of a result to a true value.*

ICH: *The accuracy of an analytical procedure expresses the closeness of agreement between the value which is accepted either as a conventional true value or an accepted reference value and the value found.*

ISO 3534-1: *It is closeness of a result to a true value.*

IUPAC: *Trueness is the closeness of agreement between a test result and the accepted reference value of the property being measured.*

NATA: *Accuracy is a measure of the quality of a result, i.e. how useful the result is to the customer or other stakeholders. It has two components, precision and trueness.*

The accuracy of an analytical method is given by the extent to which the value obtained deviates from the true value. It shows the proximity of measured results to the actual value. In other words, it is the degree of agreement between experimental values and true value.

Since the reference value is termed as true value, Accuracy is often termed as trueness. Fundamental of trueness is closely associated with fundamental of measurement of error. Trueness is also known as percentage of error.

Measurement of error includes gross error, determination of bias and random error in terms of "bias". Thus, Trueness is measured quantitatively in terms of 'bias', which are determined by comparing method response with a reference material of known purity. Trueness defines the systematic bias of the method.

Organizations such as IUPAC, NATA and ISO (ISO 5725-1), use 'closeness' of agreement between a test result and the accepted reference value of the property being measured to define 'bias' or 'trueness' and the term accuracy as the combination of trueness (defines the systematic error of the method) and precision (defines the random error of the method). These authorities require precision studies with trueness determination for accuracy studies (Total error).

150% to pre-quantified sample solutions. The amount of drug 'A' was estimated by applying values of peak area to the regression equations of the calibration graph. Three replicate samples of each concentration level were prepared.

Preparation of sample solution

Twenty tablets were powdered; powder equivalent to 3.5 mg of drug was dissolved in 5 ml solvent. This solution was spiked with 50% of the estimated drug concentration (1.75 mg). To achieve this, 1.75 ml of standard drug solution (of 1 mg/ml concentration) was added to it. The final volume was made up to 25 ml. Similarly, the samples with 100% and 150% standard drug spiking were prepared. These three solutions were applied in triplicate (2 μL) on the plate. Results may be tabulated as follows (Table 2.8):

Table 2.8: Accuracy Study of the Proposed Method for Drug 'A'

Amount of sample taken (ng/spot) drug	Amount of standard added (ng/spot)	Amount of drug recovered* (ng/spot)	% Recovery*
286.7	150	439.86 ± 0.60	100.72 ± 0.138
286.7	300	587.41 ± 3.79	100.12 ± 0.64
286.7	450	739.74 ± 3.29	100.41 ± 0.44

* Mean ± standard deviation (SD, n = 3)

Result

Since % recovery is under acceptance limits, Method may be considered as Accurate.

PRECISION

AOAC/ICH: *The precision of an analytical procedure expresses the closeness of agreement (degree of scatter) between a series of measurements obtained from multiple sampling of the same homogeneous sample under the prescribed conditions. Precision may be considered at three levels: repeatability, intermediate precision and reproducibility.*

EURACHEM: *Precision is the closeness of agreement between independent test results obtained under stipulated conditions.*

ISO: *Closeness of agreement between quantity values obtained by replicate measurements of a quantity under specified condition.*

IUPAC: *'A measure for the reproducibility of measurements within a set, that is, of the scatter or dispersion of a set about its central value.*

NATA: *The precision of a method is a measure of the closeness expected between independent replicate test results conducted under specified conditions.*

'Precision' is normally determined for specific circumstances which may be having wide variability. It indicates 'degree of scatter' or expresses the closeness of agreement between a series of measurements obtained from multiple sampling of the same homogeneous sample (Figs. 2.4 and 2.5). It is usually expressed as the variance, standard deviation or coefficient of variation of a series of measurements. It should be investigated using homogeneous, authentic or artificially prepared samples. An analyst must understand that despite of all the recommendations provided by different regulatory bodies, acceptable precision for a particular method may be defined differently. It depends on the requirement and design of the method. It should incorporate acceptance limits for analytical and manufacturing variability.

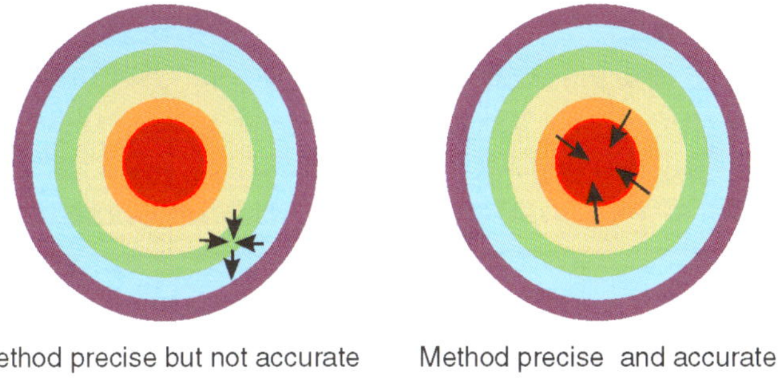

Fig. 2.5: Precision and Accuracy.

Australian Standard 2850 (1986) provides guidance on this aspect of method validation. ISO 3534-1 state that the precision depends critically on the stipulated conditions. It depends only on the distribution of random errors and does not relate to the true value or specified value.

Repeatability and Reproducibility are particular sets of extreme conditions. As per AOAC the purpose of a collaborative study is to determine estimates of the attributes of a method, particularly the "precision" of the method that may be expected when the method is used in actual practice. The AOACI uses two terms to define the precision of a method under two circumstances of replication: repeatability and reproducibility. AOAC defines repeatability as a measure of the variation, s_r^2, between replicate determinations by the same analyst. It help us to know, how well an analyst can check himself using the same method on blind replicates of the same material or split levels (Youden pairs, ±5% difference), under the same conditions (e.g., same laboratory, same apparatus, and same time). It defines reproducibility as a composite measure of variation, s_R^2, which includes the between-laboratory and within-laboratory variations. It help us to know, how well an analyst in a given laboratory can check the results of another analyst in another laboratory using the same method to analyze the same test material under different conditions (e.g., different apparatus and different time). The between-laboratory variation represents a systematic error that reflects variation arising from environmental conditions (e.g., condition of reagent and instruments, variation in calibration factors, and interpretations of the steps of the method) associated with the laboratories used in the study. If these factors are not identified and controlled, they will add up into s_R^2.

The IUPAC perspective is little different. IUPAC suggests that for single-laboratory validation, two sets of conditions should be studied. Here, analyst should use test material in duplicate and test it in successive runs. Both sets include study of sources of error. First condition include the study of *precision under repeatability conditions*, describing variations observed during a single run as expectation 0 and standard deviation s_r. Second condition includes *precision under run-to-run conditions*, describing variations in run bias d_{run} as expectation 0, and standard deviation s_{run}. Since both of these are sources of error for the method, they must be combined. This combined precision can be expressed as follows:

$$s_{TOTAL} = [(s_r)^2/n + (s_{run})^2]^{1/2}$$

where, n = no. of repeat result averaged within a run. Variance obtained from both the sets may be calculated using one-way ANOVA test.

As per ICH guidelines, precision may be considered at three levels: repeatability, intermediate precision and reproducibility.

Repeatability

It expresses the precision under the same operating conditions over a short interval of time. It is also termed as intra-assay precision. Here, tests should be performed on identical test items in short interval of time by same operator using the same equipment in one laboratory under constant conditions. Repeatability is a useful indicator of method performance. However, one should not be confused that repeatability of instrument is a part of validation parameter. It is rather, a part of equipment qualification where multiple scans of same band should be studied for variance. Repeatability of method is a critical parameter. Analyst should be aware that the preparation errors obtained through standard solution preparation may be as high as 26 times compared to instrumental precision. Precision may vary with analyte concentration. NATA recommends that, if analyte concentration is expected to vary by more than 50% of an average value, then it should be investigated keeping this variation in mind.

Procedure for performing repeatability studies

For some tests, it may be appropriate to determine precision at only one or two concentrations of particular significance to the users of test data. As per ICH recommendations for assay of drug product, a minimum of 9 determinations (Three concentrations, i.e. 80%,100% and 120% of target concentration with three replicates each = 09 samples) covering the specified range for the procedure or a minimum of 6 determinations at 100% of the test concentration should be made.

Acceptance criteria for repeatability studies

Generally, relative standard deviation obtained should not be more than 2%. However, the minimum criteria may vary as per the nature of analytical procedure. % RSD of precision data for impurity testing varies between 5%–30% depending upon the concentration of impurity. EURACHEM recommends calculation of the standard deviation using 10 independent determinations. ICH recommends an investigation of precision for assay and quantitative determination of impurities. For unknown degradation products, it sets a limit of 0.05%, for a maximum daily dose of more than 1 gm and 0.1% for a maximum daily dose of less than 1 gm. To achieve this level of quantitation, a procedure must have sufficient accuracy and precision to provide an uncertainty of less than 10%.

Bioanalytical methods requires precision to be studied at three concentrations, five determinations each (e.g. 80%, 100% and 120% of target concentration with five replicates each = 15 samples).

Intermediate precision

It expresses intra-laboratory (within the laboratory) variations: different days, different analysts, different equipment, etc. within the same laboratory. It is also described as ruggedness. Robustness and ruggedness are two different parameters of method validation. Many times ruggedness and robustness are used interchangeably i.e., NATA guideline defines it as a measure of robustness. But it should be used as separate parameter. Ruggedness is evaluation of consistency of result when method under normal test conditions is used but external factors like analyst, instrument, laboratory are varied deliberately. In some guidelines Ruggedness (USP and ISO 17025) is not defined separately, but termed as intermediate precision or reproducibility (ICH). The definition of NATA says 'The ruggedness (a measure of robustness) of a method is the degree to which results are unaffected by minor changes from the experimental conditions described in the procedure'; for example, small changes in temperature, pH, reagent concentration, chamber saturation, flow rates, extraction times, composition of mobile phase. Ruggedness is investigated by measuring the effects on the results of small, planned changes to the method conditions. In some cases, information may be available from studies conducted during in-house method development. Intra-laboratory reproducibility investigations, by their nature, take into account some aspects of a method's ruggedness. Ruggedness is now commonly accepted as intermediate precision. The USP definition of robustness is equivalent to that of the ICH. It says, "*The ruggedness of an analytical method is the degree of reproducibility of test results obtained by the analysis of the same sample under a variety of normal test conditions, such as different laboratories, different analysts, different instruments, different lots of reagents, different elapsed assay times, different assay temperatures, different days, etc.*". In fact, this definition is equivalent to that for intermediate precision (within-laboratory experimental set-up) or reproducibility (between-laboratory experimental set-up), for which ISO guidelines exist. The ICH guidelines also state that "*One consequence of the evaluation of robustness should be that a series of system suitability parameters (e.g. resolution tests) is established to ensure that the validity of the analytical procedure is maintained whenever used*". Basically the study should include the followings:

1. Identification/selection of the variables (or factors) most likely to affect method performance;
2. Selection of the number of levels for each variable (generally 2 to 3);
3. Selection of the most appropriate experimental design;
4. Establishment of the response value that evaluate the changes in the factors and experimentation;
5. Computation of the effects of individual parameters over method performance, including due to interaction amongst the factors; and,
6. A statement of the conclusions.

Procedure for performing intermediate precision studies

It requires determination of three concentrations, six determinations each, for three days (e.g. 80%, 100% and 120% of target concentration with six replicates each = 18 samples for three times = 54 samples).

Acceptance criteria for Intermediate precision studies

Generally the acceptance criteria for *Intermediate precision* ranges between 1.3 to 1.7 times the percent RSD of the repeatability study.

Reproducibility

It is an interlaboratory study. As per ICH guideline, it expresses the precision between laboratories. It is an important parameter and includes collaborative studies using more than one laboratory. Reproducibility data is not required for marketing authorization dossier, but should be considered for standardization of analytical procedures such as pharmacopoeial procedures.

Procedure and acceptance criteria for reproducibility studies

AOAC recommends using at least three laboratories to conduct pilot study and extend it up to 8–10 laboratories for obtaining valid data. It ensures standardization of methodology and generally used as final test of the method. It ensures that the variability of results remains constant in different conditions and variation amongst the factors doesn't contribute significantly in variability. For qualitative analyses, a minimum of 10 laboratories are recommended; collaborative study should include 2 analyte levels per matrix, 6 test samples per level, and 6 negative controls per matrix. David-Test may be performed to test the normal distribution of precision data. Cochran test, Grubbs test and Dixon test may be used to test the outliers present in the data. *Cochran test* should be performed for removal of laboratories or individual outlier value showing significantly greater variability among replicate, when compared with the data obtained of similar test but from different laboratory. Computation of *Cochran test* should be done using a 1-tail test at a probability value of 2.5%. *Grubbs tests* (if n > 6–8) may also be used for the same. AOAC recommends that computation should be made using single value test (2-tail; P = 2.5%); then if no outlier is found, apply pair value test (2 values at the highest end, 2 values at the lowest end, and 2 values, one at each end, at an overall P = 2.5%). A relative standard deviation value facilitates comparison of variabilities at different concentrations. When the RSD increases rapidly with decreasing concentration it reduces the limit of reliable measurement or usefulness of the method. Another indicator is *HORRAT value*, which determines the acceptability of the method. It is the ratio of the reproducibility relative standard deviation, expressed as a percent (RSDR, %) to the predicted reproducibility relative standard deviation, expressed as a percent (PRSDR, %). Acceptable HORRAT values lies between 0.5 to 1.5. HORRAT values below 0.5 don't indicate reproducibility of the method while values above 1.5 indicate higher reproducibility and requires investigation. The limits for performance acceptability are 0.5 to 2. These results should be displayed as control chart or bar chart. Relative standard deviation value of 0.5 to 0.6 times the theoretical values determined by *Horwitz function* is acceptable for repeatability study. For reproducibility study, relative standard deviation value of 0.5 to 2.0 times the theoretical values determined by *Horwitz function* is acceptable. *Neumann test* may also be used to check the trend analysis of the data. For Quantitative estimation of herbal drugs using HPTLC, Reich *et al.* (2008) have recommended that the botanical reference material should be used in three different portions with three aliquots applied on three separate plates. The plates should be chromatographed in freshly prepared portions of the mobile phase, one by one using the same chamber. The fingerprints of all tracks on a plate must be identical and any inhomogeneity such as waves, "banana fronts," etc. should be absent. It should be followed by study of variability of R_f on each plate (n = 3) and, all the three plates (n = 9) should be evaluated. The same experiment should be repeated, with one sample on three days for the study of intermediate precision and another laboratory for reproducibility study. The acceptance criteria is fulfilled if the R_f value of three markers do not exceed 0.01 across each plate, 0.02 for repeatability, 0.05 for intermediate precision, and 0.07 for reproducibility.

Example

Objective

Perform repeatability studies of Drug 'A' having labelled strength of 25 mg using HPTLC method.

Procedure

Drug was obtained as gratis sample along with certificate of analysis indicating the purity of drug equivalent to 98.5%. This means, that 101.52 mg of the drug is equivalent to 100 mg. One should keep the application volume constant. It may be set as 6 μL band/8 mm band. One stock solution was prepared as follows:

Preparation of stock solution

10.15 mg drug (purity = 98.5%) was dissolved in solvent and the volume was made up to 100 mL to get a stock solution of 100 μg/mL.

Method 1: As per ICH requirements, six replicates at 100% concentration should be studied.

Twenty tablets were powdered; powder equivalent to 25 mg of drug was dissolved in 5 ml solvent. Volume was made up to 25 ml using solvent to produce a solution of estimated 1 mg/ml concentration. When 6 μL of solution was spotted on the plate, the estimated concentration was 200 ng/band. The solution was applied nine times and results may be tabulated as follows:

Table 2.9: Repeatability Measurements (Method Precision) of Drug

Particulars	Peak area*
Trial 1	2133
Trial 2	2143
Trial 3	2156
Trial 4	2165
Trial 5	2158
Trial 6	2146
Mean Peak Area	2150
S.D. of Peak Area	10.63
Method Precision (RSD)	0.49

*Concentration, 200 ng/band

Method II: As per ICH requirements, three replicates at 80%, 100%, 120% concentration each should be studied.

Particulars	Peak area		
Concentration (ng/band)	160	200	220
Trial 1	1716	2133	2557
Trial 2	1722	2143	2563
Trial 3	1744	2156	2584
Mean Peak Area	1727	2144	2568
S.D. of Peak Area	12.03	9.41	11.57
Method Precision (RSD)	0.69	0.43	0.45

Result

Since % RSD is below 2, Method may be considered as precise.

SELECTIVITY AND SPECIFICITY

AOAC: *Selectivity is the degree to which the method can quantify the target analyte in the presence of other analytes, matrices, or other potentially interfering materials.*

EURACHEM: *The ability of a method to determine accurately and specifically the analyte of interest in the presence of other components in a sample matrix under the stated conditions of the test.*

ICH/USP: *Specificity is the ability to assess unequivocally the analyte in the presence of components which may be expected to be present. Typically these might include impurities, degradants, matrix, etc.*

IUPAC: *Selectivity is the degree to which a method can quantify the analyte accurately in the presence of interferent.*

NATA: *The selectivity of a method is the accuracy of its measurement in the presence of interferences.*

Western European Laboratory Accreditation Conference (WELAC): *Selectivity of a method refers to the extent to which it can determine particular analyte(s) in a complex mixture without interference from other components in the mixture.*

Specificity and selectivity are important indicators of method reliability. Unfortunately, international unanimity over their definitions is absent. Literature survey revealed that these definitions are often used interchangeably by many authors which is a wrong practice. Kaiser made important contributions in spectrometry by defining *'selektivitaët'* and *'spezifcitaët'* and identified ways of calculating the degree of interferences. USP 28 defines 'specificity' as the ability to assess the analyte unequivocally in the presence of other components such as impurities, degradation products, and the matrix. A method is said to be 'specific' if it provides a response for only single analyte, while the term 'selective' means that the method provides responses for a number of analytes which can be distinguished from each other. It means that method is able to measure an analyte accurately in presence of interference. According to Eurachem, both terminologies reflect the same characteristics and are related so closely that, specificity indicate 100% selectivity or 0% interference. This explains in other ways that method should be termed specific, if it is 100% selective. It means that specificity is an absolute term and what we measure is selectivity, which may not be 100% and may be described as good selectivity, high, excellent or even low selectivity. In other words, *Specific method is absolutely selective.* IUPAC also defines it similarly, '*Specificity is the ultimate of selectivity*'. IUPAC and AOAC have preferred the use of the term 'selectivity' over 'specificity' for methods that are completely selective, while USP, USFDA and ICH used the term 'specificity'. As per ICH guideline, specificity may be demonstrated in different ways depending upon the type of analysis. It classifies two types of procedures namely, identification tests and quantitative (assay & impurity) tests. This procedure may still differ depending upon the availability or unavailability of standard impurity component.

Procedure for performing specificity/selectivity studies

In Identification tests, method is said to be specific only, if it has an ability to discriminate between the compounds of closely related structures. Here, peak purity and identity is crucial.

In case of assay (purity tests) or impurity tests, method is said to be specific only if it can determine the analyte in presence of interference. The sample may be spiked with degradation products or possible interfering components. In purity testing, specificity may be demonstrated by isolation of the analyte through selective solvent extraction, chromatographic separation, by application of biochemical reactions (antibodies, enzymes) or instrumentation techniques. This helps in reducing any interference by matrix; further, chromatography or solid phase extraction technique may be used for better separation. Here, appropriate resolution of the peak is crucial.

Assay procedure requires method to be specific for active component only, without being separated from each other. Ideally, all substances available or capable of interference should be applied in purified state or as pure reference with test substance on the same chromatographic plate and results must be recorded (Figs. 2.6 and 2.7).

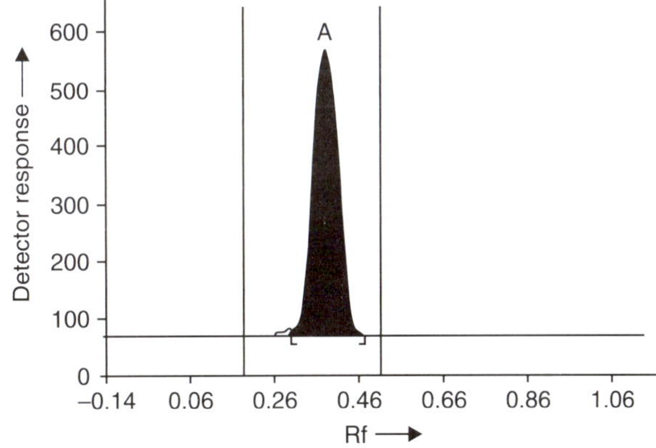

Fig. 2.6: Chromatogram showing Peak of Reference Compound (A).

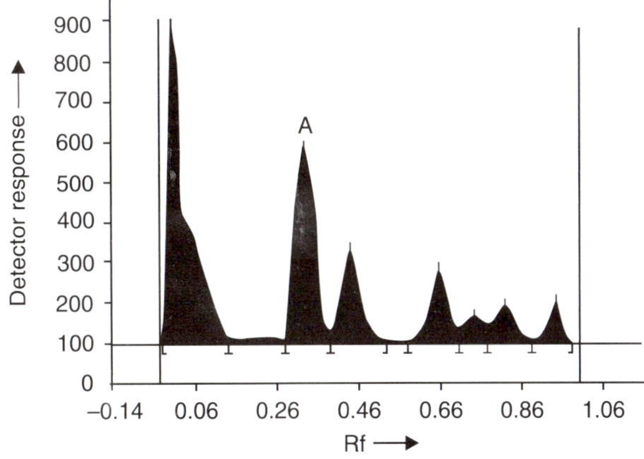

Fig. 2.7: Chromatogram showing Peak of Analyte (A) in Actual Sample Matrix.

For Quantitative estimation of herbal drugs using HPTLC Reich et al (2008) have recommended that the botanical reference material should include at least 3 authenticated samples of each species, preferably from different locality or habitat. This will help to identify the natural variability in the sample. It is advisable to use homogenized samples that include more than one specimen. Specificity is demonstrated only if fingerprint of sample is identical to botanical reference material and samples representing other species give different fingerprints.

The concentration of sample applied should be sufficiently high (100–200 μg/band) in order to optimally detect the presence of any impurity even in low quantities. This will help in identifying any extraneous peak. USFDA recommends that the baseline should be *on-scale* as *off-scale* baseline can hide minor peaks.

Generally diffuse reflectance UV spectra of the standard with sample peak are compared at the start, middle and end positions of the bands to determine peak purity and only the middle one for identity (Figure 2). This may be done by determining correlation coefficient 'r ' if you are using CATS software of CAMAG.

Precaution: Flow of mobile phase decreases with increase in distance on the HPTLC plate, therefore optimum development time may vary from 7 mins to 20 mins. Best resolution is usually obtained at a maximum developing distance of 6 cm. Mobile phase must be optimized so that the minimum R_f values of the analyte lies in the range of 0.3 to 0.5 or higher, but not below this range.

Acceptance criteria for specificity/selectivity studies

The criteria determining specificity/selectivity of method includes peak resolution, peak identity, peak purity and slope of calibration function. The USFDA suggests resolution of at least 2 for all compounds accompanying active drug dosage forms, including hydrolytic, photolytic, and oxidative degradation products. In addition, the isolated analyte should show no evidence of peaks of other compounds. Another approach suggests a minimum resolution of 1.25 so that near baseline resolution may be achieved.

However, poor resolution of the peak is a serious drawback of this practice as it can't demonstrate peak purity or identity. The effect on the measurement of a primary peak due to the presence of a secondary peak with a response ratio of 16:1 would be an error of about 0.5%, If reference material is spiked with 6.25% of impurity, then any response showing less than 0.5% level of error should be acceptable.

If slope of the calibration function (sensitivity) is denoted by or b_{an} and b_{int} be the slope of the response produced by a potential interferent, then their relation may be used as indicator of selectivity. IUPAC suggests use of selectivity index b_{an}/b_{int} as it provides quantitative measure of interference. For determination of slope of the response produced by a potential interferent (b_{int}), a matrix blank may be spiked with interfering agent of appropriate concentration. It is advisable to determine the same in the absence of drug analyte for better results in order to avoid matrix effect.

Frequent Failures and ways to avoid them

It is observed that authors used to report chromatogram of single peak to demonstrate specificity. Instead two additional chromatograms should be presented, namely, chromatogram of placebo prepared similarly to the sample and blank chromatogram of solvent used. In addition to this, chromatogram of known and related substance should be provided. Another practice includes identification of unknown degradation product by stress testing/forced degradation studies. If reference degradation products are not available then they may be generated using simulated stress conditions, and method should be compared with available reference standard method. Degradation products generated by the effect of light, humidity, acidity, basicity, oxidative -reductive conditions or accelerated temperature are chromatographed with original analyte of unstressed condition on same chromatographic plate. Here, most of the times authors end up by giving unrealistic excessive stress conditions, a logical choice is to induce and limit to approximately 5%–10% degradation in sample matrix. Any further stress will have a catastrophic effect on sample matrix which is not at all useful (Please refer section 14 for details).

LIMIT OF DETECTION AND LIMIT OF QUANTITATION

Definitions: Limit of Detection

AOAC: *The lowest content that can be measured with reasonable statistical certainty.*

ICH: *The detection limit of an individual analytical procedure is the lowest amount of analyte in a sample which can be detected but not necessarily quantitated as an exact value.*

ISO/DIS 11843-1: *'The true net concentration or amount of the analyte in the material to be analysed which will lead with probability (1-b), to the conclusion that the concentration of the analyte in the analysed material is larger than that of the blank matrix.'*

performed at a single concentration equal to about twice the LOQ. *Decision Limit (CCa)* as per European commission directives may be established using calibration curve procedure according to ISO 11843, which similarly involve estimation using spiking of analyte in blank sample matrix. The corresponding concentration at the y-intercept plus 2.33 times (a = 1 %) (or 1.64 times, a = 5% with specified permitted limits) the standard deviation of the within-laboratory reproducibility of the intercept equals the decision limit. Alternatively, 20 blank samples with spiked analyte may be analyzed similarly.

Limit of quantification or limit of determination

It is the lowest concentration of analyte that can be determined with an acceptable level of repeatability precision and accuracy. This level of precision is around 10%. Eurachem also defines it as, analyte concentration corresponding to the sample blank value plus 5, 6 or 10 standard deviations of the blank mean. It cautions that, the LOQ is an indicative value and should not normally be used in decision making. ICH describes it as quantitation limit. It is also termed as limit of reporting. NATA defines it as lowest concentration of analyte, that can be determined with an acceptable level of uncertainty. The most common recommendation is to quote the LOQ as 3 times the LOD. Similar parameter is defined as Detection capability (CC_a) as per European commission directives and, it should be below minimum specified performance level. It is also considered as signal 10 times the background signal or noise and often referred as signal to noise ratio of 10:1. It is noteworthy that the determination of signal to noise ratio is a compromise between analyte concentration and performance limit of method; as precision increases, LOQ decreases. It simply indicates towards the fact that measurement of concentration is possible even below this level but uncertainty of the quantitation will become too high for a reliable quantitative measurement. However, it should not be confused with sensitivity of the method.

Three basic approaches are recommended by ICH to estimate LOD of a method.

1. **Determination of LOQ on the basis of visual evaluation:** This approach is used for non-instrumental and instrumental methods. Solutions with known concentrations of analytes are chromatographed and minimum level of concentration which may be reliably (with acceptable accuracy and precision) detected is established.

2. **Determination of LOQ on the basis of Signal-to-Noise:** As per ICH recommendations signal-to-noise ratio may be determined by comparing the analytical signals at known low concentrations with those of blank sample up to the concentration which produces a signal to noise ratio equivalent to ten

times. Similarly, IUPAC considers the LOQ to be expressed as the signal or analyte value that will produce estimates having a specified relative standard deviation (RSD), of 10%. It may be represented as Quantification Limit, $L_Q = k_Q\ s_Q$ (where, s_Q is the standard deviation and kQ is the multiplier whose reciprocal equals the selected quantifying RSD with a default value of 10.

3. Determination of LOQ on the basis of Standard Deviation of the Response and the Slope: As per the ICH, limit of quantitation may be expressed as 10 s/S, where s is the standard deviation of the response and S is the slope of the calibration curve. Here, standard deviation of the response (s) may be calculated as follows:

A. **Using standard deviation of the blank:** Appropriate numbers of blank samples are analyzed and magnitude of background response is calculated on the basis of their standard deviations.

B. **Using calibration curve:** Appropriate concentrations close to the expected detection limits are prepared and a calibration curve is prepared. An informed judgement should be made by the analyst as ranges of determination may vary as per the requirement of the method. The residual standard deviation of a regression line or y-intercepts may be used as the standard deviation.

Detection capability (CC_b) as per European commission directives may be established using calibration curve procedure according to ISO 11843, which similarly involve estimation using spiking of analyte in blank sample matrix around and below the required performance level of the method. The corresponding concentration at the decision level plus 1.64 times (b = 5%) the standard deviation of the within-laboratory reproducibility of the mean analyte concentration at decision limit equals the detection capability. Alternatively, 20 blank samples with spiked analyte at decision limit may be analyzed similarly.

Example 1

Calculate LOD using parameters of calibration curve of data set 1. Also check the correctness of LOD determination.

Solution

Parameters	Values
Residual Standard Deviation	28.86
Intercept	54.97
Slope	11.78
Standard Deviation of Intercept	11.47

appropriate range in HPTLC is very crucial. This is one of the most critical points of the validation of quantitative TLC/HPTLC procedures. One must be clear that this range is different from 'range' which is evaluated using samples in specification range in drug product. Linearity may be established for all active substances, preservatives, and expected impurities.

The linearity of the detector (system precision) can be obtained by diluting the analyte stock solution, while the linearity of the analytical method can be determined by making a series of concentrations of the analyte from independent preparations (weighing, spiking) and not by samples that have been prepared by dilution and spotted on one HPTLC plate (Fig. 2.11). The concentration of band should be optimized to keep the peak area in the range of 500 to 5000 A.U.

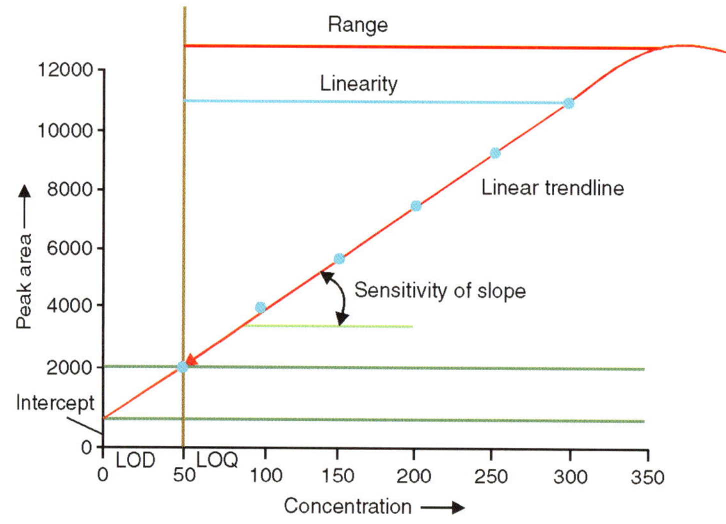

Fig. 2.10: Graphical representation of different terms used in linearity

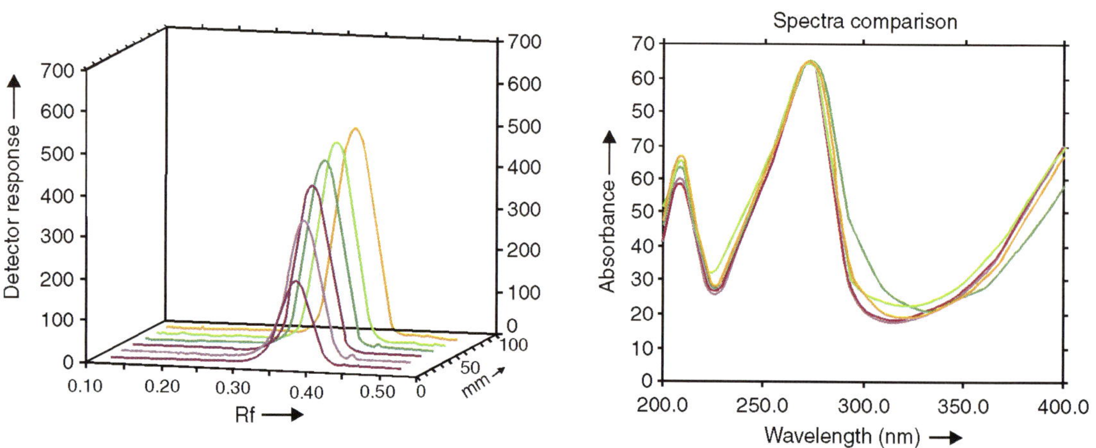

Fig. 2.11: Spectral comparison of various aliquots of same drug during linearity studies

Statistical evaluation of linearity and calibration function

Selection of technique

Statistical evaluation of linearity may be generally carried out using two techniques, generating a calibration function or best fit equation/curve.

Ordinary least squares estimation: The method of least squares is a general method of curve fitting. The best-fitting curve minimizes the sum of squares of the data points from the fitted curve. The least squares method is used extensively in many economic applications, for example, in estimating secular trend and for calculating the relationship between two or more variables for comparison purposes. It is also referred to as ordinary least squares to distinguish it from the method of weighted least squares.

Regression analysis: It is a method of fitting a regression line to data values in a scatter diagram in such a way, that the sum of the squares of the vertical deviations between the line and the individual data plots is minimized. One important thing, since we have discussed a lot about number of replications like n = 6 or 9 or so, it will be a wrong practice to calculate mean of the data and then plotting curve using mean values. Rather, one should enter all the raw replicate data, because each data has independent error and serves as separate point to devise a better fit. It may be of two types: *unweighted linear regression analysis* and *weight linear regression analysis.*

Unweighted linear regression analysis requires x and y variables to compute a best fit equation for a regression line. Here, the value of x variable, which is independent variable is supposed to be error free and vertical residuals are minimised. In this case, concentration of standard solution should be prepared by standardized material (certified reference material) of known purity with utmost care. On the other hand, *y* variable is dependent variable and supposed to be randomly distributed. This only applies to concentration range where response data has comparable variability (homogeneity of variance, when SD of data do not vary by more than 1.5–3).

Weight regression should be applied, if large concentration range is to be used. Weighted regression incorporate extra nonnegative constants, or estimated weights, associated with each data point, into the fitting criterion. The size of the weight indicates the precision of the information contained in the associated observation. The weighted fitting criterion may be optimized to find those parameter estimates, which allow the weights to determine the contribution of each observation in the final parameter estimates. One should be aware that the estimated weight for each observation is given relative to the weights of the other observations; so different sets of absolute weights can have identical effects. It is useful especially when the standard deviation of the random errors in the data is not constant across all levels of the explanatory variables. It yields the most precise parameter estimates possible, because here weights are inversely proportional to the variance at each level of the variables. i.e. the homogeneity of variations of residuals.

Calculation of confidence interval and prediction interval

Once a best fit equation is generated, the variability of equation should be proved using confidence and prediction interval. First step is to calculate the confidence interval of the calibration function. The prediction interval and statistical confidence *P* may also be used to investigate data using outlier test. Prediction interval is useful to identify variability or uncertainty in the determination. Here, regression is repeated without the suspected data pair and if it is now outside the new prediction interval, it may be regarded as outliers. The inverse of calibration function is used to calculate the analyte concentration. The intersection of this line with regression line at *x axis* estimates the concentration, further upper and lower limits of prediction interval with this intersection identify the *range of uncertainty* for the concentration. Now, confidence interval of the calibration function should be calculated. The confidence interval of intercept of a linear regression without bias includes the origin ("zero"). In HPTLC method, intercept should not be passed through origin. It is extremely important to properly select the correct calibration and working range as both values depend upon it. Ones the equation of regression analysis is completed the parameters generated are utilized to understand the correlation and dependence of y on x.

Recommendations for linear relations are available in ISO 11843 series, USFDA, USP and EMEA guidance which is based on the 'Text on Validation of Analytical Procedures' issued by the ICH. The guide line recommends that the correlation coefficient, slope of regression line, y-intercept and residual sum of squares should be submitted when evaluating a linear relationship and that the linearity, should be evaluated by 'appropriate statistical methods'.

It is a common practice to check the linearity of a calibration curve by inspection of the value of *correlation coefficient* (*r*) or *regression coefficient (coefficient of determination)* (r^2 or R^2), which should be close to unity and slope of regression line at 1.0 ± 0.1. Correlation coefficient describes the relation between two random parameters showing how well they are connected. It also indicates the sensitivity of the analysis. Regression coefficient indicates the effect of independent variable on response (positive or negative). Some statisticians define it as '*Square of correlation coefficient*'. It is a wrong practice to consider it as sufficient evidence to conclude that the experimenter has a perfect linear calibration. Hence, it is extremely important to emphasise that an "r-test or r^2 test" to check for linearity does not exist. We cannot say that $r^2 = 0.999$ is more linear than $r^2 = 0.997$.

The second step to prove linearity, is to show that the intercept is not significantly different from zero ($p > 0.05$) or at least it must be about 2 to 5% of the target concentration.

Additionally, *standard error of slope or regression* and *residual sum of square* are important parameters for describing method performance. It measures the deviation of experimental values from regression line and thus precision of regression. When expressed as percentage, it is comparable to relative standard deviation of precision studies. Residual sum of square should also be reported for regression analysis, which must also be near to unity. Detailed discussion of regression parameters obtained using Microsoft Excel[â] software is available in example 1.

Still, one must realize that generally linear regression calculations are not sufficient and several other statistical parameters should be used, such as the relative process standard deviation value (Vxo), Mandel-test, Hartley-test, the Xp value, the plot of response factor against concentration, analysis of variance (ANOVA) or the residual plot, to demonstrate the linearity of calibration function.

Preliminary statistical evaluation of linearity starts with graphical evaluation of deviations of experimental data from the assumed response model (residual analysis) residual plots. Further evaluation using numerical parameters is required, only if random errors exist.

Graphical evaluation includes:

1. Testing the residuals (the differences between the measured and the calculated values): only a residual plot without any tendency proves the linearity of the calibration. This is the simplest linearity test suggested for TLC/HPTLC methods.
2. Other non-numerical tool helps to evaluate sensitivity.

The Numerical tests, for example:

1. F-test for comparison of the standard deviations of the residuals for different, linear and nonlinear, models (Mandel test)
2. Testing homoscedasticity (homogeneity of variations of residuals: Hartley test)

Residual plot is the simplest method of linearity test for HPTLC methods. Residuals are smallest possible differences, which may be obtained by minimising the distance between the experimental points and regression line (i.e Residual values represent the differences between the actual y value and predicted y value for each x value from the curve). In other words, residuals are the difference between the experimental response and calculated response obtained from regression line. Residuals are distributed randomly at both sides of the straight-line. Positive and negative deviations would cancel each other, and square of residuals will be summarised and minimised giving its name 'least square regression'. Linearity may be confirmed, if residual values are randomly distributed around the regression line (no lack of fit). Nonlinearity is indicated, if systematic trends are observed (lack of fit). In such cases, where systematic trends are observed, data must be treated by weighted regression. Fig. 2.12 indicates comparative residual plots obtained from data set 1, 2 and 3 (these data sets are shown in later part of text as part of exercise). Data set 1 indicates good fit when compared to residual plots of data set 2 and 3. Normal probability plots are also a visual test to see, if the residuals are normally distributed. Straight line is a benchmark here, and residuals should follow it closely, if they are normally distributed. Fig. 2.13 indicates comparative normal probability plots obtained from data set 1, 2 and 3. Data set 1 indicates good fit when compared to residual plots of data set 2 and 3.

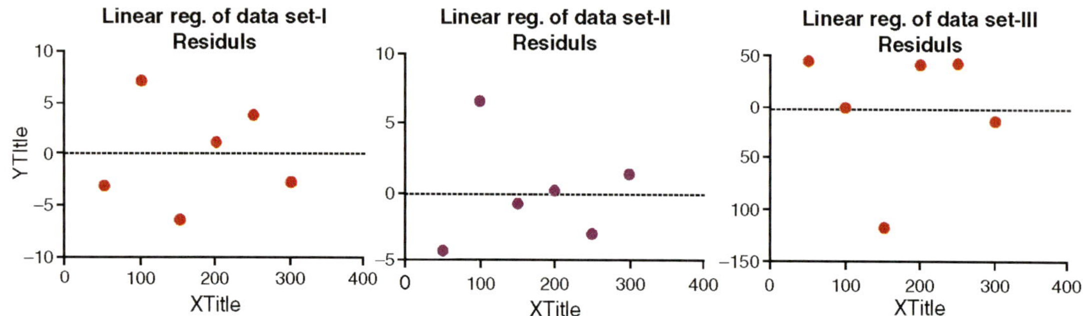

Fig. 2.12: Residual plots obtained from data sets 1, 2 and 3.

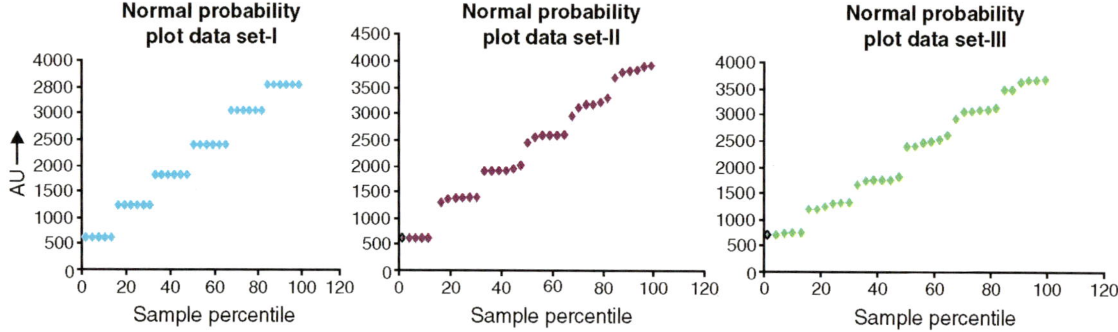

Fig. 2.13: Normal probability plots obtained from data sets 1, 2 and 3.

Another tool to evaluate linearity even with small number of data points is estimation of sensitivities. Sensitivity is a gradient of response curve. It corresponds to slope of the curve. Sensitivity may be defined as ratio of analytical signal and corresponding concentration (response factor) as function of concentration. ASTM recommends a 5% interval around sensitivity average at zero intercept.

If the calibration is non-linear, the residuals will show clear tendency, (such as a bow shaped trend) then statistical test should be used to evaluate linearity. In this case, models such as polynomial regression (for low concentration with wide range), Michaelis–Menten (for high concentration with wide range), or weighted regression should be selected. Further, other statistical tests, like lack of fit test by ANOVA or testing homoscedasticity, quadratic equation may be used for the calculation.

Mandel test uses F-test for comparison of standard deviations of the residuals for linear and nonlinear models. Larger concentrations with large response value will have a greater influence on this type of regression, due to higher effect on minimisation of the sum of squares. Hartley test checks the homogeneity of variations of residuals; which is termed as homoscedasticity. If, homoscedasticity is observed, weighting factors (i.e., 1/*concentration* or 1/*concentration*^{2}) may be used. Generally standard deviation of data should not be more than a factor of 3. The variance homogeneity (homoscedasticity) over the whole range of the linear calibration line should also be proved using the F-test. When heteroscedasticity is confirmed, and the calibration range cannot be reduced, weighting factor should be used, e.g., equal to 1/C or 1/C2, where C¼ concentration or other weighting factors.

CAMAG[â] described other parameters, such as "*sdv*" (residual standard deviation of the standard point), for expressing the fit of a calibration curve for HPTLC by using its CATS software. The lower the value means, the closer the points to the curve. The *sdv* value is a measure for the quality of all types of calibration curves. The acceptance criterion of *sdv* (according to our experiences) is not more than 5.0. The *sdv* can be calculated from the deviation between each measured standard value and the calibration curve. Ideally, the smallest value of *sdv* should be selected to determine the most suitable regression model that will be used for the calibration.

Choice of linearity range

The choice of linearity range depends on the objective of the method. Generally, it is kept at 80%–120% of the target concentration. Alternatively, it may be 0–50% or 50%–150% of analyte concentration likely to be encountered. For uniformity assays, the range would be 70%–130% of the target concentration. For impurity methods, the range would start from its lower limit of quantitation and extends to 120% of the target concentration. The recommended range for dissolution studies lies between 80 % to 120% of specified range. For degradation studies, the range would start from its lower limit of quantitation and extends

Solution

Drug was obtained as gratis sample along with certificate of analysis indicating the purity of drug equivalent to 98.5%. This means, that 101.52 mg of the drug is equivalent to 100 mg. One should keep the application volume constant. It may be set as 6 μL/8 mm. Six independent stock solutions were prepared as follows:

Preparation of stock solution: 10.15 mg drug (purity = 98.5%) was dissolved in solvent and the volume was made up to 100 mL to get a stock solution of 100 μg/mL. Solutions were further diluted to achieve 100 ng/band concentration in 6 μL. 6 μL of solution was spotted on the plate to get 100 ng/band concentrations. Similarly other five independent stock solutions (drug equivalent to 20 mg/100 ml to 60 mg/100 ml) were prepared to achieve concentration ranging from 100–600 ng/band. Peak area was recorded and tabulated as follows:

Tabulation of data:

HPTLC calibration plot data and linearity measurements of drug

	Peak area					
Concentration (ng/band) / Particulars	100	200	300	400	500	600
Trial 1	931	1814	2738	3578	4539	5429
Trial 2	939	1797	2678	3658	4479	5387
Trial 3	949	1804	2698	3648	4498	5456
Trial 4	944	1844	2725	3597	4532	5378
Trial 5	952	1838	2758	3645	4527	5443
Trial 6	942	1784	2738	3617	4563	5432
Mean Peak Area	943	1813	2722	3623	4523	5420
S.D. of Peak Area	7.64	23.52	29.41	31.83	30.04	31.30
(RSD) of Peak Area	0.81	1.29	1.08	0.87	0.66	0.57

Calibration curve was plotted using all data set and various parameters may be calculated as discussed in section on Linearity.

Example 2

Six concentrations of Drug A were subjected to linearity studies using six replicates each and peak areas were recorded. Calculate the Regression parameters of data set-one generated for preparing calibration curve of Drug A using data analysis tool from Excel® (Microsoft Office®, 2007).

Concentration (ng/band) / Particulars	Peak area					
	50	100	150	200	250	300
Replica 1	627	1219	1838	2411	3033	3524
Replica 2	621	1223	1828	2462	3045	3544
Replica 3	631	1232	1822	2438	2998	3531
Replica 4	630	1230	1829	2432	3024	3564
Replica 5	626	1238	1818	2418	3052	3582
Replica 6	622	1224	1832	2437	3043	3548

Solution

Mean, standard deviation and % RSD of the data set was found to be as follows:

Concentration (ng/band) / Particulars	50	100	150	200	250	300
Mean	626	1228	1828	2434	3033	3549
Standard deviation	4.246	6.893	7.185	17.83	19.76	21.39
% RSD	0.68	0.56	0.39	0.73	0.65	0.60

Note: Microsoft Office, 2007, data analysis tool pack is required to be installed from source file as follows: Microsoft Excel > Office button > Excel option > Add-in > Analysis toolpack > double click or press GO. Excel will install the analysis toolpack and now can be used from Data > Data analysis > Regression. The typical output will include the following:

ANOVA®

Model		Sum of Squares	df	Mean Square	F	Sig.
1	Regression	(A) 34211367	1	(D) 34211367	(F) 41059.25	(G) 1.17E-52
	Residual	(B) 27496.24	33	(E) 833.2195		
	Total	(C) 34238863	34			

(a) Predictors: Concentration

(b) Variable: Peak area

Regression Statistics		
Multiple R	0.999598	
R Square	0.999197	(H)
Adjusted R Square	0.999173	(H)
Standard Error	28.86554	(I)
Observations	35	(J)

	Coefficients	Standard	t Stat (O)	P-value (P)	Lower 95% (Q)	Upper 95%
Intercept	54.97475 (K)	11.47277 (M)	4.791758	3.4E-05	31.63322	78.31629
50	11.78256 (L)	0.058148 (N)	202.6308	1.17E-52	11.66426	11.90086

(A) Model sum of squares (MSS): Closer to TSS, better the fit.
(B) Residual sum of squares (RSS).
(C) Total sum of squares (TSS).
(D) Average Model sum of squares (AMSS)=MSS/(k – 1), k is the no. of predictors.
(E) Average Residual sum of squares (ARSS) = RSS/(n – k), n is the no. of observations.
(F) The F-*statistics*, evaluates, whether R^2 is different from zero.
(G) Indicate the significance of predictor; should be close to zero.
(H) R^2 values should be close to 1.0. Adjusted R^2 values are obtained by adjusting it using no. of data and variables, it is a better estimation of relation between X and Y.
(I) Residual standard deviation of data.
(J) No. of samples studied.
(K) Intercept.
(L) Slope.
(M) Standard deviation (Standard error) of intercept
(N) Standard deviation (Standard error) of Slope.
(O) Significance of the slope of regression line is determined from t- statistics, it is a probability that the observed correlation coefficient occurred by chance if the true correlation is zero. Checks, whether coefficient is different from zero. Here, t- values should be greater than 1.96 at 95% confidence interval. It is calculated by dividing coefficient by its standard error. Here results are significant, indicating good fit.
(P) P-value checks whether coefficient is different from zero. *P-value* should be less than 0.05 (at a 0.10). So, the results are significant, indicating good fit.
(Q) It indicates upper and lower values at 95% confidence interval.

Residual plot of data set 1 is given as Figure 12 and 13, indicating good fit. Further, RSD values are lower than 2, which indicate acceptable variation in data. On the basis of above discussion, we may consider the data set as linear, indicating a good fit.

For better understanding of all these *stat*-stuff reader is requested to go through the paragraphs below. But mind well, the discussion here, is *very subjective* to our data sets, specifically linearity in HPTLC method data. Any statement given here may not hold good in other contexts, You may refer detailed literature available, but for all those, who don't want a PhD. in linearity, here is some common *stat* sense.

Quick glance fundamental of linear/non-linear regression analysis for non-statistician

Oh! Don't be afraid I am just telling you very important values amongst the values or parameters thrown over you by your stat software. Only the useful ones.

Nonlinear regression is used to fit data to a model that defines Y as a function of X. Y must be a variable like concentration in our case, It is dependent variable. X is independent variable, peak area or absorbance in our case. Linear regression calculation keeps *FOUR* basic assumptions; *First*, X values (independent variable) do not contain errors or uncertainties (much less than Y) as analysts control it, and *Second*, Y values (dependent variable) have all of it. *Third*, the scatter of points around the line follows a Gaussian (normal, bell shaped) distribution and *fourth* that the standard deviation of the scatter is the same for every value of X. One should note that linear regression is only a simpler, special case of nonlinear regression, and results will be similar if we use a nonlinear regression model to fit linear model.

Generally one assume that the average scatter of data around the curve is the same all the way along the curve, one should instruct the nonlinear program to minimize the sum of the squared distances of the points from the curve. We may choose to minimize the sum-of-squares with no weighting. One important thing, repeating again, it will be a wrong practice to calculate mean of the data and then plotting curve using mean values. Please, enter all the raw replicate data to devise a better fit.

'Curve fit' and interpretation of the 'best-fit' parameter values

1. Nonlinear regression programs report the standard error of each parameter, standard error values of slope and intercept is used to compute the 95% confidence interval.
2. 95% confidence interval of intercept should be statistically indistinguishable from zero. Slope of regression line should be checked using *F-ratio*.
3. The *sum of squares* (SS) is the sum of squares of the vertical distances of the points from the curve. Least square nonlinear regression works by varying the values of model parameters to minimize SS.

4. Distance of the points from the line is known as *residuals.* If it is above the curve it is said to be positive and below the curve, negative. Using SS and degree of freedom, we can calculate *standard deviation of residuals.*
5. When one variable is changed it affects the other variable, since this change can be correlated, we can quantify the direction and magnitude of correlation using Correlation coefficient r. Even If you exchange the labels and make X, the Y and vice versa, values of r^2 will not change. Coefficient of determination is traditionally known as R^2 for non-linear regression and r^2 for linear regression, but both of them are same!!!!! And, one more absurd stuff, R^2 or r^2 is not even a square of anything, only convention. r^2 is the fraction of variation that is shared between X and Y. One should not be confused between two types of coefficients that are frequently encountered during regression analysis. The quantity r, is termed as *linear correlation coefficient.* It measures the strength and the direction of a linear relationship between two variables. It is also known as *Pearson product moment correlation coefficient* in honour of its developer Karl Pearson, r is a dimensionless quantity; that is, it does not depend on the units employed. The other type of coefficient is known as *coefficient of determination,* r^2. It is also known as *r squared.* It is the ratio of the explained variation to the total variation. It is a measure that allows us to determine how certain one can be in making predictions from a certain graph or how well the regression line represents the data. It gives the proportion of the variance of one variable that is predictable from the other variable. It represents the percent of the data that is the closest to the line of best fit. The example data set 1 shows the r^2 = 0.998, which means that 99.8% of the total variation in y can be explained by the linear relationship between x and y .The other 0.2% of the total variation in *y* remains unexplained.
6. One should not force the line to pass through the origin (X = 0, Y = 0) or set the intercept to zero. Better fit will be obtained by not constraining the line.
7. Sum of the squares (SS) value of the distances of the points from best fit curve is known as SS_{reg}, and the values obtained through normalization to SSreg from a horizontal line through the mean of all Y values is called SS_{tot}. Do you know that here, If the curve fits the data well, SS_{reg} will be much smaller than SS_{tot}.
8. Data should be randomly distributed around the curve (Gaussian). The average distance of points from curve should be same for all parts of the curve. Data points should not be clustered even above and below the curve.

9. *Residuals* and *runs* tests will help to evaluate if curve deviates systematically from data. A run is a series of points (*residuals*) which are either above or below the regression curve. Suppose we have a data set with nine replicates (n = 10), so number of runs that should be present would be (n/2 + 1) = 6. If you observe less *runs* than expected , it means curve deviates systematically from data and P values will be lower than 0.5. It indicate that the model is inappropriate and data were fit to wrong equation, or data don't follow a straight line. If more runs than expected are observed the P values will be higher than 0.5, indicating good fit.
10. The z-score should indicate clusters of data around 0 (not calculated here).

Example 3

Calculate and compare linear regression parameters and Nonlinear regression parameters including computation of 95% confidence interval of slope and intercept of Data Set 1. Further Apply runs test to check deviation from linearity.

Solution

Parameters were computed using Graph Pad prism5 software. As per discussion in the section parameters indicate similar results, data set 1 indicate good fit.

Data obtained from Graph Pad 5	Linear regression	Nonlinear regression
Best-fit values		
Slope	10 ± 0.06	11.79
Y-intercept when X = 0.0	50 ± 10	53.12
X-intercept when Y = 0.0	–5	—
1/slope	0.08	—
95% Confidence Intervals		—
Slope	10 to 10	11.68 to 11.90
Y-intercept when X = 0.0	30 to 80	31.03 to 75.20
X-intercept when Y = 0.0	–7 to –2	—
Goodness of Fit		—
r^2	1	0.9992
Sy.x	30	28.57
Is slope significantly non-zero?		
F	40000	—
DFn, DFd	1,30	—
P value	<0.0001	—
Deviation from zero?	Significant	—
Runs test		
Points above line	3	—
Points below line	3	—

(*Contd.*)

Data obtained from Graph Pad 5	Linear regression	Nonlinear regression
Number of runs	5	—
P value (runs test)	0.300	—
Deviation from linearity	Not Significant	—
Normality of Residuals		—
D'Agostino & Pearson omnibus K2	—	0.5794
P value	—	0.7485
Kolmogorov-Smirnov distance	—	0.09073
P value	—	>0.10

Example 4

Data Set 1, Data Set 2 and Data Set 3 (peak area) were generated during linearity estimation of drug A using different mobile phase composition for HPTLC method. Compare the data set using regression parameters and identify, which data set indicate linearity using Graph Pad prism 5 software.

Data Set 1

Concentration (ng/band)	50	100	150	200	250	300
Replica 1	627	1219	1838	2411	3033	3524
Replica 2	621	1223	1828	2462	3045	3544
Replica 3	631	1232	1822	2438	2998	3531
Replica 4	630	1230	1829	2432	3024	3564
Replica 5	626	1238	1818	2418	3052	3582
Replica 6	622	1224	1832	2437	3043	3548

Data Set 2

Concentration (ng/band)	50	100	150	200	250	300
Replica 1	628	1394	1998	2580	3173	3684
Replica 2	607	1374	1878	2558	3211	3814
Replica 3	621	1365	1909	2588	2948	3831
Replica 4	657	1296	1895	2592	3114	3894
Replica 5	674	1395	1908	2438	3295	3792
Replica 6	612	1384	1928	2577	3163	3908

Data Set 3

Concentration (ng/band)	50	100	150	200	250	300
Replica 1	682	1214	1788	2538	3173	3754
Replica 2	731	1344	1768	2458	3211	3794
Replica 3	682	1267	1798	2568	3198	3601
Replica 4	744	1204	1795	2602	3244	3604
Replica 5	707	1328	1858	2698	3035	3822
Replica 6	752	1354	1698	2467	3163	3798

Solution

Data sets were compared using Graph Pad Prism 5 software (ver. 5.01, 2007) observed linear regression parameters are tabulated below. Based on the discussion in previous section Data set 1 indicate good fit and was found to be linear.

Parameters	Data Set 1	Data Set 2	Data Set 3
Best-fit Values			
Slope	10 ± 0.06	10 ± 0.1	12.28 ± 0.1744
Y-intercept when X = 0.0	50 ± 10	50 ± 30	58.14 ± 33.96
X-intercept when Y = 0.0	–5	–4	–4.734
1/slope	0.08	0.08	0.08143
95% Confidence Intervals			
Slope	10 to 10	10 to 10	11.93 to 12.63
Y-intercept when X = 0.0	30 to 80	–7 to 100	–10.91 to 127.2
X-intercept when Y = 0.0	–7 to –2	–10 to 2	–12.85 to 3.084
Goodness of Fit			
r^2	1	1	0.9932
Sy.x	30	70	89.34
Is Slope Significantly Non-zero?			
F	40000	8000	4959
DFn, DFd	1, 30	1, 30	1.000, 34.00
P value	<0.0001	<0.0001	<0.0001
Deviation from zero?	Significant	Significant	Significant
Data			
Number of X values	6	6	6
Maximum number of Y replicates	6	6	6
Total number of values	36	36	36
Number of missing values	0	0	0
Runs test			
Points above line	3	3	3
Points below line	3	3	3
Number of runs	5	6	4
P value (runs test)	0.9000	1.0000	0.7000
Deviation from linearity	Not significant	Not significant	Not significant

Example 4

Data Set 1, Data Set 2 and Data Set 3 (peak area) were generated during linearity estimation of drug A using different mobile phase composition for HPTLC method. Compare the data set using regression parameters and identify which data set indicate linearity using Microsoft excel 2007 software.

Solution

Data sets were compared using Microsoft excel 2007 software. Observed linear regression parameters are compared and tabulated below. Analysis of regression parameters gives various parameters to estimate whether deviation from linearity is significant or not.

Based on the discussion in previous section Data set 1 indicate good fit and was found to be linear.

(Hint: r^2 close to 1; High *F* values, low *significance F* value, High t-stat values, *P* values <0.05, observed *runs* more than expected)

Parameters	Data Set 1	Data Set 2	Data Set 3
n	36	36	36
mean %RSD	0.60	2.87	3.47
r^2	0.9991	0.9990	0.9962
F-values	3401.687	3186.235	791.1927
Significance F	1.11E-05	1.22E-05	9.86E-05
t-stat	1.777039	2.350043	–0.04561
t (Slope)	58.32	56.45	28.13
p-value	0.0000340	0.069102	0.12392
Runs test			
Observed runs test	5	6	4
P value (runs test)	0.900	1.0	0.700

RANGE

EURACHEM: *'Set of values of measurands for which the error of a measuring instrument is intended to lie within specified limits.'*

ICH: *The range of an analytical procedure is the interval between the upper and lower concentration (amounts) of analyte in the sample (including these concentrations) for which it has been demonstrated that the analytical procedure has a suitable level of precision, accuracy and linearity.*

IUPAC: *The validated range is the interval of analyte concentration within which the method can be regarded as validated.*

NATA: *The working range of a method is defined as the concentration range within which results will have an acceptable level of uncertainty.*

The range of determinations is generally identified through linearity studies and depends on the intended application of the procedure. It should be noted that this range is not necessarily identical to the useful range of the calibration curve. Here, calibration may cover a wide concentration range, but the validation study may be limited to a more restricted range (Fig. 2.14). It may be considered as the

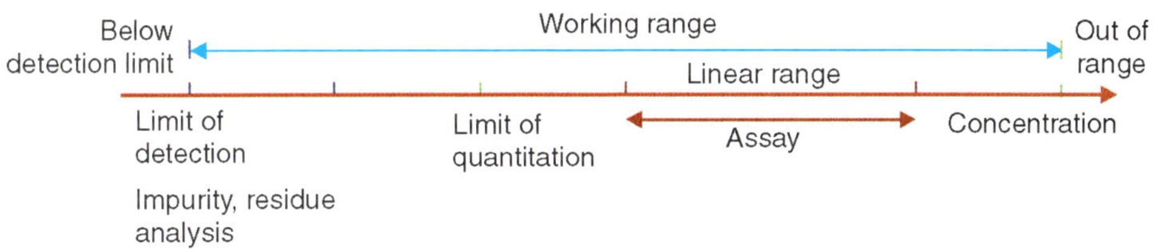

Fig. 2.14: Graphical representation of range.

concentration range within which results will have an acceptable level of uncertainty. Generally it may be as low as limit of quantitation and may extend to the upper limit of linear calibration or highest concentration studied during validation. Range should confirm that the method provides an acceptable degree of linearity, accuracy and precision when applied to samples having concentrations within the range. Many types of ranges are reported by authors, such as analytical range, linear range, dynamic range, calibration range or working range. They may be broadly categorized as analytical/ working range or linear/calibration range. Linear range is shorter than the working range. As per ICH recommendations, range of assay procedures and dissolution testing should include 80 to 120% percent of the test concentration; for content uniformity, range may be 70 to 130% percent or more of the test concentration, for impurity it ranges from detection limits to 120% of specification. However, the range should encompass 0–150 % or 50–150 % of the concentration likely to be encountered.

ROBUSTNESS

IUPAC: *The ruggedness of an analytical method is the resistance to change in the results produced by an analytical method when minor deviations are made from the experimental conditions described in the procedure.*

ICH: *The robustness of an analytical procedure is a measure of its capacity to remain unaffected by small, but deliberate variations in method parameters and provides an indication of its reliability during normal usage.*

USP (ruggedness): *The ruggedness of an analytical method is the degree of reproducibility of test results obtained by the analysis of the same sample under a variety of normal test conditions, such as different laboratories, different analysts, different instruments, different lots of reagents, different elapsed assay times, different assay temperatures, different days, etc.".*

Robustness evaluates the effect of internal factors, while ruggedness evaluates the effect of external factors over method performance.

The robustness of a method is determined to find the influence of slight changes of *internal* conditions such as mobile phase composition, chamber saturation, temperature etc. over the output of a method. If the effect of slight changes over method performance is higher, then an analyst should make efforts for maintaining these parameters at a stable level. This parameter indicates the reliability of the method during routine usage. Planner chromatography being '*open*' system is more vulnerable to external stimuli. Environmental and analytical conditions affecting the performance of method should be carefully identified in order to develop a reliable method. Many guidelines such as IUPAC harmonized guidelines for single laboratory validation of methods of analysis; NATA guidelines for the validation and verification of chemical test methods, AOAC guideline for single laboratory validation of chemical methods for dietary supplements and botanicals do not describe this parameter. Robustness evaluates the effect of internal factors while ruggedness evaluates the effect of external factors over method performance. In other words if the variables considered belong to the method of analysis, the study will check robustness. However, if the variables studied are environmental in nature such as different analyst, laboratory temperature, different suppliers of the reagents, ruggedness will be examined. Robustness is related to the stability of the method of analysis, practicability and the intrinsic variables; while ruggedness is related to the inter-laboratory method transferability. Robustness and ruggedness testing should be carried out during or nearly at the end of the method development since it may help in identifying critical variables of the method and evaluating the precision of the analytical method which may influence the performance of the analytical method. However, both aims at demonstrating reproducibility of test results. Reproducibility is defined as ruggedness in USP and ISO 17025. Robustness is Included as method development activity while ruggedness is defined as reproducibility in ICH.

Procedure for performing robustness studies and acceptance criteria

Various factors that may be used for robustness studies in HPTLC may be as follows:

Parameters	Deviation in condition	Acceptance criteria
1. pH of the mobile phase	±5% variation	No new spot on same R_f. A deviation of R_f <0.05 may be acceptable. No change in resolution. Shape of band intact. Precision of peak area NMT 2% RSD.
2. Development distance	±5 mm variation	A deviation of R_f <0.05 may be acceptable. No change in resolution. Shape of band intact. Precision of peak area NMT 2% RSD.

(*Contd.*)

Parameters	Deviation in condition	Acceptance criteria
3. Spot size and shape	Minor variation	Shape of band intact. Precision of peak area NMT 2% RSD.
4. Drying conditions	Drying at normal temperature and using a heating source such as dryer	Selectivity of separation is not affected, no change in resolution. Precision of peak area NMT 2% RSD.
5. Temperature	±5 °C	A deviation of R_f <0.05 may be acceptable. Shape of band intact. Precision of peak area NMT 2% RSD.
6. Time	Chamber saturation time	A deviation of R_f <0.05 may be acceptable. Shape of band intact. Precision of peak area NMT 2% RSD.
7. Composition of the mobile phase	Minor change in composition, may be ±5%	A deviation of R_f <0.05 may be acceptable. Shape of band intact, no solvent front. Precision of peak area NMT 2% RSD.
8. Batch of the plates	At least two batches	No change in resolution, A deviation of R_f <0.05 may be acceptable Shape of band intact. Precision of peak area NMT 2% RSD.
9. Volume of sample	0.5 to 5 µL for TLC plate; 2 to 10 µL for HPTLC plate	No band broadening. Precision of peak area NMT 2% RSD.
10. Chamber design	Minimum of two chambers of diffe-rent dimensions. Camag twin trough chambers for 10 × 10, 20 × 10, 20 × 20 cm plates	A deviation of R_f <0.05 may be acceptable, No change in resolution. Precision of peak area NMT 2% RSD.
11. Stability of analyte on plate	Time period for which analyte is stable (in hrs).	No new spot on same R_f. A deviation of R_f <0.05 may be acceptable. No change in resolution. Shape of band intact. Precision of peak area NMT 2% RSD.

Most of the times authors conducting robustness studies choose too few non significant parameters that don't affect the method performance and it becomes an intermediate precision reporting. Ideally the purpose should be the risk assessment. Chamber type may be studied using different dimension of chamber, usually one or two types of chambers may be sufficient. Variation in developing distance of 5 mm may be sufficient. A deviation of R_f <0.05 may be acceptable. In HPTLC, each plate is a new chromatographic system. Its performance may vary with prior humidity exposure due to environmental condition. Most of the time humidity control may not be available in the laboratory, therefore system suitability testing should include critical assessment of each plate to see whether development includes critical separation zones or not. Ultimate objective of this parameter involves selection of the suspected sources of variation and the experimentation, estimating the effects and the statement of the conclusions. An automated developing chamber with humidity control is very highly desirable in QC labs.

Evaluation of robustness can be achieved through two ways, one-variable-at-a-time procedure or an experimental design procedure using a nested design or nested Analysis of Variance (ANOVA). The *one-variable-at-a-time procedure* (OVAT) varies the levels of a given factor while keeping the other factors at nominal levels, to evaluate the effect of the former factor on the method response(s). When applying an experimental design, the effect of a given factor is calculated at several level combinations of the other factors, while with the OVAT approach this is only at one level. In the *experimental design procedure*, many parameters are evaluated. They may be qualitative factors or quantitative factors. Usually, the factors are examined at two extreme *levels*, and interval between them represents the variability arising due to change of laboratories, instruments or analysts. Selection of factor should be based on the uncertainty with which a level can be set and reset. Selection of an experimental design, factors and their levels and responses are critical choices based on experience and requirements.

One should be cautious to add several measurements at the central point to estimate the method repeatability and to be sure that the response surface has no curvature. If the response surface presents an important curvature, two-level screening designs Plackett and Burman or fractional factorial (FF) designs are not suitable to check robustness and Star designs which are "one factor at a time" designs may be used. Plackett–Burman (PB) designs are applied. These designs are based on Hadamard matrices and the mathematical model used to interpret the results is a first degree polynomial model. They examine the f selected factors in Ne > f + 1 experiments. Two-level full factorial designs (N = 2f) may also can be used. Usually two small, but deliberately introduced variations (in the low (–1) and a high (+1) level which are situated around the nominal (0) levels) may be sufficient. Nominal levels are conditions mentioned in the assay procedure. However three level desigr is sufficient where it is expected that the effects between [–1, 0] differ from those between [0, +1], with –1 and +1 the extreme levels and 0 the nominal. Many commercial software are available for carrying out such functions. The estimated effects are then usually graphically and/or statistically interpreted, to determine their significance. Graphical methods consist of drawing, for example, normal probability or half-normal probability. The most important outcome of this exercise is the derivation of system suitability limits from robustness test results. This helps in identification of worst case conditions and the worst case conditions should not affect the quantitative results. These worst-case conditions are predicted from the calculated effects. The worst-case situation is then the factor (level) combination giving for instance the lowest resolution. To define the worst-case conditions only the statistically significant factors (at a = 0.05) and the ones that come close to it (significant at a = 0.1) are considered. The factors not significant at a = 0.1 are considered negligible and their effects are considered to originate only from experimental error.

SYSTEM SUITABILITY DETERMINATION

HPTLC is an analytical system. Components of this analytical system include the plate, Instrumentation, software, chamber, reagents including mobile phase and lab environment. The objective of system suitability testing is to evaluate all components of the system performs as per specifications of the method through meaningful parameters variation. HPTLC system suitability determination is based on precision of R_f and peak areas, resolution, tailing or capacity factors and comparison with certified standards. The relative standard deviation associated with the repeatability of the R_f should be less than or equal to 1%, the R_f should be between 0.3-0.8, the tailing factor (T) should be greater than 0.9 and less than 1.1 and the resolution should be greater than or equal to 1.0 . These parameters should be documented with observed values for any trend analysis in retrospective validation. In case of herbal material separation of two critical zones specific to the herbal material may be used to check the adequacy of the plate.

FILTER RETENTION STUDIES

Filter retention studies are especially important during cleaning validation or residual determination, when analyte is available in very low concentration and study of its retention is required. These studies should be conducted for USP methods category I, II, III and IV. Unfiltered solutions are compared with filtered solution, blank, sample solution and standard solution with respect to recovery studies and appearance of chromatogram. It should be checked, if filter is contributing any unknown peak (compound). Placebo sample in triplicate should be spiked with a dry API concentration equivalent to 100% of the assay concentration. Finished formulations of any dosage form in triplicate may also be spiked with dry API at concentration equivalent to 100% of the assay concentration .The recovery should fall in the range of 100 ± 2%. The acceptable limits for dissolution studies shall be 100 ± 3%. These solutions should be filtered through at least two filters and analyzed. The results should be compared with the solution prepared similarly but instead of filtration it should be subjected to centrifugation (i.e. at 3000 rpm for 10 mins). Resultant solution should be analyzed in triplicate and compared using appropriate analytical method. The recovery of each sample should be calculated in sample wt. with % RSD of individual results. Percent difference of average result of filtered and centrifuged sample should be compared. Filter may be considered acceptable if the % RSD of the result is below 1.5% and 2% for assay and dissolution studies respectively. If, filter retention studies are required for USP method category II (impurity and degradants), sample solution should be prepared with addition of known quantities of impurity as per limits (~0.5%) and should be evaluated similarly. Percent difference of average result of filtered and centrifuged sample should be compared. Filter may be considered acceptable if the % RSD of the result for impurity is below 5%. The recovery of each impurity should fall within the range of 100±25%.

EXTRACTION EFFICIENCY STUDIES

An optimum extraction procedure ensures economical and complete extraction of drug from its dosage form without affecting the quality of drug. Study of extraction efficiency is especially important to measure the effectiveness of the extraction procedure. These studies should be conducted for USP methods category I, III and IV methods except dissolution testing, if applicable. It is generally not performed in USP method category II (impurity and degradants) because appropriate samples are difficult to obtain. Extraction procedure is critical in dosage form related estimations. Critical variables include volume of extracting solvent, its composition, effective time required for complete extraction, optimum temperature and sonication time. A comparative study of above factors may help in development of an optimum scheme of extraction with maximum extraction efficiency. Twelve samples may be divided in four sets of three samples each. Using the given extraction protocol three sets should be extracted in such a fashion that the extraction time of first sample should be as per protocol, second set should have longer extraction time than first and third sample should be longest amongst all. The fourth set should be extracted for shorter period than that mentioned in the protocol. Percent recovery of all the sets should be documented to establish the extraction range of the sample.

FORCED DEGRADATION STUDIES

Forced degradation studies are used to evaluate an analytical method's capability to measure an active ingredient and its degradation product without interference. The studies involve degrading the sample deliberately. Samples are exposed to heat, light, acid, base and oxidizing agents to produce 10% to 30% degradation of the active analyte. Excessive degradation is unnecessary and analysts should gradually degrade the analyte, so that useful conclusions may be drawn. The hydrolytic degradation of drug may be studied in acidic or alkaline conditions by refluxing it with 0.1 N HCl or 0.1 N NaOH for 8 hr. Higher strengths and time may be used, if required. Degradation under neutral condition may be induced by refluxing the drug with water for 12 hr or more. Humidity of 75% RH or above d 1.2 million Lux hr fluorescent light and 200 W hr/m^2 UV may be used to study effect of humidity and photo degradation. To observe the effect of oxidation, a 3–30% solution of hydrogen peroxide may be used. Appropriate detector settings should be applied so that degradation products even at 0.1% concentration may produce a peak with feasible area count. The objective here is restricted to the identification of degradation peak and not the characterization, in addition it helps to identify whether peak of the analyte is still resolved. This method doesn't demonstrate presence of impurities, any by-product, any excipients or any other material, what so ever.

Note:

1. 10–30% decomposition of analyte should be taken as reasonable for different stress conditions.
2. If no decomposition occurs, stress conditions to be increased.
3. If 100% decomposition occurs, reduce the stress level.

"Key to maintaining constant and reliable results with low uncertainty remains strongly attached to validation of method and calibration of analytical instruments."

GLOSSARY OF TERMS RELATED TO HPTLC METHOD VALIDATION

Acceptance criteria: Limits to determine acceptability of obtained analytical results.

Accuracy: The degree of closeness of the determined value to the nominal or known true value under prescribed conditions. This is sometimes termed *trueness*.

Analyte: A specific chemical moiety being measured, which can be intact drug, biomolecule or its derivative, metabolite, and/or degradation product in a analytical matrix.

Analytical run (or batch): A complete set of analytical and study samples with appropriate number of standards and QCs for their validation. Several runs (or batches) may be completed in one day, or one run (or batch) may take several days to complete.

Biological matrix: A discrete material of biological origin that can be sampled and processed in a reproducible manner. Examples are blood, serum, plasma, urine, feces, saliva, sputum, and various discrete tissues.

Bias: It is an effect generated due to the presence of a systematic error in the analysis. It shifts the results to a greater or lower value than expected. It is particularly difficult to identify the bias because unlike random error repeated analysis does not expose bias.

Blank: A sample of an analyte matrix to which no analytes have been added, that is used to assess the specificity of the method.

Calibration standard: Calibration standards are used to construct calibration curves from which the concentrations of analytes in QCs and in unknown study samples are determined.

Chromatogram: It is a relationship profile generated during a separation between the detector response and time.

Chromatography: It is a series of techniques that are used to separate multiple components in a samples based on relative affinities of these components between the mobile phase and the stationary phase.

Derivatization: It indicates a process of chemical modification of a functional group to improve its detection specificity or sensitivity. It may be also brought by alteration in the polarity of the packing material surface.

Drift: It may be considered as the mean slope of the detector baseline during a run in an analysis. It may be attributed to the system leaks, impurity, contamination or temperature changes.

Effective plates: The calculation of the number of effective plates generated by an analyte is determined by correcting for the system void volume t_0:

$$N_{eff} = 5.54\ [(t_r - t_o)/w_{1/2}]^2$$

where $w_{1/2}$ is the peak width at half-height and t_r is the retention time of the analyte.

Elution: When an analyte travels as band along stationary phase with help of mobile phase.

Fronting: The condition in which the elution profile of a peak is non symmetrical before the peak maximum. It is indicative of a elution profile varying from a symmetric Gaussian distribution.

High-performance thin-layer chromatography (HPTLC): It is a technique that requires a stationary phase of small particles (5–15 mm) with approximately 150 mm thickness applied over supporting material. The sample is applied to the stationary phase that is contained in a sealed container known as development chamber. The mobile phase and thus the sample moves using capillary action through the stationary phase on the basis of selective affinity between the stationary phase and mobile phase. Reduced thickness of the stationary phase produce faster separation and the smaller particle diameter helps to produce higher efficiency.

Internal standard: Test compound(s) (e.g. structurally similar analogue, stable labelled compound) added to both calibration standards and samples at known and constant concentration to facilitate quantification of the target analyte(s).

Least squares: It identifies the best fit for the data termed as the least-squares fit (regression) of the line. It minimizes the sum of the squares of the dependent variable value from that of the determined line. The resulting relationship is expressed as y = mx + b, where y is the dependent variable, m is the slope of the line, x is the independent variable and b is the y-intercept value.

Limit of detection (LOD): The lowest concentration of an analyte that the analytical procedure can reliably differentiate from background noise.

Lower limit of quantification (LLOQ): The lowest amount of an analyte in a sample that can be quantitatively determined with suitable precision and accuracy.

Matrix effect: The direct or indirect alteration or interference in response due to the presence of unintended analytes (for analysis) or other interfering substances in the sample.

Method: A comprehensive description of all procedures used in sample analysis.

Precision: The closeness of agreement (*degree of scatter*) between a series of measurements obtained from multiple sampling of the same homogenous sample under the prescribed conditions.

Quality control sample (QC): A spiked sample used to monitor the performance of a analytical method and to assess the integrity and validity of the results of the unknown samples analyzed in an individual batch.

Quantification range: The range of concentration, including upper and lower limit of quantitation that can be reliably and reproducibly quantified with accuracy and precision through the use of a concentration-response relationship.

Recovery: The extraction efficiency of an analytical process, reported as a percentage of the known amount of an analyte carried through the sample extraction and processing steps of the method.

Reproducibility: The precision between two laboratories. It also represents precision of the method under the same operating conditions over a short period of time.

Resolution: It is a measure of efficiency of peak separation (>1.5)., which is required for reliable quantitation

Sample: A generic term including original material, controls, blanks, unknowns, and processed analyte matrix.

Selectivity: The ability of the analytical method to measure and differentiate the analytes in the presence of components that may be expected to be present. These could include metabolites, impurities, degradants, or matrix components.

Stability: The chemical stability of an analyte in a given matrix under specific conditions for given time intervals.

Standard: A material of known identity and purity to compare the unknown. It may be having certificate of analysis.

Standard curve: The relationship between the experimental response value and the analytical concentration (also called a *calibration curve*).

System suitability: Determination of instrument performance (e.g., sensitivity and chromatographic retention) by analysis of a reference standard prior to running the analytical batch.

Tailing factor: It is the distance from upslope of the peak to the down-slope divided by twice the distance from the centre line of the peak to the front slope with all measurements made at 5% of maximum peak height. The accuracy of quantitation decreases with increase in peak tailing.

Unknown: A sample that is the subject of the analysis.

Validation:

Full validation: Establishment of all validation parameters to apply to sample analysis for the analytical method for each analyte.

Partial validation: Modification of validated analytical methods that do not necessarily call for full revalidation.

Cross-validation: Comparison validation parameters of two analytical methods.

EXAMPLE

Typical Example of Development and Validation of HPTLC Method for Drug A

Steps for method development

1. Purpose of the method
2. Identification of the analyte.
3. Procurement of a reference standard of analyte
4. Deriving the analytical profile of analyte.
5. Selecting a suitable solvent for the analyte.
6. Stability of analyte in solution.
7. Designing sample preparation method to obtain the sample for analysis and assessment of the stability of sample solution.
8. Trial run of the TLC to understand the behaviour of analyte with various mobile phase and optimization.
9. Performing HPTLC to finalize the mobile phase, and to determine stability of analyte on plate, before and after development.
10. To study system suitability parameters: Rf, peak purity, identity, resolution, theoretical plate and tailing factor.
11. Steps of validation.
12. Determination of LOD and LOQ.
13. Determination of linearity.
14. Determination of precision.
15. Accuracy determination.
16. Robustness studies.
17. System suitability studies.
18. Forced degradation studies.
19. Filter retention studies.
20. Extraction efficiency studies.

Purpose

Development and validation of HPTLC method for assay of drug A in tablet dosage form containing 5 mg of drug, total weight of tablet is 100 mg.

Desired Analyte: Drug A

Reference standard for Drug A: Drug A was obtained as gratis sample along with certificate of analysis indicating the purity of drug equivalent to 99.5%. This means, that 100.50 mg of the drug is equivalent to 100 mg of 100% pure drug.

Analytical profile of Drug A:

Name of the drug: Drug A
CAS No.: XXXXXXX
Chemical Name: XXXXXXXXXX
Melting range: 90–92°C
Solubility: soluble in methanol, sparingly soluble in Acetonitrile.
Storage: Room temperature.

1. Selecting a suitable solvent for the analyte

Drug A is having good solubility in methanol, so methanol can be selected as solvent for Drug A. Methanol is also selected for extraction of Drug A based on solubility and reported literature.

2. Preparation of stock solution of reference standard Drug A

10.5 mg drug (purity = 99.5%) was dissolved in solvent methanol and the volume was made up to 100 mL to get a stock solution of 100 µg/mL.

3. Preparation of stock solution of sample (sample preparation protocol)

Tablet powder (100 mg) was homogenated and extracted using extraction solvent (methanol, 30 ml) at 30°C for 15 mins. The mixture was centrifuged at 2000 rpm for 15 min at 4°C and the supernatant was collected. The residue was resuspended in extraction solvent and the extraction was repeated three times. The supernatants were pooled and concentrated under vacuum at room temperature and made up to a known volume (100 ml) using solvent (methanol). The extracts were filtered through 0.45 µm filter and sample analysis was performed under the conditions optimized for the reference Drug A.

4. Trial run

Trial run of TLC to understand the behaviour of analyte with various mobile phase and optimizing the mobile phase:

***Chromatographic conditions*:** CAMAG HPTLC system was used to perform the analysis. Instrument details were as follows:

1. Make: CAMAG, Switzerland.
2. Applicator: Camag Linomat 5, semi-automatic application, band application by spray on technique (2–500 mL).
3. Syringe: Hamilton 100 ml HPTLC syringe.
4. Stationary Phase: Silica Gel 60 G F_{254} coated on aluminium sheet. (Merck, Germany)
5. Chamber: Camag twin trough glass chamber (10 cm × 10 cm and 20 cm × 10 cm).

6. Scanner: Camag TLC Scanner 3, scan speed up to 100 mm/s, Spectral range 190–800 nm.
7. Software: WinCATS Planner Chromatography Manager, version 1.3.4.
8. Documentation: Camag Reprostar 3 with digital camera for 254 nm, 366 nm and visible light source.
9. UV Cabinet: Camag UV cabinet with dual wavelength UV lamp 254 & 366 nm.

The analysis was performed at 22° C (±2°C) and 55% (±5%) relative humidity. Two μl of the sample solutions were spotted as bands of 6 mm width, at least 11.6 mm apart, 8 mm from the lower edge and at least 15 mm from left and right edge of the plate by spray-on technique using the auto sampler fitted with a 100 μl Hamilton syringe. The plates were developed to a distance of 85 mm using mobile phase in a CAMAG twin—trough plate development chamber which was lined with a filter paper and presaturated with 30 ml mobile phase in trough opposite to the plate. The developed plates were dried using warm air of hair dryer and scanned at 254 nm. A spectro-densitometer (Scanner 3, CAMAG) equipped with 'win CATS' planar chromatography manager (version 1.3.0) software was used for the densitometry measurements, spectra recording and data processing at 290 nm. Absorption/remission were measured at a scan speed of 20 nm/s.

(***Note:*** One should keep the application volume constant throughout the studies within the range of 1–8 μL/band. In the present example, it was set at 2 μL).

Mobile phase selection and optimization

Trial runs involved different combination of polar and non polar mobile Phases, acid or base may be included, whenever required. Movement of spots in sample, their resolution and tailing was observed with change in mobile phase, while change in R_f of standard (within range of 0.3–0.8) is observed with change in mobile phase.

Mobile phase, toluene: ethyl acetate (70:30, %v/v) produced well resolved bands of drug A in sample matrix at R_f of 0.4. Band could be visualized at 254 nm in UV chamber and at 366 nm in florescence mode (Fig. A), thus no derivatization was required.

U.V spectra (Fig. B) of the standard indicated, λ_{max} of the drug A at 290 nm. Identity and purity of the band of drug A in sample matrix was confirmed by comparing R_f, using overlain UV spectra (Fig. B) of the drug A in sample with that of standard drug A. Spectra of drug A was also compared with spectra of excipients and other impurity. Chromatogram for standard and sample were recorded at 290 nm (Figs. C & D). Resolution, tailing factor and number of theoretical plates were calculated.

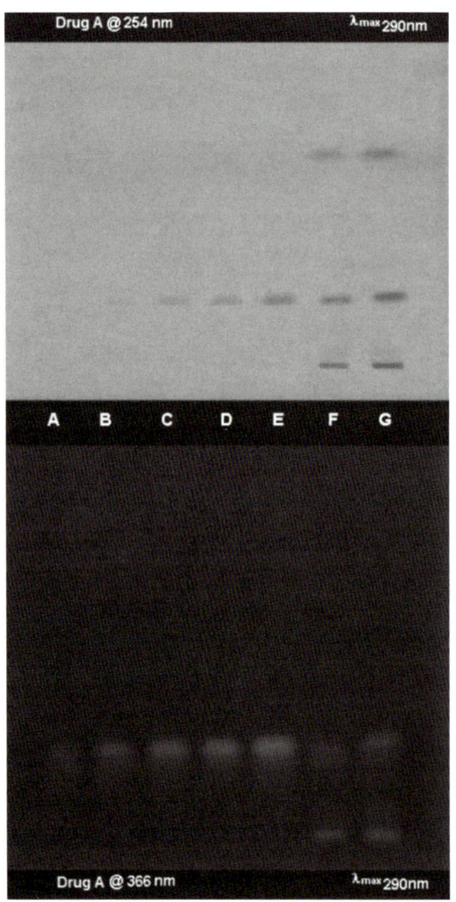

Fig. A: Well-resolved bands of drug A visualized under UV-254. Mixture of toluene – ethyl acetate (7 : 3 v/v) used as MP.

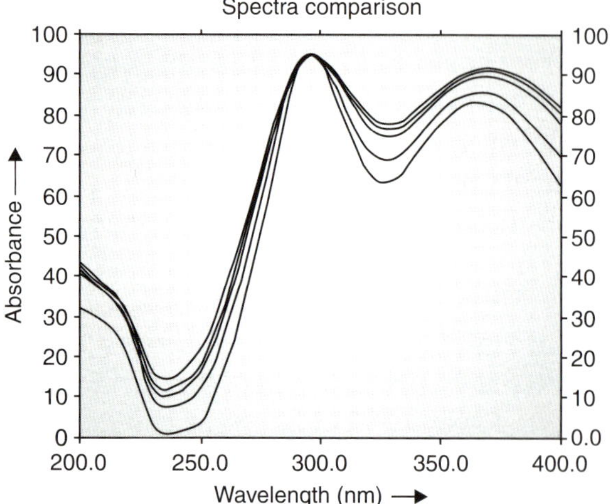

Fig. B: UV-spectra of the drug in sample matrix for identity and puriry of peak (λ_{max} 290 nm).

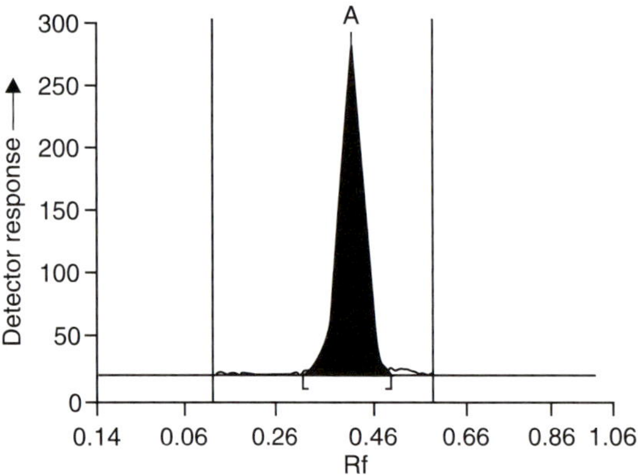

Fig. C: Densitogram of the standard scanned at 290 nm.

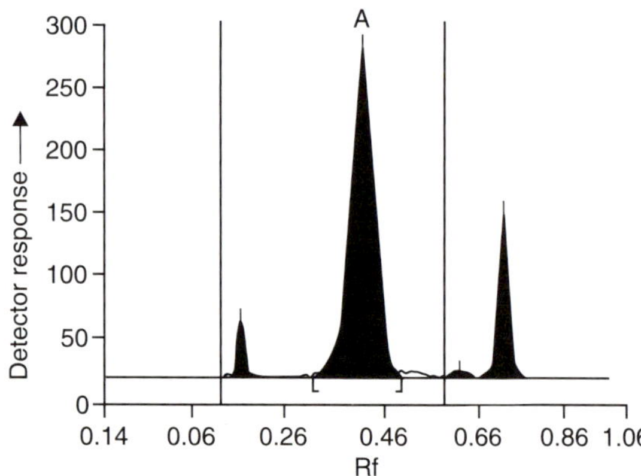

Fig. D: Densitogram of the sample scanned at 290 nm.

Tips on development

- Tailing of band may be due to the higher concentration of bands applied, in such conditions further dilution of standard and sample may be required.
- Concentration of standard stock and sample during trial run can be varied by varying the spotting volume within 1–10 μl.
- Once a well resolved sample band was obtained, final spotting volume should be adjusted such that, the sample band provide a peak area between 700–900.
- The concentration of standard stock solution for system suitability studies should be decided on the basis of concentration of sample band as per label claim. Here, 2 μl band of sample was equivalent to approximate 50 ng/band (assumed based on label claim). Thus, standard stock solution should be such that 2 μl produce a band of 100 ng/band.

Performing HPTLC to finalize the mobile phase and chromatographic conditions

Above procedure was repeated with optimized mobile phase and sample application volume. HPTLC Chromatogram was recorded at 290 nm. Overlain UV spectra of band for standard and band of drug A in sample was obtained for peak purity and identity. R_f, resolution, theoretical plate and tailing factor was noted for the band of Drug A in standard and sample. Photograph were recorded at 254 nm and 366 nm.

Parameter	Drug A
R_f [c]	0.43 ± 0.01
Resolution	1.8
Area (average)	3232 ± 51
Peak purity	0.9991

5. Study of system suitability parameters

Standard stock solution equivalent to 100% test concentration was considered as system suitability standard solution (In present studies 100 μg/ml). It was used for the determination of system suitability test parameters. Duplicate bands of 2 μL of standard solution for system suitability and test sample were applied on plate and subjected to development. Analysis was repeated in triplicate (2 × 3, Total six replicates). Peak area, R_f, resolution, was noted for the band of drug A in standard and sample solution. Further, peak purity was evaluated for sample. The following minimum criteria should be met for the assay standard: Resolution must be equal to or greater than 1.5 and %RSD of peak area should not be more than 2% for at least five replicate standard and sample solutions.

However, the system suitability test parameter ranges were finalized after completion of validation based on the history of values observed. Thus the values were also recorded for each run during validation experimentation.

System suitability Standard Conc. (50 ng/band)	Peak area	R_f
Replicate 1	1662	0.42
Replicate 2	1658	0.44
Replicate 3	1667	0.44
Replicate 4	1654	0.41
Replicate 5	1668	0.42
Replicate 6	1659	0.42

Test sample	Peak area	R_f	Peak purity	Resolution
Replicate 1	1672	0.43	0.9994	1.57
Replicate 2	1652	0.42	0.9993	1.56
Replicate 3	1677	0.42	0.9994	1.62
Replicate 4	1666	0.44	0.9991	1.56
Replicate 5	1674	0.43	0.9992	1.55
Replicate 6	1665	0.43	0.9991	1.58

6. Stability studies for the solution

Both system suitability standard stock solution (100 ml) and working sample solution (100 ml) were prepared freshly as mentioned above. Solutions were divided into four portions. The freshly prepared standard stock solution (S) and working sample solution (T) were analyzed in triplicate, as per the developed method. A part of solution (S1, T1) was store in clear glass container at room temperature (25 ml). A part of solution (S2, T2) was store in clear glass container in refrigerator (25 ml). A part of solution (S3, T3) was store in amber glass container at room temperature (25 ml). The stored sample were analyzed in duplicate, every 8 hrs for first 24 hrs and than at end of 2 days. The HPTLC chromatogram were compared for % recovery with that of freshly prepared standard analyzed initially. The results were as shown in table. No changes in the peaks of the chromatogram was observed, % peak area variation was NMT ± 1.5% for sample, and NMT ±1% for standard.

Band analysed	Time of analysis	Peak area± SD
S	0 hrs	1672
S1	8 hrs	1652
S2	8 hrs	1677

(Contd.)

Band analysed	Time of analysis	Peak area± SD
S3	8 hrs	1666
S1	16 hrs	1674
S2	16 hrs	1665
S3	16 hrs	1672
S1	24 hrs	1652
S2	24 hrs	1677
S3	24 hrs	1662
S1	48 hrs	1658
S2	48 hrs	1659
S3	48 hrs	1662

Band analysed	Time of analysis	Peak area± SD
T	0 hrs	1657
T1	8 hrs	1659
T2	8 hrs	1653
T3	8 hrs	1666
T1	16 hrs	1657
T2	16 hrs	1654
T3	16 hrs	1652
T1	24 hrs	1654
T2	24 hrs	1653
T3	24 hrs	1649
T1	48 hrs	1652
T2	48 hrs	1648
T3	48 hrs	1652

Method validation

7. Specificity and selectivity

Overlain spectra of sample and standard for drug A are not sufficient to prove specificity. Spectrum and chromatogram of blank, placebo , and impurities must be provided to prove Specificity. Further, resolution of analyte from other bands should be provided. Diagonal development can be done to evaluate purity of band.

Parameter	Drug A
R_f [c]	0.43
Resolution	1.62
Area (average)	1656
Peak purity	0.9991

8. Determination of LOD and LOQ using calibration curve parameters

Bands of blank (methanol), 5 ng/band, 10 ng /band, 20 ng/band, 50 ng/band, 100 ng/band drug A on the plate were applied using standard stock solutions. (If response is not obtained, the range of analysis should be increased). Therefore, bands of Blank, 100 ng/band, 150 ng/band, 200 ng/band, 250 ng/band and 300 ng/band were applied. 10 ng/band produces a response. Bracketed concentration range (which will include three times the concentration producing the lowest response) was selected on the basis of above results. Three levels were included in the studies. Here, 20 ng/band, 40 ng/band and 60 ng/band concentrations were selected . Standard stock solution was used to apply bands for each concentration in duplicate on 10 × 10 cm plate. The analysis was repeated in triplicate. Regression parameters based on peak area were as follows:

Parameters		Observation
n	n	18
Slope	b	32.30
Intercept	a	37.94
Residual standard deviation	SD*xy*	38.40
Standard deviation	SD	0.15
Standard deviation	SD*a*	15.26
Regression coefficient	r	0.9998

The LOD value was determined using the equation:

LOD = 3.3S D/b
LOD (SDxy) = 3.92 ng
LOD (SDa) = 1.55 ng
LOD (mean) = 2.73 ng

The correctness of LOD determination was confirmed according to the following equations:

LOD was greater than the minimum concentration of bracketed concentration range studied, and Secondly, the ten times of the calculated LOD was higher than the lowest concentration of solution used in calibration

Thus, the determined LOD value was correct.

LOQ may be calculated on the basis of following relationship:

LOQ = 3 × LOD
The LOQ value was found to be:
LOQ = 8.21 ng

Linearity and working range

Based on the observations during LOD and LOQ studies and working sample concentration as per label claim, a range of concentration was carefully selected (peak area from 500–5000 AU). Trial run with broad range of concentration from 20, 500 ng/band are preformed. Based on observations in trail, Range of 25–150 ng/band was selected for linearity studies. Experimental determination of linearity involved preparation of independent stock solutions of standard in the range of 25–150 ng/band (2 μl). Six replicate analysis were performed, and the results were as follows (Fig. E):

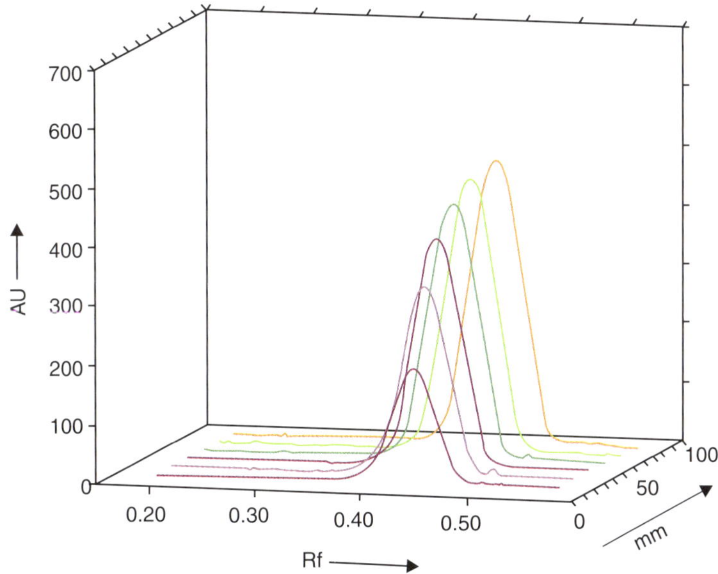

Fig. E: Chromatogram of the standard solutions of drug A (25–150 ng) for linearity profile.

	Peak area					
Concentration (ng/band)	25	50	75	100	150	200
Trial 1	832	1665	2434	3257	4109	4911
Trial 2	821	1684	2453	3134	4078	4863
Trial 3	824	1698	2525	3272	4045	4889
Trial 4	836	1680	2465	3257	4024	4846
Trial 5	838	1668	2459	3216	4087	4921
Trial 6	828	1671	2514	3259	4121	4938
Mean peak area	829	1677	2475	3232	4077	4894
STD DEV	6.70	12.30	36.17	51.84	37.13	35.33
RSD	0.80	0.73	1.46	1.60	0.91	0.72

The linearity was assessed as discussed earlier, some of the observed parameters are as follows (Fig. F):

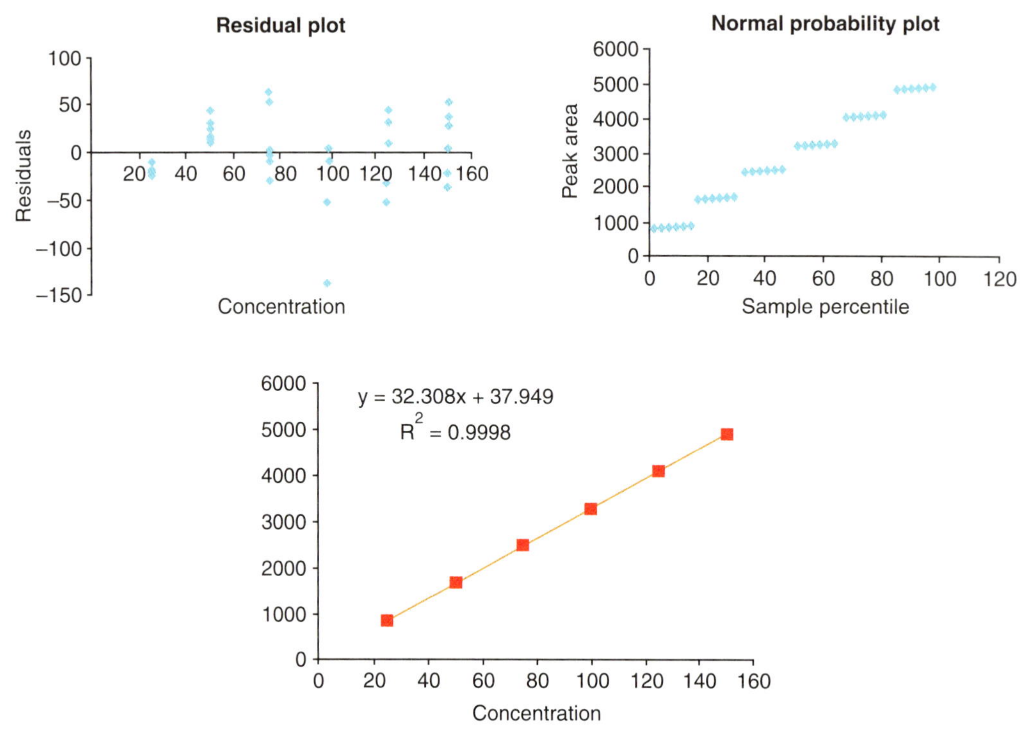

Fig. F

Best-fit values	
Slope	32 ± 0.15
Y-intercept when X = 0.0	36 ± 14
X-intercept when Y = 0.0	–1.1
1/slope	0.031
95% Confidence Intervals	
Slope	32 to 33
Y-intercept when X = 0.0	7.1 to 66
X-intercept when Y = 0.0	–2.4 to 0.14
Goodness of Fit	
r^2	1.0
Sy.x	38
Is slope significantly non-zero?	
F	48000
DFn, DFd	1.0, 34
P value	<0.0001
Deviation from zero?	Significant

Data	
Number of X values	6
Maximum number of Y replicates	6
Total number of values	36
Number of missing values	0
Runs test	
Points above line	4
Points below line	2
Number of runs	4
P value (runs test)	0.8000
Deviation from linearity	Not significant

The calibration plot was found to be linear.

Note: The 100% test concentration in sample to be tested, should be approximately the second level concentration of the working range of at least six levels linearity studies.

Precision

Repeatability Studies (Method Precision)

20 tablets were powdered. Powdered sample equivalent to 80%, 100% and 120% of test concentration (40 mg, 50 mg, 60 mg) was withdrawn in triplicate (total 9 samples withdrawn). Test samples were prepared using the sample preparation protocol. Otherwise, six independent test samples at 100% concentrations may also be analyzed. Each test sample was spotted in duplicate. Data obtained as mean peak area (of duplicate bands) were as follows:

Cons. (ng/band)	40	50	60
Peak Area			
Trial 1	1358	1677	1979
Trial 2	1378	1634	1922
Trial 3	1362	1681	1951
Parameters			
Mean	1366	1664	1950.667
S.D.	10.58	26.05	28.50
R.S.D.	0.77	1.56	1.46

Intermediate precision

It requires determination of three concentrations levels, six determinations each, on three different days (e.g. 80%, 100% and 120% of target concentration with six replicates each = 18 samples for three times = 54 samples). 20 tablets were powdered. Powdered sample equivalent to 80%, 100% and 120% of test concentration (40 mg, 50 mg, 60 mg) was withdrawn. Test samples were prepared using the sample preparation protocol. Six replicate analysis were performed. The same procedure was repeated on three different days. RSD values were less than 2%.

Cons.	Cons. (40 ng/band)			Cons. (50 ng/band)			Cons. (60 ng/band)		
Days	Day 1	Day 2	Day 3	Day 1	Day 2	Day 3	Day 1	Day 2	Day 3
Peak Area	1389	1387	1369	1667	1663	1672	1966	1963	1968
	1377	1381	1359	1665	1658	1684	1970	1959	1965
	1381	1379	1393	1682	1671	1671	1973	1953	1958
	1380	1382	1380	1666	1683	1674	1979	1970	1959
	1384	1385	1376	1672	1662	1668	1965	1969	1957
	1379	1381	1385	1673	1667	1664	1966	1960	1969
Mean		1380	1670	1969					
SD		7.50	7.27	6.46					
RSD		0.54	0.43	0.32					

Reproducibility

Reproducibility is determined when a method is transferred from one laboratory to other laboratory, thus it does not form part of single laboratory validation.

Instrument precision studies

Standard stock solution of drug used for system suitability determination was applied on the plate in triplicate and developed. Each developed band was scanned nine times. Dataset obtained was as follows:

Concentration	Mean Peak area ± RSD, (n = 18)
50 ng/band	1669 ± 0.2

Accuracy

Accuracy should be determined, after determination of precision, linearity, specificity, LOD, and LOQ. 20 tablets were powdered. Powdered sample equivalent to 100% of test concentration was withdrawn (total 9 samples of 50 mg). Three test samples were spiked with standard equivalent to 50% of the test concentration (1.25 mg). Spiking of standard was done in powdered form (dry API) to the test samples. Similar procedure was repeated for spiking with standard equivalent to 100% (2.5 mg) and 150% (5 mg) of the test concentration. Test samples were subjected to sample preparation protocol. Nine samples were applied in triplicate and analyzed. The data obtained indicate accuracy of the method.

Cons. of Sample (ng/band)	Cons. of Std. Spiked (ng/band)	Mean Peak Area ± SD	Cons. Recovered (ng/band)	% Recovery
49.5	0	1645 ± 0.32	49.74158	100.488
49.5	25	2474 ± 0.54	75.40086	101.2092
49.5	50	3206 ± 0.23	98.05779	98.55054
49.5	75	4104 ± 0.76	125.8528	101.0866
49.5	0	1645 ± 0.22	49.74158	100.488
49.5	25	2474 ± 0.43	75.40086	101.2092

Robustness

Studies were performed using the standard solution as discussed in system suitability studies.

Variation of mobile phase composition was kept ±5% and ±10% for major components and, ±15% and ±10% for minor components. Other parameters were varied by ±10%. Analysis was performed in triplicate. Method was found to be robust as % RSD were less than 2%. Results obtained were as follows:

Parameters Variation	Mcan Peak Area± RSD	R_f	Resolution	Peak Purity
Toluene: ethyl acetate, (73.5:30, v/v)	3248 ± 1.34	0.42	1.51	0.9991
Toluene: ethyl acetate, (66.5:30, v/v)	3211 ± 0.89	0.43	1.61	0.9991
Toluene: ethyl acetate, (63:30, v/v)	3274 ± 0.67	0.41	1.43	0.9996
Toluene: ethyl acetate, (70:27, v/v)	3255 ± 1.44	0.42	1.49	0.9995
Toluene: ethyl acetate, (70:33, v/v)	3268 ± 1.43	0.43	1.51	0.9991
Toluene: ethyl acetate, (70:24, v/v)	3231 ± 0.43	0.41	1.61	0.9993
Toluene: ethyl acetate, (70:36, v/v)	3259 ± 0.56	0.44	1.54	0.9992
Temperature, 25°C	3288 ± 0.76	0.42	1.65	0.9999
Temperature, 30°C	3241 ± 0.34	0.41	1.73	0.9998
Temperature, 20°C	3189 ± 0.51	0.43	1.81	0.9993
Chamber size (10 × 20 cm)	3131 ± 0.32	0.43	1.76	0.9993
Relative Humidity, 70%	3174 ± 1.01	0.44	1.55	0.9995
Relative Humidity, 80%	3229 ± 0.78	0.41	1.88	0.9997
Developing Distance, 80 mm	3248 ± 0.43	0.43	1.76	0.9992
Developing Distance, 90 mm	3189 ± 0.66	0.41	1.43	0.9991
Chamber Saturation Time, 18 min	3222 ± 1.33	0.42	1.77	0.9998
Chamber Saturation Time, 22 min	3272 ± 1.47	0.44	1.69	0.9991

Extraction efficiency test

The test sample was spiked with standard at 100% test concentration. Extraction time was varied from 10 mins to 25 mins. The analysis was done in duplicate, and % recoveries were as follows. The studies confirmed that the extraction time of 15 minutes was sufficient to ensure complete extraction.

Extraction time (Mins)	Peak area*	% Recoveries
15	3254	100.68
20	3262	100.92
25	3259	100.83
10	3144	97.27

* n = 2, Mean Peak Area

Filter retention studies

The test sample was subjected extraction step. Extracted solution was spiked with standard at 100% test concentration. The percentage recoveries and chromatograms for bands of unfiltered, single filtered and double filtered solution were compared. Analysis was done in duplicate. The data obtained were as follows:

Sample analyzed	Peak area.*	R_f and system suitability parameters	% Recoveries
Unfiltered Solution	3289	Within range	101.76
Solution after first Filtration	3257	Within range	100.77
Solution after Second Filtration	3198	Within range	98.94

Validated method needs monitoring for its analytical performance by control samples through its entire life-cycle.

Bibliography

Anonymous, Camag bibliography services, Accessed dated 28.03.2012, (http://www.camag.com/v/literature/parameter_hints.html)

Dejaegher, Y. Vander Heyden, J. Chromatogr. A 1158 (2007) 138.

B. Dejaegher, Y. Vander Heyden, LC–GC Europe (July) (2006) 418.

B. Renger, H. Jehle, M. Fischer, W. Funk, J. Planar Chromatogr. 8 (1995) 269.

B. Renger, H. Jehle, M. Fischer, W. Funk, Pharm. Ind. 56 (1994) 993.

B. Renger, J. Chromatogr. B 745 (2000) 167.

CDER reviewer guidance: Validation of chromatographic methods, US Food and Drug Administration, Centre for Drugs and Biologics, Department of Health and Human Services. http://www.fda.gov/downloads/Drugs/GuidanceCompliance Regulatory Information/ Guidances /UCM134409.pdf, November 1994.

D.M. Blisner, Validating Chromatographic Methods -A practical guide, John Wiley & Sons, Inc., Hoboken, New Jersey, 2006.

D.L. Massart, B.G.M. Vandeginste, S.N. Deming, Y. Michotte, L. Kaufman,

Chemo-metrics: A Textbook, Elsevier, Amsterdam, 1988.

Draft guidance analytical procedures and method validation. US Food and Drug Administration, Centre for Drugs and Biologics, Department of Health and Human Services. http://www.fda.gov/downloads/Drugs/GuidanceComplianceRegulatory Information/Guidances/ucm122858.pdf, August 2000.

Reich, A. DeBarr, J. AOAC Int. 91 (2009) 13.

EN ISO/IEC 17025, General Requirements for the Competence of Testing and Calibration Laboratories, EN Management Centre, Brussels, 2005.

EURACHEM: the fitness for purposes of analytical methods. A laboratory guide to method validation and related topics. http://www.eurachem. org/guides/pdf/valid.pdf, 1998.

G. Indrayanto, M. Yuwono, in: J. Cazes (Ed.), Encyclopedia of Chromatography, 2nd ed., Francis & Taylor LLC, 2005, p. 1759.

G. Szepesi, J. Planar Chromatogr. 6 (1993) 187.

G.A. Shabir, W.J. Lough, A.A. Shafique, T.K. Bradshaw, J. Liq. Chromatogr. Related Technol. 30 (2007) 311.

Guide to the Expression of Uncertainty in Measurement, ISO, Geneva, 1993. ISBN 92-67-10188-9 (Reprinted 1995).

ICH harmonised tripartite guideline: impurities in new drug substances, Q3A (R1), Geneva.

http://www.ich.org/LOB/media/MEDIA422.pdf, 2006 (Parent Guideline dated 16 September 1992).

J. Ermer, in: J. Ermer, J.H.McB. Miller (Eds.), Method Validation in Pharmaceutical Analysis. A Guide to Best Practice, Wiley-VCH Verlag GmbH & Co, KGaA, Weinheim, 2005.

J.W. Einax, M. Reichenbächer, Anal. Bioanal. Chem. 384 (2006) 14.

K. Ferenczi-Fodor, B. Renger, Z. Végh, J. Planar Chromatogr. 23 (2010) 173.

K. Ferenczi-Fodor, Z. Végh, A. Nagy-Turák, B. Renger, M. Zeller, J. AOAC Int. 84 (2001) 1265.

K. Ferenczi-Fodor, Z. Végh, B. Renger, J. Chromatogr. A 1218 (2011) 2722.

K. Ferenczi-Fodor, Z. Végh, Zs. Pap-Sziklay, J. Planar Chromatogr. 6 (1993) 198.

Monograph 2.02.27, Thin-Layer Chromatography, European Pharmacopoeia (suppl. 6.8), 6th ed., European Pharmacopoeia Commission, Strasbourg, France, 2010, p. 43.

Nagy-Turák, Z. Végh, K. Ferenczi-Fodor, J. Planar Chromatogr. 8 (1995) 188.

P Konieczka, J Namie´snik, Quality Assurance and Quality Control in the Analytical Chemical Laboratory, A Practical Approach (Analytical chemistry series), CRC press, 2009.

S. Ebel, Analytical Chemistry Progress, Springer, Berlin-Heidelberg, 1984, p. 71.

S.L.R. Ellison, M. Rösslein, A. Williams (Eds.), Eurachem/CITAC Guide: Quantifying Uncertainty in Analytical Measurement, 2nd ed., 2000. http://www.eurachem.org/guides/pdf/QUAM2000-1.pdf.

Shabir, J. Chromatogr. A 987 (2003) 57.

United States Pharmacopeia 30, General Chapter <1225>, Validation of Compendial Methods, US Pharmacopoeial Convention, Rockville, MD, 2007, p. 680.

United States Pharmacopeia 32, General Chapter <466>, Ordinary Impurities, US Pharmacopoeial Convention, Rockville, MD, 2009, p. 162.

V.R. Meyer, J. Chromatogr. A 1158 (2007) 15.

W. Funk, V. Damman, C. Vonderheid, G. Oehlmann, Statistische Methoden in der Wasseranalytik, VCH, Weinheim, 1985.

W. Funk, V. Damman, G. Donnevert, Qualitätssicherung in der Analytischen Chemie, VCH, Weinheim, 1992.

Validation requirements are not universal, have to be tailored to meet particular application's needs and characteristics.

W. Funk, V. Damman, G. Donnevert, Quality Assurance in Analytical Chemistry, VCH, Weinheim, 1995.

ICH harmonised tripartite guideline: validation of analytical procedures: text and methodology, Q2 (R1), Geneva. http://www.ich.org LOB/media/MEDIA417.pdf, 2005 (Parent Guideline dated 27 October 1994, Complementary Guideline on Methodology dated 6 November 1996 incorporated in November 2005).

Harmonized guidelines for single laboratory Validation of methods of analysis (IUPAC technical report), international union of pure and applied chemistry, *pure appl. Chem.*, Vol. 74, No. 5, pp. 835–855, 2002.

Acceptance criteria for different validation parameters should be set in advance before starting the experiment. This will provide guidance to the analyst on the range of acceptability of validation results, otherwise the analyst shall have the tendency to vary experimental conditions.

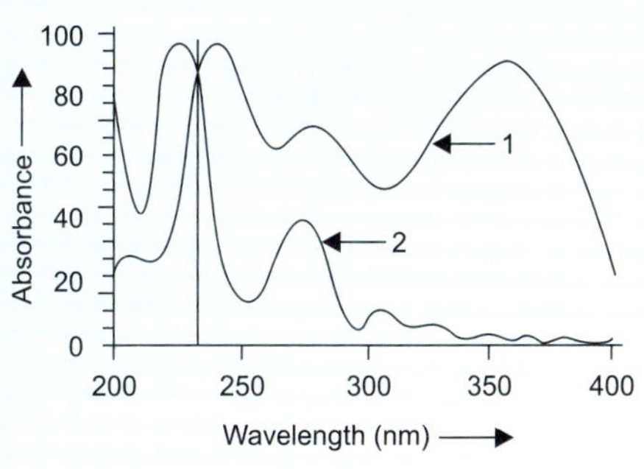

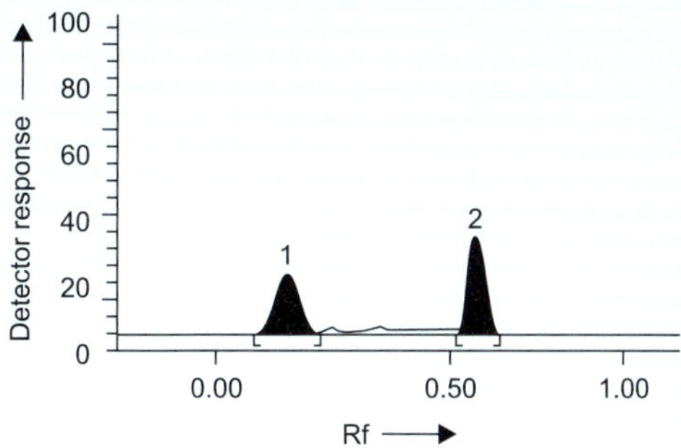

3

Cardiovascular System

- Beta-blockers
- Antiarrhythmic drugs
- Anti-anginals
- Anti-hypertensives
- Diuretics

Protocols and Densitograms from 1 to 120

Knowledge comes from taking things apart, wisdom from putting things together.

HPTLC : High Performance Thin Layer Chromatography
HPTLC DENSITOGRAM

No. 1

NH
Cl, N, CONHCNH$_2$
HCl
H_2N, N, NH_2

Amiloride hydrochloride

COOH
NH — CH_2, O
NH_2SO_2
Cl

Frusemide

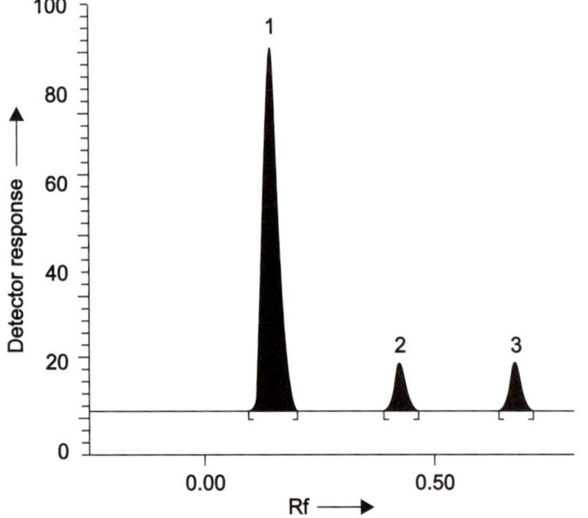

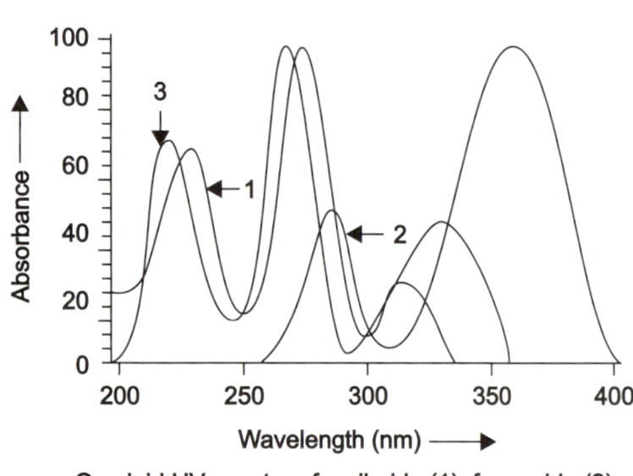

Overlaid UV-spectra of amiloride (1), frusemide (2) and hydrochlorothiazide (3) for selection of suitable wavelength for densitometric scanning

Typical densitogram of the sample containing amiloride hydrochloride and frusemide. For detailed experimental and chromatographic conditions, refer to Protocol No.1. Peaks identification: 1. Frusemide; 2. Amiloride; 3. Hydrochlorothiazide (IS).

PROTOCOL FOR HPTLC ANALYSIS OF PHARMACEUTICAL FORMULATION

Protocol No. 1

Formulation: Amiloride hydrochloride, Frusemide

Classification: Cardiovascular System **Dosage form:** Tablets

Standard preparation: 25 mg of amiloride hydrochloride and 100 mg of frusemide dissolved in methanol to produce 50 ml. 2 ml of the resulting solution was further diluted with methanol to 100 ml for analysis.

Sample preparation: Powdered sample equivalent to 25 mg of amiloride suspended in 10 ml of water, sonicated for 10 min, diluted to 50 ml with methanol, filtered and 2 ml of the filtrate diluted to 100 ml with methanol for application.

Chromatographic equipments:

Sample applicator: Camag Linomat–IV

Development chamber: Camag twin-trough glass chamber, 10 × 10 cm

Densitometric scanner: Camag TLC Scanner–II

Chromatographic conditions:

1. Stationary phase: Silica gel $60F_{254}$ pre-coated HPTLC plates, 10 × 10 cm (200 μm) – Merck
2. Mobile phase (MP): Ethyl acetate–methanol–25% ammonia (7.5 : 1 : 0.8 v/v)
3. Standard/Sample application:

   Band length: 50 mm Volume applied: 3 μl Spacing: 50 mm
4. Chamber saturation: 30 min (MP)
5. RH (%): 55 ± 5
6. Temperature °C: 25 ± 2
7. Separation technique: Ascending
8. Quantity of mobile phase: 9 ml
9. Migration distance: 70 mm
10. Migration time: 30 min

Densitometric evaluation:

Wavelength: UV–285 nm Scanning mode: Reflectance/Absorbance

HRF: Frusemide—14; Amiloride hydrochloride—43; Hydrochlorothiazide (IS)—67

Linearity (ng/band): Amiloride HCl—20–120; Frusemide—240–320

Recovery (%): 99.37–100.10 for both the compounds.

References: A.P. Argekar, S.V. Raj and S.U. Kapadia, *Indian Drugs*, **32(4)**, 166–171, 1995.

Comments: The method validated for accuracy, precision, linearity, LOD and LOQ.

HPTLC : High Performance Thin Layer Chromatography
HPTLC Densitogram

No. 2

Amiloride hydrochloride

Frusemide

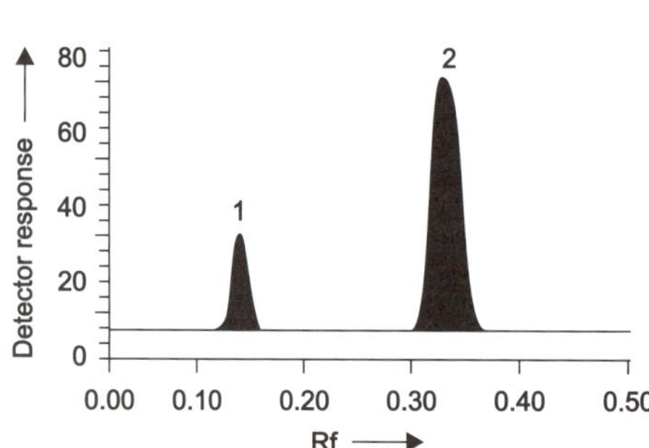

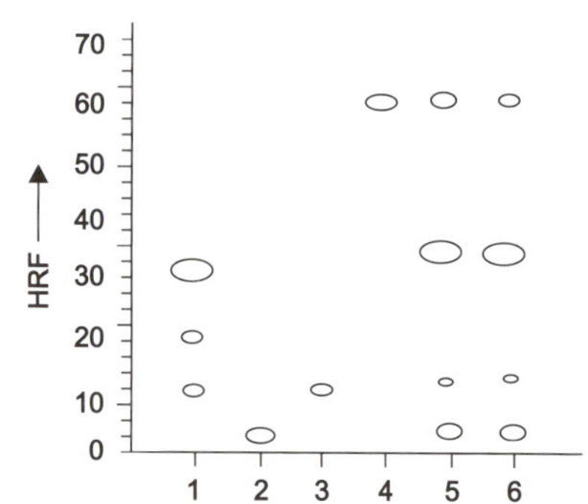

Thin layer chromatogram of (1) 1% Frusemide; (2) 0.14% Amiloride HCl; (3) 0.05% 4-Chloro-5-sulphamoyl-anthranilic acid (free amine); (4) 0.000625% 3,5-Diamino-6-chloropyrazine-2-carboxylate; (5 and 6) commercial samples (tablets) under analysis.

Typical densitogram of the standard containing amiloride hydrochloride and frusemide. For detailed experimental and chromatographic conditions, refer to Protocol No. 2. Peaks identification: 1. Amiloride HCl; 2. Frusemide.

PROTOCOL FOR HPTLC ANALYSIS OF PHARMACEUTICAL FORMULATION

Protocol No. 2

Formulation: Amiloride hydrochloride, Frusemide, Impurities

Classification: Cardiovascular System **Dosage form:** Tablets

Standard preparation: Prepare 1% solution of frusemide, 0.14% solution of amiloride hydrochloride, 0.005% solution of free amine and 0.000625% solution of carboxylate – all in methanol. Apply 10 µl of each solution for determination of impurities.

Sample preparation: Powdered sample equivalent to 5 mg of amiloride hydrochloride suspended in 40 ml of methanol, sonicate for 5 min, dilute to 50 ml, filter and dilute 1 ml to 10 ml with methanol to use for assay.

Chromatographic equipments:

Sample applicator: Camag Linomat–IV

Development chamber: Camag twin-trough glass chamber, 10 × 10 cm

Densitometric scanner: Camag TLC Scanner–II

Chromatographic conditions:

1. Stationary phase: Silica gel 60F_{254} pre-coated HPTLC plates, 10 × 10 cm (200 µm) – Merck
2. Mobile phase (MP): Chloroform–methanol–glacial acetic acid (8.5 : 1.5 : 0.05 v/v) or (9 : 0.5 : 0.5 v/v) or (45 : 2.5 : 2.5 v/v)
3. Standard/Sample application:
   Band length: 80 mm Volume applied: 10 µl Spacing: 100 mm
4. Chamber saturation: —
5. RH (%): —
6. Temperature °C: —
7. Separation technique: Ascending
8. Quantity of mobile phase: 50 ml
9. Migration distance: 120 mm
10. Migration time: 60 min

Densitometric evaluation:

Wavelength: UV–254 nm, Vis-550 nm Scanning mode: Reflectance/Absorbance

HRF: Amiloride HCl—15; Frusemide—35

Linearity (ng/band): Amiloride HCl—10–100; Frusemide—20–200

Recovery (%): 96.85–103.0 for both the compounds

References: —

Comments:

- The above chromatographic conditions are suitable for determination of impurities (4-chloro-5-sulphamoyl-anthranilic acid – free amine) and 3,5-diamino-6-chloropyrazine-2-carboxylate) in the finished formulation.
- The chromatogram was first scanned at 254 nm, then the plate dipped in 0.3% $NaNO_2$ solution (IS), dried, dipped in NED solution, dried in oven (60°C) and scanned at 550 nm.

HPTLC : High Performance Thin Layer Chromatography
HPTLC Densitogram

No. 3

Atenolol

Nifedipine

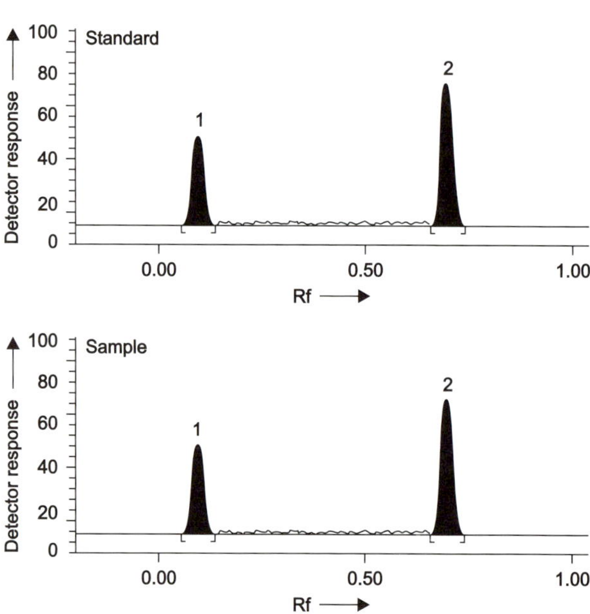

Typical densitogram of the sample and standard containing atenolol and nifedipine. For detailed experimental and chromatographic conditions, refer to Protocol No. 3. Peaks identification: 1. Atenolol; 2. Nifedipine.

PROTOCOL FOR HPTLC ANALYSIS OF PHARMACEUTICAL FORMULATION

Protocol No. 3

Formulation: Atenolol, Nifedipine

Classification: Cardiovascular System **Dosage form:** Tablets

Standard preparation: Prepare 250 μg/ml solution of atenolol and 100 μg/ml solution of nifedipine, both in methanol and use for chromatographic analysis.

Sample preparation: Powdered sample equivalent to 25 mg of atenolol or 10 mg of nifedipine suspended in 70 ml of methanol, sonicated, diluted to 100 ml, filtered and used for analysis.

Chromatographic equipments:

Sample applicator: Camag Linomat–IV

Development chamber: Camag twin-trough glass chamber, 10 × 10 cm

Densitometric scanner: Camag TLC Scanner–II

Chromatographic conditions:

1. Stationary phase: Silica gel $60F_{254}$ pre-coated HPTLC plates, 10 × 10 cm (200 μm) – Merck
2. Mobile phase (MP): Toluene–2-propranolol–25% ammonia (7.5 : 2.5 : 0.1 v/v)
3. Standard/Sample application:
   Band length: 5 mm Volume applied: 5 μl Spacing: 22 ± 2
4. Chamber saturation: 20 min (MP)
5. RH (%): 55 ± 5
6. Temperature °C: 22 ± 2
7. Separation technique: Ascending
8. Quantity of mobile phase: 10 ml
9. Migration distance: 50 mm
10. Migration time: 23 min

Densitometric evaluation:

Wavelength: UV–235 nm Scanning mode: Reflectance/Absorbance

HRF: Atenolol—10; Nifedipine—70

Linearity (μg/band): Atenolol—10–50; Nifedipine—5–50

Recovery (%): 98.07–101.70 for both the compounds

References: —

Comments:

- The method was optimized and analytical work carried out at **Anchrom's HPTLC Application Laboratory**, Mumbai, India.
- All the experimental work was carried out in dark using actinic glass.
- The method was suitable for impurity profile and content uniformity.

HPTLC : High Performance Thin Layer Chromatography
HPTLC Densitogram

No. 4

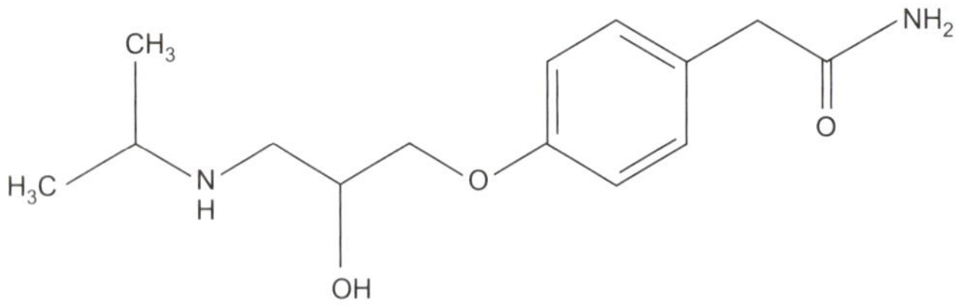

Atenolol

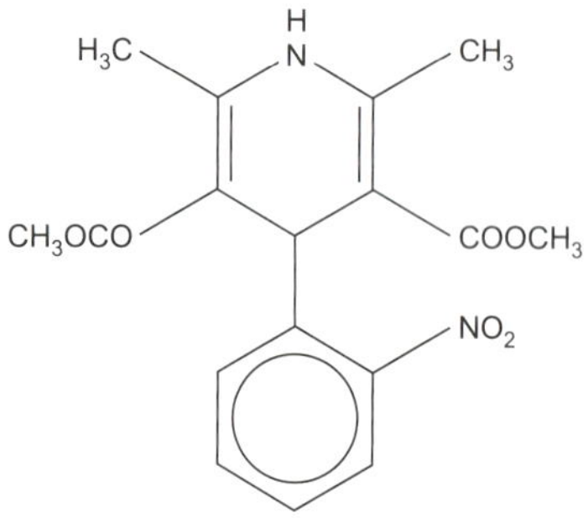

Nifedipine

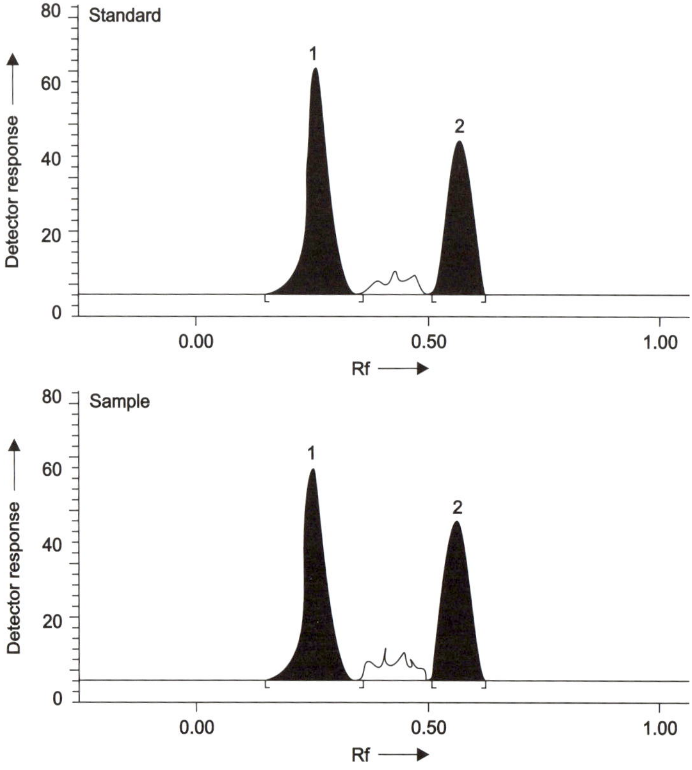

Typical densitogram of the sample and standard containing atenolol and nifedipine. For detailed experimental and chromatographic conditions, refer to Protocol No. 4. Peaks identification: 1. Nifedipine; 2. Atenolol.

PROTOCOL FOR HPTLC ANALYSIS OF PHARMACEUTICAL FORMULATION

Protocol No. 4

Formulation: Atenolol, Nifedipine

Classification: Cardiovascular System **Dosage form:** Tablets

Standard preparation: Dissolve 25 mg of atenolol and 10 mg of nifedipine in 100 ml of methanol and use for chromatographic analysis.

Sample preparation: Weigh powdered sample equivalent to 25 mg of atenolol or 10 mg of nifedipine, suspend in 70 ml of methanol, sonicate for 10 min, dilute to 100 ml, filter.

Chromatographic equipments:

Sample applicator: Camag Linomat–IV
Development chamber: Camag twin-trough glass chamber, 10 × 10 cm
Densitometric scanner: Camag TLC Scanner–II

Chromatographic conditions:

1. Stationary phase: Silica gel 60 RP–18F_{254s} pre-coated HPTLC plates, 10 × 10 cm (200 μm) – Merck
2. Mobile phase (MP): 0.5 M sodium chloride–methanol–acetonitrile–glacial acetic acid (5 : 2 : 3 : 0.1 v/v)
3. Standard/Sample application:
   Band length: 5 mm Volume applied: 5 μl Spacing: 10 mm
4. Chamber saturation: 40 min (MP)
5. RH (%): 55 ± 5
6. Temperature °C: 22 ± 2
7. Separation technique: Ascending
8. Quantity of mobile phase: 10 ml
9. Migration distance: 50 mm
10. Migration time: 25 min

Densitometric evaluation:

Wavelength: UV–235 nm Scanning mode: Reflectance/Absorbance
HRF: Nifedipine—28; Atenolol—68
Linearity (μg/band): Atenolol—10–50; Nifedipine—5–50
Recovery (%): 100.90–101.50 for both the compounds

References: —

Comments:

- The method was optimized and analytical work carried out at **Anchrom's HPTLC Application Laboratory**, Mumbai, India.
- All the experimental work carried out in dark and in actinic glass apparatus.
- The method suitable for impurity profile and content uniformity.
- The RP-chromatography resulted in reversal of retention order as compared to NP-chromatography.
- The RP-chromatography carried out in laboratory-made RP-HPTLC plates (impregnated with 5% silicon oil in pet. ether).

HPTLC : High Performance Thin Layer Chromatography
HPTLC Densitogram

No. 5

Atenolol

Nifedipine

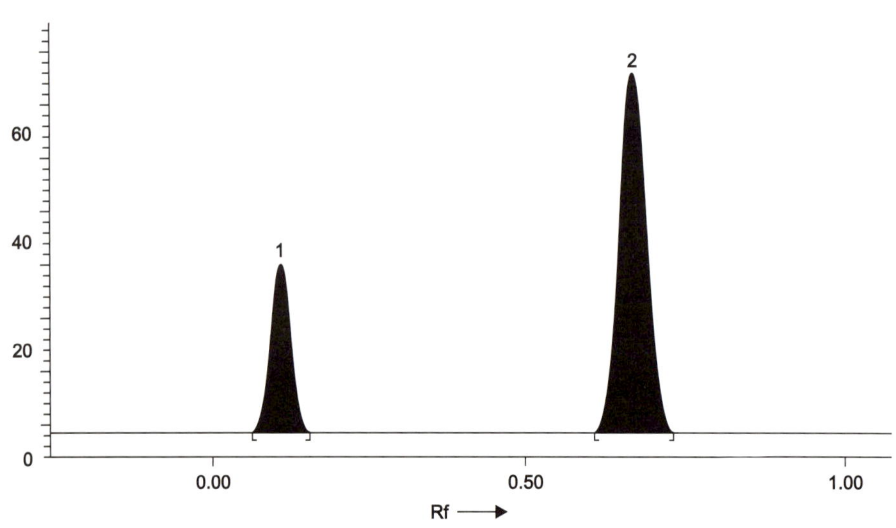

Typical densitogram of the sample containing atenolol and nifedipine. For detailed experimental and chromatographic conditions, refer to Protocol No. 5. Peaks identification: 1. Atenolol; 2. Nifedipine.

PROTOCOL FOR HPTLC ANALYSIS OF PHARMACEUTICAL FORMULATION

Protocol No. 5

Formulation: Atenolol, Nifedipine

Classification: Cardiovascular System **Dosage form:** Tablets

Standard preparation: Prepare 1 mg/ml solution of each drug in methanol separately. Solution of nifedipine was further diluted to get 400 μg/ml concentration. Apply 3–2 μl of each solution for linearity studies.

Sample preparation: Powdered sample equivalent to 50 mg of atenolol suspended in 25 ml of methanol, shaken for 10 min, diluted to 50 ml with methanol and filtered. The filtrate was suitably diluted and used for chromatographic evaluation.

Chromatographic equipments:

Sample applicator: Camag Linomat–IV

Development chamber: Camag twin-trough glass chamber, 10 × 10 cm

Densitometric scanner: Camag TLC Scanner–III

Chromatographic conditions:

1. Stationary phase: Silica gel 60F_{254} pre-coated HPTLC plates, 10 × 10 cm (200 μm) – Merck
2. Mobile phase (MP): Cyclohexane–methanol–ethyl acetate–25% ammonia (5 : 15 : 3 : 0.5 v/v)
3. Standard/Sample application:
   Band length: 6 mm Volume applied: 3–21 μl Spacing: 10 mm
4. Chamber saturation: 15 min (MP)
5. RH (%): 55 ± 5
6. Temperature °C: 25 ± 5
7. Separation technique: Ascending
8. Quantity of mobile phase: 10 ml
9. Migration distance: 70 mm
10. Migration time: 18 min

Densitometric evaluation:

Wavelength: UV–230 nm Scanning mode: Reflectance/Absorbance

HRF: Atenolol—07; Nifedipine—69

Linearity (μg/band): Atenolol—3–21; Nifedipine—1.2–8.4

Recovery (%): 99.98–100.44 for both the drugs

References: Madhuri Ramteke, Avinash Kasture and Narendra Dighade, *Asian J. Chem.*, **22(8)**, 5951–5955, 2010.

Comments: The method validated for accuracy, precision, linearity, LOD, LOQ, specificity, robustness and ruggedness.

HPTLC : High Performance Thin Layer Chromatography
HPTLC Densitogram

No. 6

Nitrendipine

Atenolol

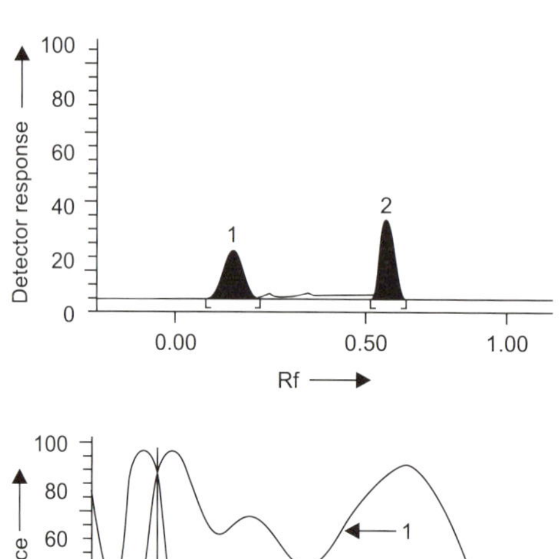

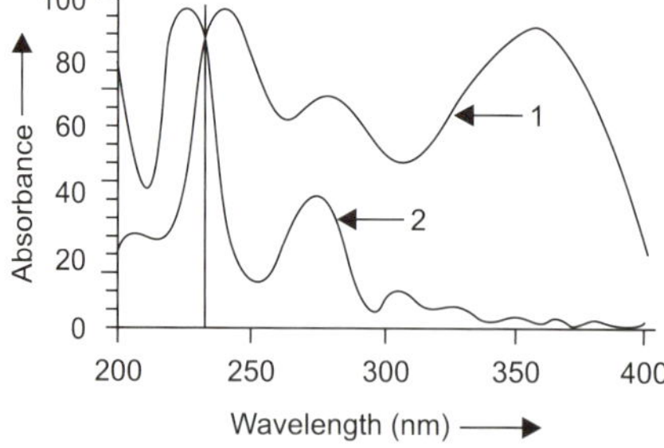

In-situ UV-spectra of atenolol (1) and nitrendipine (2) for selection of suitable wavelength for densitometric scanning

Typical densitogram of the standard containing atenolol and nitrendipine. For detailed experimental and chromatographic conditions, refer to Protocol No. 6. Peaks identification: 1. Atenolol; 2. Nitrendipine.

PROTOCOL FOR HPTLC ANALYSIS OF PHARMACEUTICAL FORMULATION

Protocol No. 6

Formulation: **Atenolol, Nitrendipine**

Classification: Cardiovascular System **Dosage form:** Tablets

Standard preparation: Prepare 5 mg/ml solution of atenolol and 2 mg/ml solution of nitrendipine both in methanol. Mix 6 ml of each solution and dilute to 25 ml with methanol for analysis.

Sample preparation: Powdered sample equivalent to 60 mg of ATN and 20 mg of NIT suspended in 20 ml of methanol, sonicated for 10 min, dilute to 25 ml with methanol, filter through Whatman No. 42 filter paper and dilute 5 ml of filtrate to 10 ml with methanol for assay.

Chromatographic equipments:

Sample applicator: Camag Linomat–IV

Development chamber: Camag twin-trough glass chamber, 10 × 10 cm

Densitometric scanner: Camag TLC Scanner–II

Chromatographic conditions:

1. Stationary phase: Silica gel $60F_{254}$ pre-coated HPTLC plates, 10 × 10 cm (200 μm) – Merck
2. Mobile phase (MP): Chloroform–methanol–toluene–25% ammonia (2 : 2.5 : 5.5 : 0.1 v/v)
3. Standard/Sample application:
   Band length: 6 mm Volume applied: 5 μl Spacing: 10 mm
4. Chamber saturation: —
5. RH (%): 55 ± 5
6. Temperature °C: 22 ± 2
7. Separation technique: Ascending
8. Quantity of mobile phase: 10 ml
9. Migration distance: 50 mm
10. Migration time: 30 min

Densitometric evaluation:

Wavelength: UV–233 nm Scanning mode: Reflectance/Absorbance

HRF: Atenolol—17; Nitrendipine—54

Linearity (μg/band): Atenolol—4–10; Nitrendipine—1.6–4

Recovery (%): Atenolol–100.5–101.90; Nitrendipine—96.93–99.34

References: A.P. Argekar and J.G. Sawant, *J. Liq. Chromatogr. and Rel. Technol.*, **22(10)**, 1571–1578, 1999.

Comments: The method validated for accuracy, precision, linearity, LOD and LOQ.

HPTLC : High Performance Thin Layer Chromatography
HPTLC Densitogram

No. 7

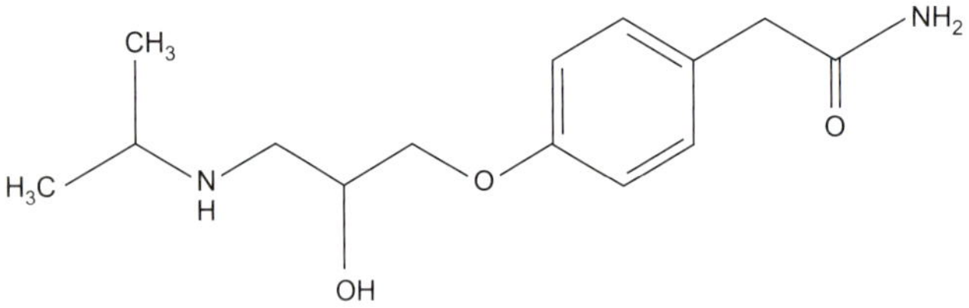

Atenolol

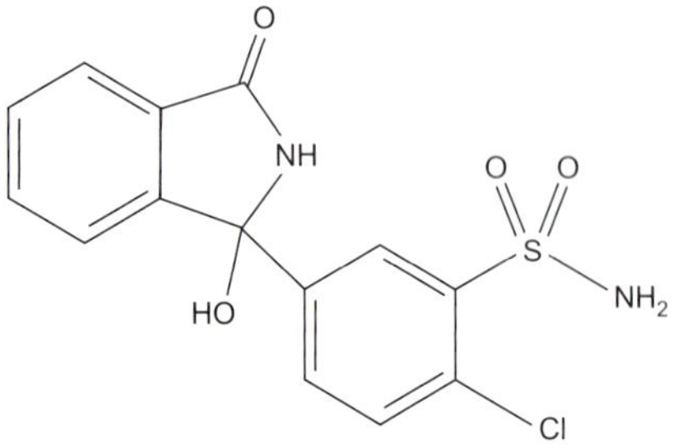

Chlorthalidone

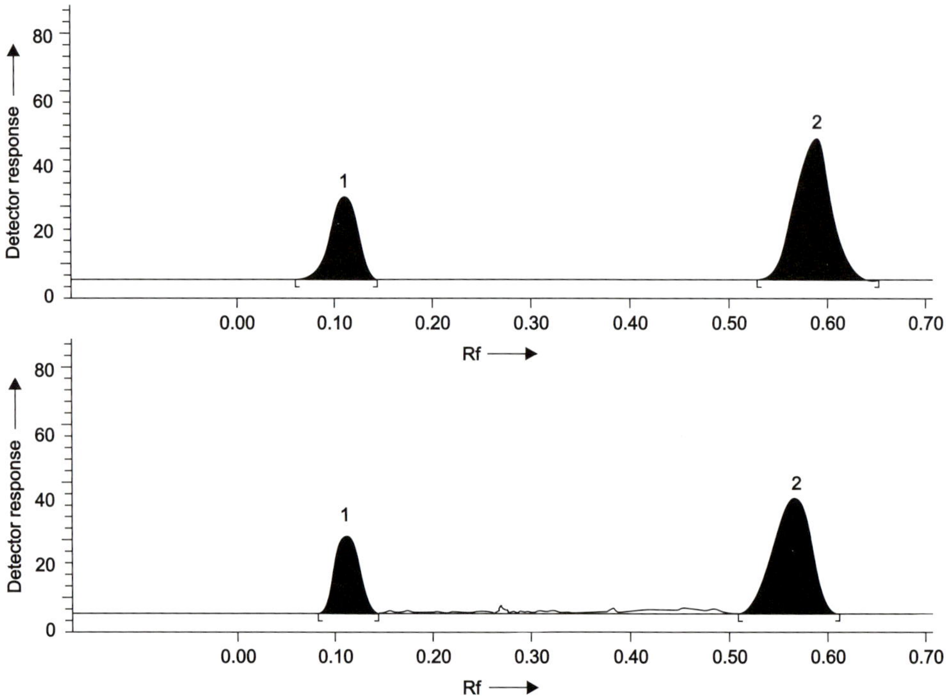

Typical densitogram of the sample and standard containing atenolol and chlorthalidone. For detailed experimental and chromatographic conditions, refer to Protocol No. 7. Peaks identification: 1. Atenolol; 2. Chlorthalidone.

PROTOCOL FOR HPTLC ANALYSIS OF PHARMACEUTICAL FORMULATION

Protocol No. 7

Formulation: Atenolol, Chlorthalidone

Classification: Cardiovascular System **Dosage form:** Tablets

Standard preparation: Prepare 1 mg/ml solution of chlorthalidone in methanol. Weigh 20 mg of atenolol, add 5 ml of chlorthalidone solution, dilute to 100 ml with methanol and use for analysis.

Sample preparation: Powdered sample equivalent to 20 mg of atenolol suspended in 60–70 ml of methanol, sonicate for 10 min, dilute to 100 ml with methanol, filter to use for application.

Chromatographic equipments:

Sample applicator: Camag Linomat–IV

Development chamber: Camag twin-trough glass chamber, 10 × 10 cm

Densitometric scanner: Camag TLC Scanner–II

Chromatographic conditions:

1. Stationary phase: Silica gel $60F_{254}$ pre-coated HPTLC plates, 10 × 10 cm (200 μm) – Merck
2. Mobile phase (MP): Toluene–2-propanol–25% ammonia (6.5 : 3.5 : 0.02 v/v)
3. Standard/Sample application:

   Band length: 5 mm Volume applied: 5 μl Spacing: 7 mm
4. Chamber saturation: 20 min (MP)
5. RH (%): 55 ± 2
6. Temperature °C: 22 ± 2
7. Separation technique: Ascending
8. Quantity of mobile phase: 10 ml
9. Migration distance: 50 mm
10. Migration time: 20 min

Densitometric evaluation:

Wavelength: UV–254 nm Scanning mode: Reflectance/Absorbance

HRF: Atenolol—11; Chlorthalidone—56

Linearity: Atenolol—100–400 ng; Chlorthalidone—20–200 ng

Recovery (%): 99.13–103.52 for both the compounds

References: —

Comments: The method was optimized and analytical work carried out at **Anchrom's HPTLC Application Laboratory**, Mumbai, India.

HPTLC : High Performance Thin Layer Chromatography
HPTLC Densitogram

No. 8

Atenolol

Chlorthalidone

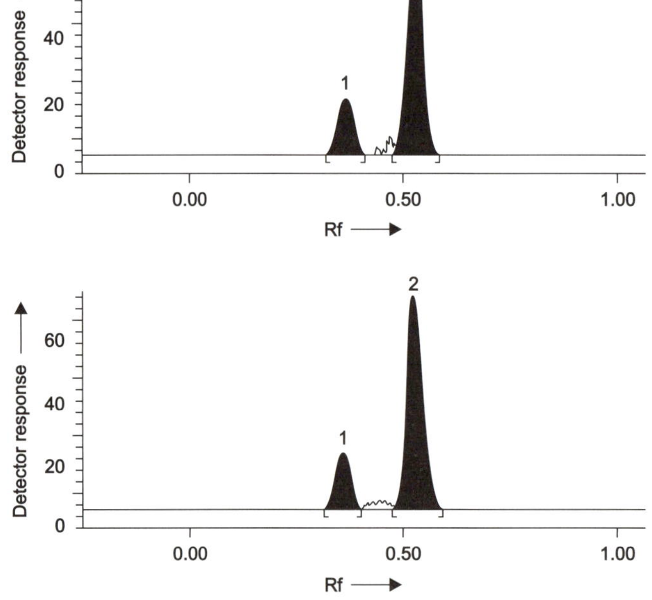

Typical densitogram of the sample and standard containing atenolol and chlorthalidone. For detailed experimental and chromatographic conditions, refer to Protocol No. 8. Peaks identification: 1. Atenolol; 2. Chlorthalidone.

PROTOCOL FOR HPTLC ANALYSIS OF PHARMACEUTICAL FORMULATION

Protocol No. 8

Formulation: Atenolol, Chlorthalidone

Classification: Cardiovascular System **Dosage form:** Tablets

Standard preparation: Prepare 1 mg/ml solution of chlorthalidone in methanol. Weigh 20 mg of atenolol, add 5 ml of chlorthalidone solution, dilute to 100 ml with methanol and use for analysis.

Sample preparation: Powdered sample equivalent to 20 mg of atenolol suspended in 60–70 ml of methanol, sonicate for 10 min, dilute to 100 ml with methanol, filter to use for application.

Chromatographic equipments:

Sample applicator: Camag Linomat–IV

Development chamber: Camag twin-trough glass chamber, 10 × 10 cm

Densitometric scanner: Camag TLC Scanner–II

Chromatographic conditions:

1. Stationary phase: Silica gel 60 RP–18F_{254s} pre-coated HPTLC plates, 5 × 7.5 cm (200 μm) – Merck
2. Mobile phase: 0.5 M sodium chloride–methanol–acetonitrile–glacial acetic acid (10 : 4 : 6 : 0.01 v/v)
3. Standard/Sample application:
   Band length: 5 mm Volume applied: 6 μl Spacing: 7 mm
4. Chamber saturation: 40 min (MP)
5. RH (%): 55 ± 2
6. Temperature °C: 22 ± 2
7. Separation technique: Ascending
8. Quantity of mobile phase: 20 ml
9. Migration distance: 50 mm
10. Migration time: 20 min

Densitometric evaluation:

Wavelength: UV–254 nm Scanning mode: Reflectance/Absorbance

HRF: Atenolol—36; Chlorthalidone—52

Linearity (ng/band): Atenolol—100–400; Chlorthalidone—20–200

Recovery (%): 98.31–101.68 for both the compounds

References: —

Comments:

- The method was optimized and analytical work carried out at **Anchrom's HPTLC Application Laboratory**, Mumbai, India.
- The resolution in RP, HPTLC was superior to NP. HPTLC.
- The RP–HPTLC carried out on laboratory-made RP–HPTLC plates by impregnating NP plates in 5% silicon oil in pet. ether gave very good resolution.

HPTLC : High Performance Thin Layer Chromatography
HPTLC Densitogram

No. 9

Atenolol **Indapamide**

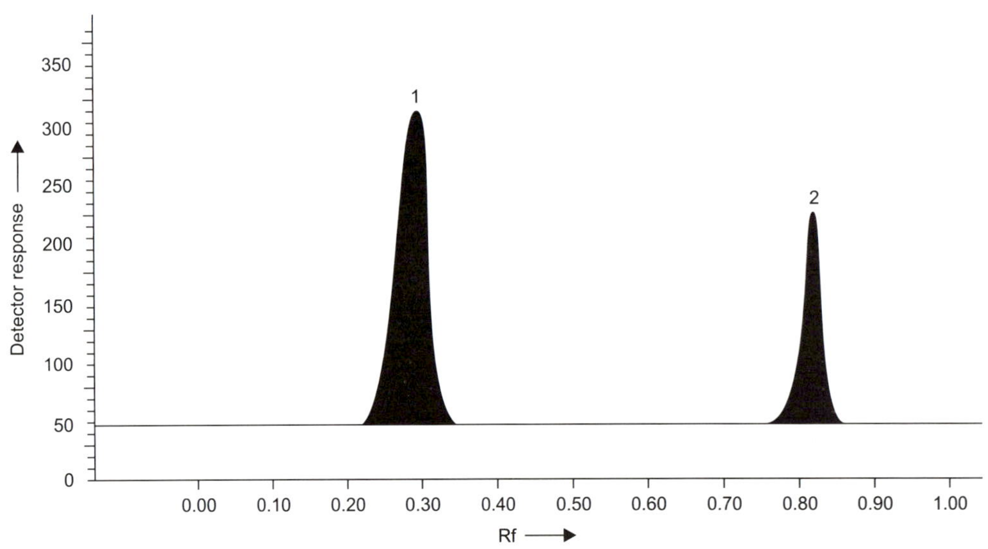

Typical densitogram of the sample containing atenolol and indapamide. For detailed experimental and chromatographic conditions, refer to Protocol No. 9. Peaks identification: 1. Atenolol; 2. Indapamide.

PROTOCOL FOR HPTLC ANALYSIS OF PHARMACEUTICAL FORMULATION

Protocol No. 9

Formulation: Atenolol, Indapamide

Classification: Cardiovascular System **Dosage form:** Tablets

Standard preparation: Prepare 1 mg/ml solution of each compound in methanol. Mix 20 ml of atenolol solution to 1 ml of indapamide solution and dilute to 25 ml with methanol. Apply 10 μl for analysis.

Sample preparation: Powdered sample equivalent to 40 mg of atenolol suspended in 20 ml of methanol, sonicated for 10 min, diluted to 25 ml with methanol, filtered, filtrate diluted appropriately for analysis.

Chromatographic equipments:

Sample applicator: Camag Linomat–IV

Development chamber: Camag twin-trough glass chamber, 10 × 10 cm

Densitometric scanner: Camag TLC Scanner–III

Chromatographic conditions:

1. Stationary phase: Silica gel 60F_{254} pre-coated TLC plates, 10 × 10 cm (250 μm) – Merck
2. Mobile phase (MP): Toluene–ethanol–acetone–25% ammonia (7 : 2.5 : 3 : 0.3 v/v)
3. Standard/Sample application:
   Band length: 4 mm Volume applied: 10 μl Spacing: 4 mm
4. Chamber saturation: 10 min (MP)
5. RH (%): 55 ± 5
6. Temperature °C: 22 ± 2
7. Separation technique: Ascending
8. Quantity of mobile phase: 12 ml
9. Migration distance: 70 mm
10. Migration time: 25 min

Densitometric evaluation:

Wavelength: UV–266 nm Scanning mode: Reflectance/Absorbance

HRF: Atenolol—27; Indapamide—82

Linearity (μg/band): Atenolol—3.8–10.9; Indapamide—0.2–0.6

Recovery (%): Atenolol—99.42–100.5; Indapamide—98.65–99.0

References: K.R. Gupta, S.B. Wankhede, M.R. Tajne and S.G. Wadodkar, *Asian J. Chem.*, **19(6)**, 4183–4187, 2007.

Comments:

- The method validated for accuracy, precision, linearity, LOD, LOQ, specificity and ruggedness.
- The method is stability indicating (acid, alkali, H_2O_2, thermal and photolytic).

HPTLC : High Performance Thin Layer Chromatography
HPTLC Densitogram

No. 10

Atenolol

Indapamide

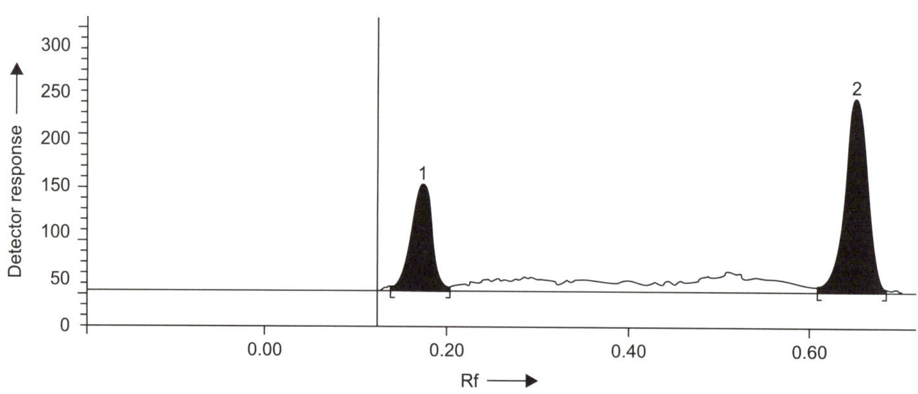

Typical densitogram of the standard containing atenolol and indapamide. For detailed experimental and chromatographic conditions, refer to Protocol No. 10. Peaks identification: 1. Atenolol; 2. Indapamide.

PROTOCOL FOR HPTLC ANALYSIS OF PHARMACEUTICAL FORMULATION

Protocol No. 10

Formulation: Atenolol, Indapamide

Classification: Cardiovascular System **Dosage form:** Tablets

Standard preparation: Prepare 1 mg/ml solution of each compound separately in methanol. Apply varying volume of each solution for linearity profile.

Sample preparation: Powdered sample equivalent to 2.5 mg of indapamide suspended is 20 ml of methanol, sonicated for 30 min, diluted, filtered. Apply 0.8 μl of the resulting solution for chromatographic evaluation.

Chromatographic equipments:

Sample applicator: Camag Linomat–V

Development chamber: Camag twin-trough glass chamber, 10 × 10 cm

Densitometric scanner: Camag TLC Scanner–III

Chromatographic conditions:

1. Stationary phase: Silica gel $60F_{254}$ pre-coated HPTLC plates, 10 × 10 cm (200 μm) – Merck, pre-washed with methanol and dried.
2. Mobile phase (MP): Toluene–ethyl acetate–methanol–25% ammonia (5 : 3 : 3 : 0.1 v/v)
3. Standard/Sample application:
   Band length: 6 mm Volume applied: — Spacing: —
4. Chamber saturation: 20 min (MP)
5. RH (%): 60 ± 5
6. Temperature °C: 25 ± 2
7. Separation technique: Ascending
8. Quantity of mobile phase: 11 ml
9. Migration distance: 80 mm
10. Migration time: 18 min

Densitometric evaluation:

Wavelength: UV–229 nm Scanning mode: Reflectance/Absorbance

HRF: Atenolol—17; Indapamide—65

Linearity (ng/band): Atenolol—200–1200; Indapamide—100–600

Recovery (%): 99.67–99.95 for both the compounds.

References: Savita S. Yadav and Janhavi R. Rao, *International J. Comprehensive Pharmacy*, **2(9)**, 1–4, 2011.

Comments: The method validated for accuracy, precision, linearity, LOD, LOQ, specificity and robustness.

HPTLC : High Performance Thin Layer Chromatography
HPTLC Densitogram

No. 11

Lercanidipine HCl

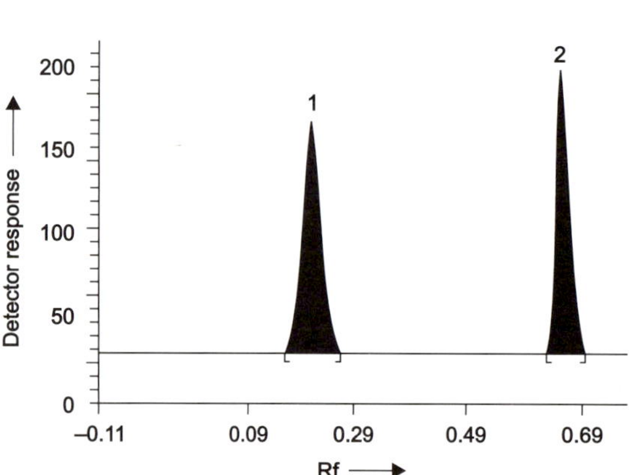

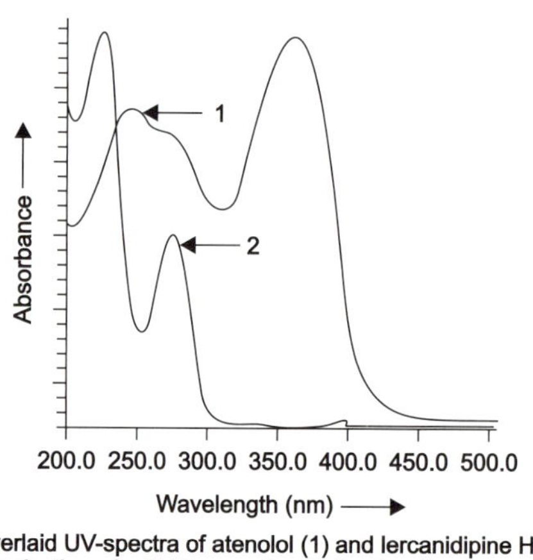

Overlaid UV-spectra of atenolol (1) and lercanidipine HCl (2) for selection of suitable wavelength for densitogram scanning

Typical densitogram of the sample containing atenolol and lercanidipine. For detailed experimental and chromatographic conditions, refer to Protocol No. 11. Peaks identification: 1. Atenolol; 2. Lercanidipine.

PROTOCOL FOR HPTLC ANALYSIS OF PHARMACEUTICAL FORMULATION

Protocol No. 11

Formulation: Atenolol, Lercanidipine hydrochloride

Classification: Cardiovascular System **Dosage form:** Tablets

Standard preparation: Prepare mixed standard solution of atenolol (5 mg/ml) and lercanidipine HCl in methanol. Further serial dilutions made for linearity studies. Apply 8 μl of each solution for analysis.

Sample preparation: Powdered sample equivalent to 50 mg of atenolol and 10 mg of lercandipine hydrochloride suspended in 50 ml of methanol, sonicated for 10 min, diluted to 100 ml, filtered through Whatman No. 41 filter paper and used for chromatographic application.

Chromatographic equipments:

Sample applicator: Camag Linomat–IV

Development chamber: Camag twin-trough glass chamber, 10 × 10 cm

Densitometric scanner: Camag TLC Scanner–III

Chromatographic conditions:

1. Stationary phase: Silica gel $60F_{254}$ pre-coated TLC plates, 10 × 10 cm (250 μm) – Merck
2. Mobile phase (MP): Toluene–methanol–triethylamine (3.5 : 1.5 : 0.1 v/v)
3. Standard/Sample application:
   Band length: 6 mm Volume applied: 8 μl Spacing: 15.4 mm
4. Chamber saturation: 25 min (MP)
5. RH (%): 60 ± 5
6. Temperature °C: 25 ± 2
7. Separation technique: Ascending
8. Quantity of mobile phase: 10 ml
9. Migration distance: 80 mm
10. Migration time: 35 min

Densitometric evaluation:

Wavelength: UV–275 nm Scanning mode: Reflectance/Absorbance

HRF: Atenolol—24; Lercanidipine HCl—68

Linearity (ng/band): Atenolol—2000–12000; Lercandipine HCl—400–2400

Recovery (%): Atenolol—98.60–100.4; Lercandipine HCl—98.98–100.31

References: P.V. Deore, A.A. Shirkhedkar and S.J. Surana, *Acta Chromatographica*, **20(3)**, 463–473, 2008.

Comments: The method validated for accuracy, precision, linearity, LOD, LOQ, specificity, ruggedness and robustness.

HPTLC : High Performance Thin Layer Chromatography
HPTLC Densitogram

No. 12

Atenolol

Losartan potassium

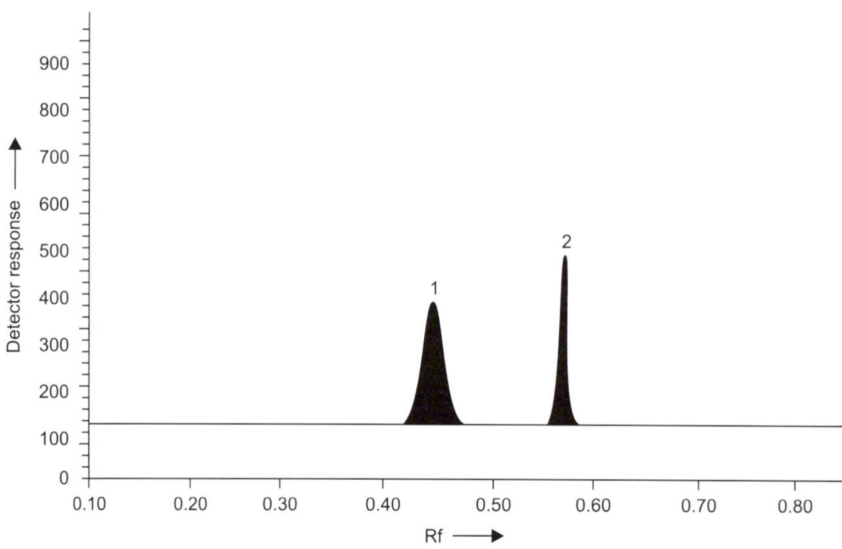

Typical densitogram of the sample containing atenolol and losartan potassium. For detailed experimental and chromatographic conditions, refer to Protocol No. 12. Peaks identification: 1. Atenolol; 2. Losartan potassium.

PROTOCOL FOR HPTLC ANALYSIS OF PHARMACEUTICAL FORMULATION

Protocol No. 12

Formulation: Atenolol, Losartan potassium

Classification: Cardiovascular System **Dosage form:** Tablets

Standard preparation: Prepare 1 mg/ml solution of each compound in methanol. Apply 1–7 μl of each solution to plate and carry out the chromatographic analysis for linearity studies.

Sample preparation: Powdered sample equivalent to 50 mg of atenolol or losartan potassium, suspended in 40 ml of methanol, sonicated for 30 min, diluted to 50 ml with methanol, filtered through Whatman No. 41 filter paper, the filtrate used for analysis.

Chromatographic equipments:

Sample applicator: Camag Linomat–IV

Development chamber: Camag twin-trough glass chamber, 10 × 10 cm

Densitometric scanner: Camag TLC Scanner–III

Chromatographic conditions:

1. Stationary phase: Silica gel $60F_{254}$ pre-coated HPTLC plates, 10 × 10 cm (200 μm) – Merck, pre-washed with methanol, dried at 50°C for 5 min, prior to use
2. Mobile phase (MP): Toluene–methanol–triethylamine (6 : 4 : 0.5 v/v)
3. Standard/Sample application:
   Band length: 6 mm Volume applied: 1.5 μl Spacing: 13 mm
4. Chamber saturation: 45 min (MP)
5. RH (%): 55 ± 5
6. Temperature °C: 25 ± 2
7. Separation technique: Ascending
8. Quantity of mobile phase: 10 ml
9. Migration distance: 70 mm
10. Migration time: 20 min

Densitometric evaluation:

Wavelength: UV–230 nm Scanning mode: Reflectance/Absorbance

HRF: Atenolol—45; Losartan K^+—57

Linearity: 1000–4000 ng/band for both the compounds

Recovery (%): 99.82–99.86 for both compounds

References: R.S. Sathe and S.B. Bari, *Indian Drugs*, **46(1)**, 79–81, 2009.

Comments: The method validated for accuracy, precision, linearity, LOD and specificity.

HPTLC : High Performance Thin Layer Chromatography
HPTLC Densitogram

No. 13

Atenolol

Losartan potassium

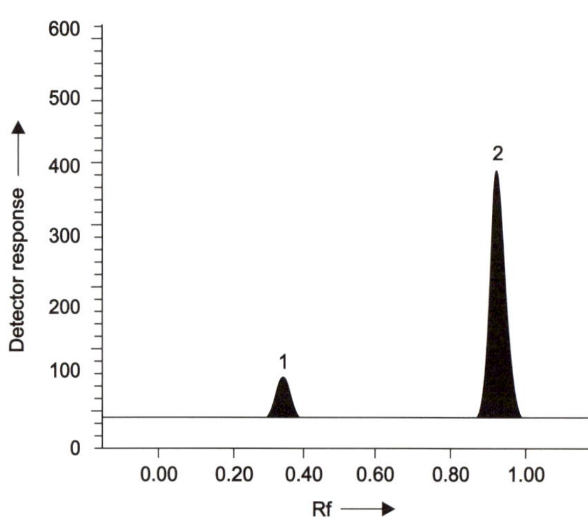

Typical densitogram of the sample containing atenolol and losartan potassium. For detailed experimental and chromatographic conditions, refer to Protocol No. 13. Peaks identification: 1. Losartan potassium; 2. Atenolol.

PROTOCOL FOR HPTLC ANALYSIS OF PHARMACEUTICAL FORMULATION

Protocol No. 13

Formulation: Atenolol, Losartan potassium

Classification: Cardiovascular System **Dosage form:** Tablets

Standard preparation: Prepare 100 μg/ml solution of atenolol and 1000 μg/ml solution of losartan potassium in methanol to use for analysis.

Sample preparation: Powdered sample equivalent to 50 mg of atenolol or losartan potassium, suspended in 40 ml of methanol, sonicated for 30 min, diluted to 50 ml with methanol, filtered through Whatman No. 41 filter paper, filtrate used for analysis.

Chromatographic equipments:

Sample applicator: Camag Linomat–IV

Development chamber: Camag twin-trough glass chamber, 10 × 10 cm

Densitometric scanner: Camag TLC Scanner–III

Chromatographic conditions:

1. Stationary phase: Silica gel $60F_{254}$ pre-coated HPTLC plates, 10 × 10 cm (200 μm) – Merck
2. Mobile phase (MP): Ethyl acetate–methanol–1,4-dioxane–25% ammonia (10 : 2 : 1 : 2 v/v)
3. Standard/Sample application:
   Band length: 5 mm Volume applied: 5 μl Spacing: 10 mm
4. Chamber saturation: 20 min (MP)
5. RH (%): 55 ± 5
6. Temperature °C: 22 ± 2
7. Separation technique: Ascending
8. Quantity of mobile phase: 15 ml
9. Migration distance: 75 mm
10. Migration time: 22 min

Densitometric evaluation:

Wavelength: UV–225 nm Scanning mode: Reflectance/Absorbance

HRF: Losartan potassium—35; Atenolol—92

Linearity (ng/band): Atenolol—400–1000; Losartan potassium—200–1000

Recovery (%): 98.92–99.46 for both the compounds

References: Swati Shenoy, Personal communication, 2009.

Comments: The method validated for accuracy, precision, linearity, LOD and specificity.

HPTLC : High Performance Thin Layer Chromatography
HPTLC Densitogram

No. 14

Atorvastatin calcium

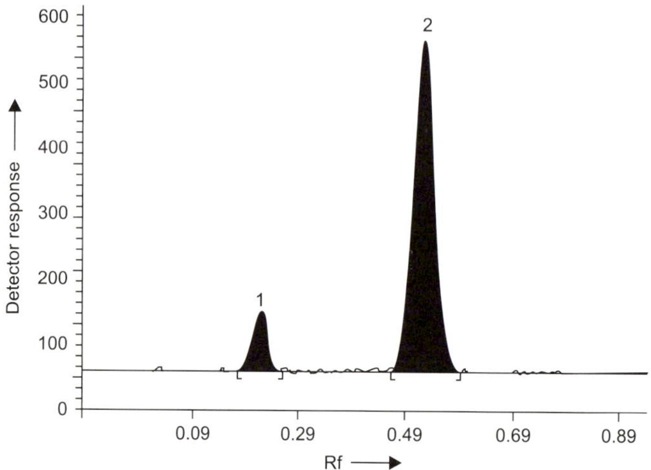

Typical densitogram of the sample containing metoprolol succinate and atorvastatin calcium. For detailed experimental and chromatographic conditions, refer to Protocol No. 14. Peaks identification: 1. Atorvastatin calcium; 2. Metoprolol succinate.

PROTOCOL FOR HPTLC ANALYSIS OF PHARMACEUTICAL FORMULATION

Protocol No. 14

Formulation: Metoprolol succinate, Atorvastatin calcium

Classification: Cardiovascular System **Dosage form:** Capsules

Standard preparation: Prepare solution of both the compounds separately in methanol to get 1000 µg/ml of metoprolol succinate and 500 µg/ml of atorvastatin calcium. Apply 1–6 µl of each solution for linearity profile of both the compounds.

Sample preparation: Powdered sample equivalent to 25 mg of metoprolol succinate suspended in 20 ml of methanol, sonicated for 10 min, diluted to 25 ml with methanol, filtered and the filtrate suitably diluted with methanol for assay. Apply 5 µl of the solution for chromatographic separation and evaluation.

Chromatographic equipments:

Sample applicator: Camag Linomat–V

Development chamber: Camag twin-trough glass chamber, 10 × 10 cm

Densitometric scanner: Camag TLC Scanner-III

Chromatographic conditions:

1. Stationary phase: Silica gel 60F_{254} pre-coated HPTLC plates, 10 × 10 cm (200 µm) – Merck, pre-washed with methanol and activated prior to use
2. Mobile phase (MP): Toluene–methanol–ethylacetate–glacial acetic acid (7 : 1.5 : 1 : 0.5 v/v)
3. Standard/Sample application:
   Band length: 5 mm Volume applied: 5 µl Spacing: 5.6 mm
4. Chamber saturation: 10 min (MP)
5. RH (%): 55 ± 5
6. Temperature °C: 25 ± 2
7. Separation technique: Ascending
8. Quantity of mobile phase: 10 ml
9. Migration distance: 80 mm
10. Migration time: 20 min

Densitometric evaluation:

Wavelength: UV–276 nm Scanning mode: Reflectance/Absorbance

HRF: Atorvastatin Ca^{++}—23, Metoprolol succinate—56

Linearity (ng/band): Metoprolol succinate—1000–6000; Atorvastatin Ca^{++}—500–3000

Recovery (%): Metoprolol succinate—98.81–100.17; Atorvastatin Ca^{++}—99.48–99.74

References: Sagar B. Wankhede, Nitin R. Dixit and Sohan S. Chitlange, *Der Pharmacia Lettre*, **3(1)**, 1–7, 2011.

Comments: The method validated for accuracy, precision, linearity, LOD, LOQ, specificity, robustness and ruggedness.

HPTLC : High Performance Thin Layer Chromatography
HPTLC Densitogram

No. 15

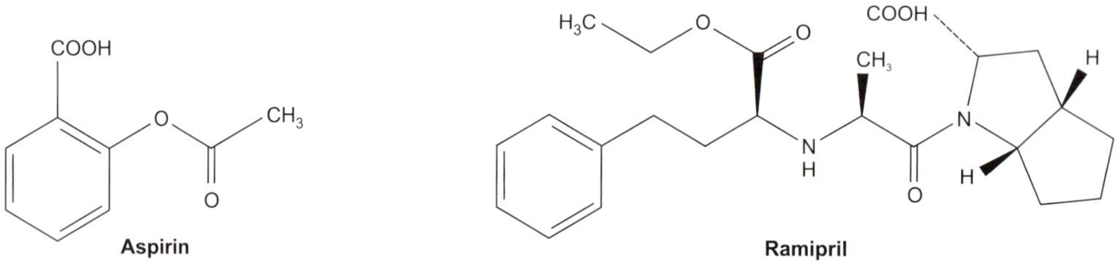

Aspirin

Ramipril

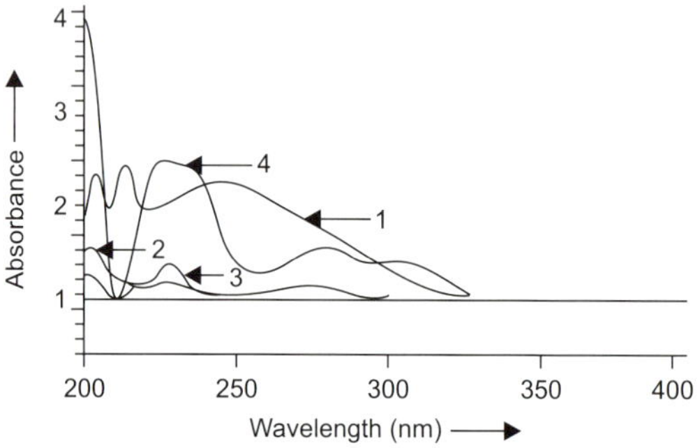

Overlaid UV-spectra of metoprolol succinate (1), ramipril (2), atorvastatin calcium (3) and aspirin (4) for selection of suitable wavelength for densitometric scanning

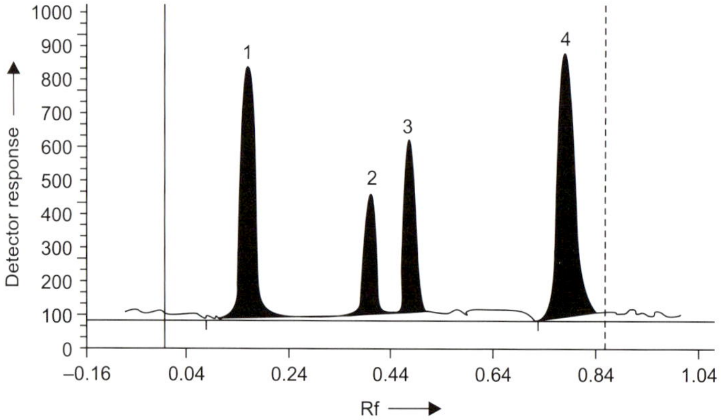

Typical densitogram of the standard containing metoprolol succinate, ramipril, atorvastatin Ca^{++} and aspirin. For detailed experimental and chromatographic conditions, refer to Protocol No. 15. Peaks identification: 1. Metoprolol succinate (MET); 2. Ramipril (RAM); 3. Atorvastatin Ca^{++} (AT); 4. Aspirin (AS).

PROTOCOL FOR HPTLC ANALYSIS OF PHARMACEUTICAL FORMULATION

Protocol No. 15

Formulation: Metoprolol succinate, Ramipril, Atorvastatin calcium, Aspirin

Classification: Cardiovascular System **Dosage form:** Tablets

Standard preparation: Prepare 1 mg/ml solution of each drug separately in methanol. Carry out further dilution to get 100 μg/ml of each. Mix 3.75 ml (AS), 0.5 ml (AT), 0.5 ml (MET) and 0.25 ml (RAM) and dilute to 10 ml with methanol. Apply varying volumes of the solution for linearity profile.

Sample preparation: Weigh accurately from composite sample equivalent to 75 mg (AS), 10 mg (AT), 50 mg (MET) and 2.5 mg (RAM), dilute to 10 ml with methanol. Apply an appropriate quantity and carry out chromatographic separation and evaluation.

Chromatographic equipments:

Sample applicator: Camag Linomat–V

Development chamber: Camag twin-trough glass chamber, 20 × 10 cm

Densitometric scanner: Camag TLC Scanner–III

Chromatographic conditions:

1. Stationary phase: Silica gel $60F_{254}$ pre-coated HPTLC plates, 10 × 10 cm (200 μm) – Merck, pre-washed with methanol, air dried and used for analysis
2. Mobile phase (MP): n-Hexane–chloroform–methanol–glacial acetic acid (2.7 : 6.4 : 0.89 : 0.01 v/v)
3. Standard/Sample application:
   Band length: 6 mm Volume applied: 50–130 μl Spacing: 10 mm
4. Chamber saturation: 15 min (MP)
5. RH (%): 55 ± 5
6. Temperature °C: Ambient
7. Separation technique: Ascending
8. Quantity of mobile phase: 20 ml
9. Migration distance: 80 mm
10. Migration time: 15 min

Densitometric evaluation:

Wavelength: UV–210 nm Scanning mode: Reflectance/Absorbance

HRF: Metoprolol succinate—18; Ramipril—39; Atorvastatin Ca^{++}—47; Aspirin—79

Linearity (ng/band): Metoprolol succinate—1250–3250; Ramipril—125–325; Atrovastatin Ca^{++}—250–650; Aspirin—1850–4810

Recovery (%): 99.65–100.37 for all the four drugs

References: K. Thumar, L. Bhatia and A. Patel, Abstract No. F-269, 63rd IPC, 2011, Data provided by Prof. Kashyap Thumar.

Comments: The method validated for accuracy, precision, linearity, LOD, LOQ, specificity and robustness.

HPTLC : High Performance Thin Layer Chromatography
HPTLC Densitogram

No. 16

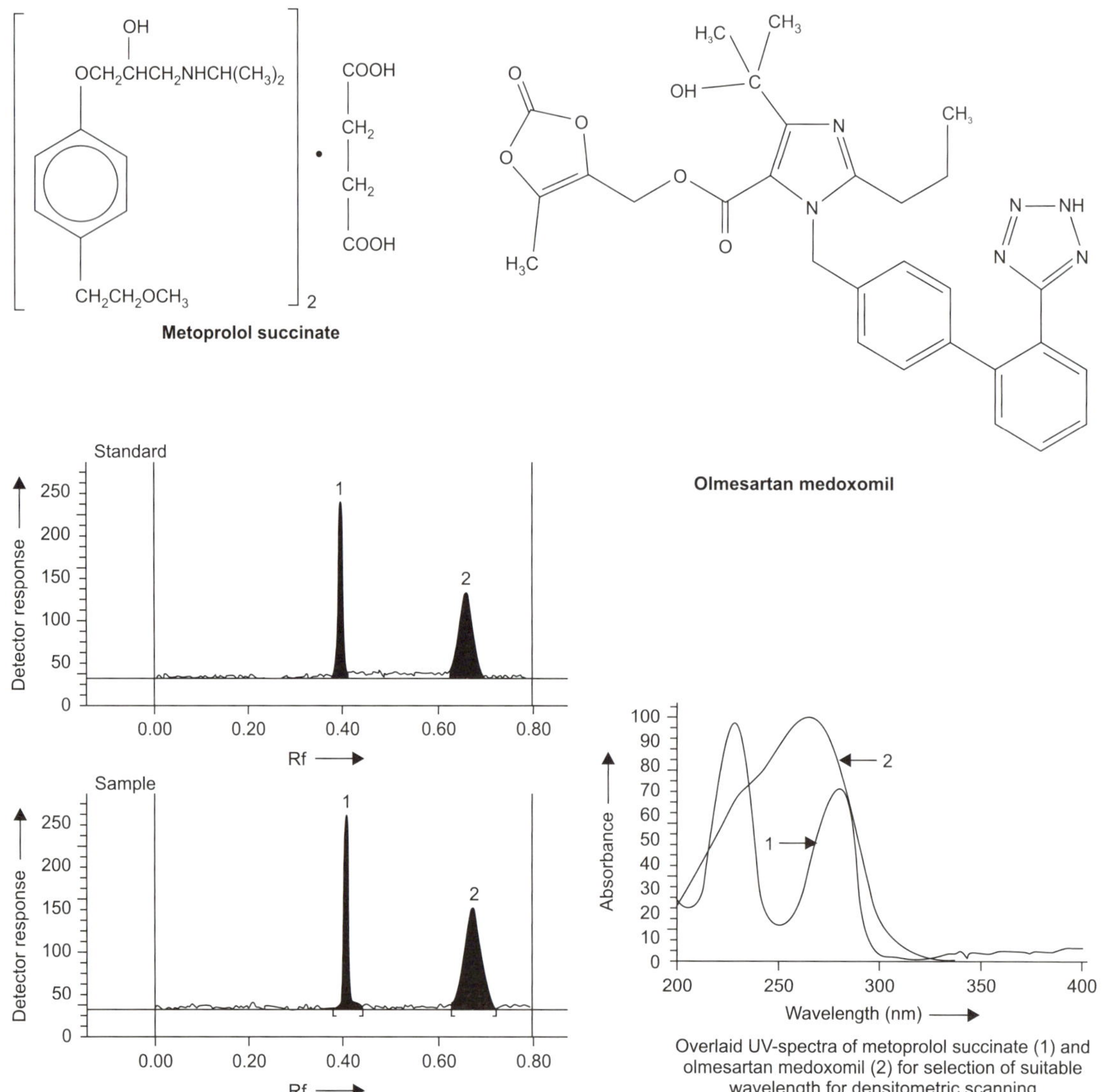

Overlaid UV-spectra of metoprolol succinate (1) and olmesartan medoxomil (2) for selection of suitable wavelength for densitometric scanning

Typical densitogram of the standard and sample containing metoprolol succinate and olmesartan medoxomil. For detailed experimental and chromatographic conditions, refer to Protocol No. 16. Peaks identification: 1. Metoprolol succinate; 2. Olmesartan medoxomil.

PROTOCOL FOR HPTLC ANALYSIS OF PHARMACEUTICAL FORMULATION

Protocol No. 16

Formulation: Metoprolol succinate, Olmesartan medoxomil

Classification: Cardiovascular system **Dosage form:** Tablets

Standard preparation: Prepare solution of both the compounds separately in methanol to get 500 µg/ml of metoprolol succinate (MS) and 200 µg/ml of olmesartan medoxomil (OM). Apply varying volume of each solution for linearity profile.

Sample preparation: Powdered sample equivalent to 5 mg of MS and 2 mg of OM suspended in 8 ml of methanol, sonicated for 10 min, diluted to 10 ml, filtered and the filtrate used for analysis.

Chromatographic equipments:

Sample applicator: Camag Linomat–V

Development chamber: Camag twin-trough glass chamber, 20 × 10 cm

Denistometric scanner: Camag TLC Scanner–III

Chromatographic conditions:

1. Stationary phase: Silica gel $60F_{254}$ pre-coated HPTLC plates, 10 × 20 cm (200 µm) – Merck, pre-washed with methanol and dried prior to use
2. Mobile phase (MP): Toluene–methanol–acetonitrile–triethylamine (4 : 2 : 4 : 0.2 v/v)
3. Standard/Sample application:
   Band length: 6 mm Volume applied: 1–6 µl Spacing: 10 mm
4. Chamber saturation: 20 min (MP)
5. RH (%): 55 ± 5
6. Temperature °C: 25 ± 2
7. Separation technique: Ascending
8. Quantity of mobile phase: 20 ml
9. Migration distance: 85 mm
10. Migration time: 20 min

Densitometric evaluation:

Wavelength: UV–254 nm Scanning mode: Reflectance/Absorbance

HRF: Metoprolol succinate—39; Olmesartan medoxomil—66

Linearity (ng/band): Metoprolol succinate—500–3000; Olmesartan medoxomil—200–1200

Recovery (%): Metoprolol succinate—99.39–100.95; Olmesartan medoxomil—99.71–100.33

References: Jasmin Chikhalia, Mihir Raval, Kashyap N. Thumar and Navin R. Sheth, Manuscript submitted for Dr. P.D. Sethi Award, 2011. Data courtesy Prof. Kashyap.

Comments: The method validated for accuracy, precision, linearity, LOD, LOQ, specificity and robustness.

HPTLC : High Performance Thin Layer Chromatography
HPTLC Densitogram

No. 17

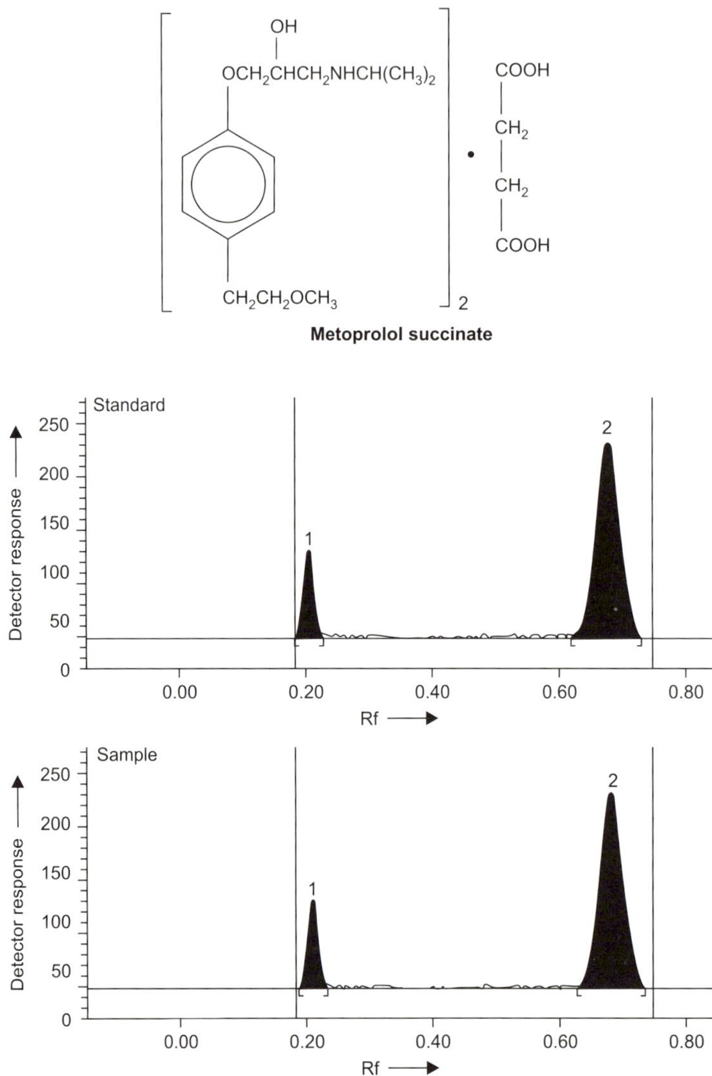

Typical densitogram of the standard and sample containing metoprolol succinate and clopidogrel bisulphate. For detailed experimental and chromatographic conditions, refer to Protocol No. 17. Peaks identification: 1. Metoprolol succinate; 2. Clopidogrel bisulphate.

PROTOCOL FOR HPTLC ANALYSIS OF PHARMACEUTICAL FORMULATION

Protocol No. 17

Formulation: Metoprolol succinate, Clopidogrel bisulphate

Classification: Cardiovascular system **Dosage form:** Tablets

Standard preparation: Prepare standard solution of both the compounds separately in methanol to get 500 μg/ml of metoprolol succinate (MS) and 75 μg/ml of clopidogrel bisulphate (CB). Apply varying volumes of each solution for linearity profile.

Sample preparation: Powdered sample equivalent to 5 mg of MS suspended in 8 ml of methanol, sonicated for 10 min, diluted to 10 ml with methanol, filtered and the filtrate used for assay of both the ingredients.

Chromatographic equipments:

Sample applicator: Camag Linomat–V

Development chamber: Camag twin-trough glass chamber, 10 × 10 cm

Denistometric scanner: Camag TLC Scanner–III

Chromatographic conditions:

1. Stationary phase: Silica gel $60F_{254}$ pre-coated HPTLC plate, 10 × 10 cm (200 μm) – Merck, pre-washed with methanol and dried prior to use
2. Mobile phase (MP): n-hexane–toluene–methanol–triethylamine (5 : 3 : 1.2 : 0.5 v/v)
3. Standard/Sample application:
   Band length: 6 mm Volume applied: 1–7 μl Spacing: 10 mm
4. Chamber saturation: 10 min (MP)
5. RH (%): 55 ± 5
6. Temperature °C: Ambient
7. Separation technique: Ascending
8. Quantity of mobile phase: 9.7 ml
9. Migration distance: 80 mm
10. Migration time: 25 min

Densitometric evaluation:

Wavelength: UV–222 nm Scanning mode: Reflectance/Absorbance

HRF: Metoprolol succinate—23; Clopidogrel bisulphate—68

Linearity (ng/band): Metoprolol succinate—1000–3500; Clopidogrel bisulphate—1500–5250

Recovery (%): Metoprolol succinate—99.57–99.99; Clopidogrel bisulphate—99.21–99.84

References: Mital Gosai, Rupal Tanna, Kashyap N. Thumar and Navin R. Sheth, Manuscript submitted for Dr. P.D. Sethi Award, 2011. Data courtesy Prof. Kashyap.

Comments: The method validated for accuracy, precision, linearity, LOD, LOQ, specificity and robustness.

HPTLC : High Performance Thin Layer Chromatography
HPTLC Densitogram

No. 18

Atenolol

Amlodipine besylate

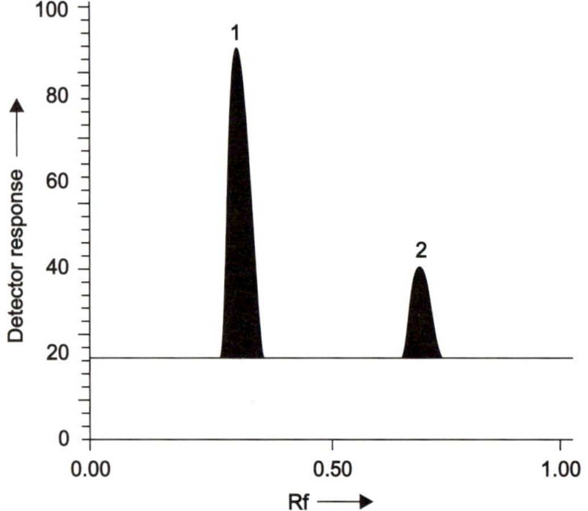

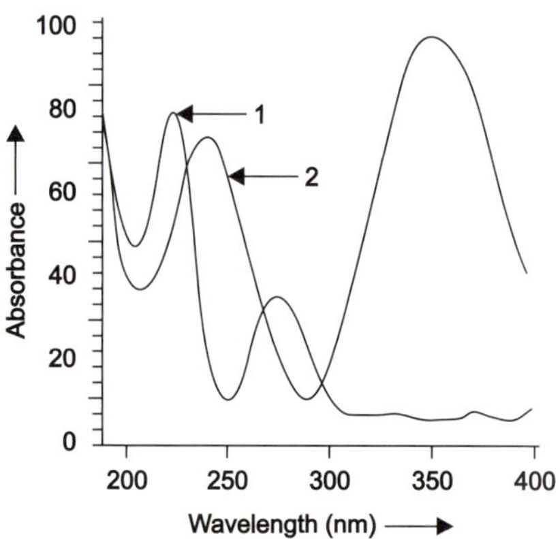

In-situ UV-spectra of atenolol (1) and amlodipine (2) for selection of suitable wavelength for densitometric scanning

Typical densitogram of the sample containing atenolol and amlodipine besylate. For detailed experimental and chromatographic conditions, refer to Protocol No. 18. Peaks identification: 1. Atenolol; 2. Amlodipine besylate.

PROTOCOL FOR HPTLC ANALYSIS OF PHARMACEUTICAL FORMULATION

Protocol No. 18

Formulation: Amlodipine besylate, Atenolol

Classification: Cardiovascular System **Dosage form:** Tablets

Standard preparation: Prepare standard solution of atenolol (10 mg/ml) and amlodipine (1 mg/ml) in methanol. Further dilute 4 ml of each solution to 100 ml with methanol to use for analysis.

Sample preparation: Powdered sample equivalent to 100 mg of atenolol and 10 mg of amlodipine suspended in 40 ml of methanol, sonicate for 40 min, dilute to 50 ml, filter through Whatman No. 1 filter paper. Dilute 2 ml of filtrate to 10 ml with methanol and use for assay.

Chromatographic equipments:

Sample applicator: Camag Linomat–IV

Development chamber: Camag twin-trough glass chamber, 10 × 10 cm

Densitometric scanner: Camag TLC Scanner–III

Chromatographic conditions:

1. Stationary phase: Silica gel $60F_{254}$ pre-coated HPTLC plates, 10 × 10 cm (200 μm) – Merck
2. Mobile phase (MP): Methylene chloride–methanol–25% ammonia (8.8 : 1.3 : 0.1 v/v)
3. Standard/Sample application:
   Band length: 8 mm Volume applied: 10 μl Spacing: 10 mm
4. Chamber saturation: —
5. RH (%): 55 ± 5
6. Temperature °C: 22 ± 2
7. Separation technique: Ascending
8. Quantity of mobile phase: 11.2 ml
9. Migration distance: 80 mm
10. Migration time: 35 min

Densitometric evaluation:

Wavelength: UV–230 nm Scanning mode: Reflectance/Absorbance

HRF: Atenolol—33; Amlodipine—73

Linearity: 10–500 μg/ml for both the compounds

Recovery (%): Atenolol—98.30–99.86; Amlodipine—98.0–99.63

References: A.P. Argekar and S.G. Powar, *J. Pharm. Biomed. Anal.*, **21**, 1137–1142, 2000.

Comments: The method validated for accuracy, precision, linearity and system suitability.

HPTLC : High Performance Thin Layer Chromatography
HPTLC Densitogram

No. 19

Atenolol

Amlodipine besylate

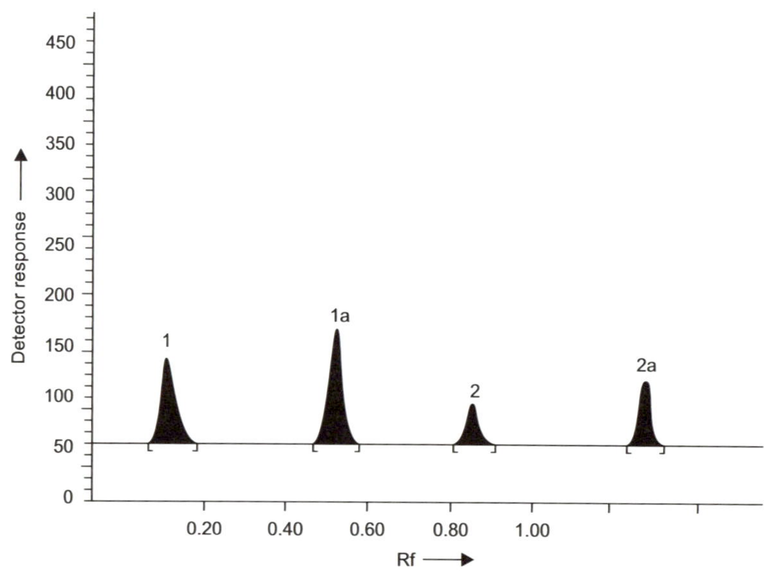

Typical densitogram of the sample containing amlodipine besylate and atenolol. For detailed experimental and chromatographic conditions, refer to Protocol No. 19. Peaks identification: 1. Atenolol (2 µg, 3 µg); 2. Amlodipine besylate (200 ng, 300 ng).

PROTOCOL FOR HPTLC ANALYSIS OF PHARMACEUTICAL FORMULATION

Protocol No. 19

Formulation: Amlodipine besylate, Atenolol

Classification: Cardiovascular System **Dosage form:** Tablets

Standard preparation: Prepare 1 mg/ml solution of each compound in methanol. Further serial dilutions made to get 200–500 ng/ml of amlodipine and 2–5 μg/ml of atenolol. Use each solution for analysis.

Sample preparation: Powdered sample equivalent to 5 mg of amlodipine and 50 mg of atenolol suspended in methanol, sonicated, diluted to get 50 μg/ml of atenolol, further dilutions suitably made for application and analysis.

Chromatographic equipments:

Sample applicator: Camag Linomat–IV

Development chamber: Camag twin-trough glass chamber, 20 × 10 cm

Densitometric scanner: Camag TLC Scanner–III

Chromatographic conditions:

1. Stationary phase: Silica gel $60F_{254}$ pre-coated HPTLC plates, 20 × 10 cm (200 μm) – Merck
2. Mobile phase (MP): Toluene–acetone–ethanol–25% ammonia (6.5 : 0.7 : 4 : 0.4 v/v)
3. Standard/Sample application:
   Band length: 5 mm Volume applied: 5 μl Spacing: 6 mm
4. Chamber saturation: 30 min (MP)
5. RH (%): 55 ± 5
6. Temperature °C: 25 ± 2
7. Separation technique: (MP)
8. Quantity of mobile phase: 23 ml
9. Migration distance: 80 mm
10. Migration time: 30 min

Densitometric evaluation:

Wavelength: UV–254 nm Scanning mode: Reflectance/Absorbance

HRF: Atenolol—16; Amlodipine—54

Linearity: Atenolol—2–3.5 μg/ml; Amlodipine besylate—200–350 ng/ml

Recovery (%): 98–102 for both the compounds

References: Kalliappan, Lango, Pabbisetty, Balashanmuga Kumar and Karunanidhi Santhana Lakshmi, *Indian Drugs*, **37(1)**, 497–499, 2000.

Comments: The method validated for accuracy, precision, linearity and system suitability.

HPTLC : High Performance Thin Layer Chromatography
HPTLC Densitogram

No. 20

Bisoprolol fumarate

Amlodipine besylate

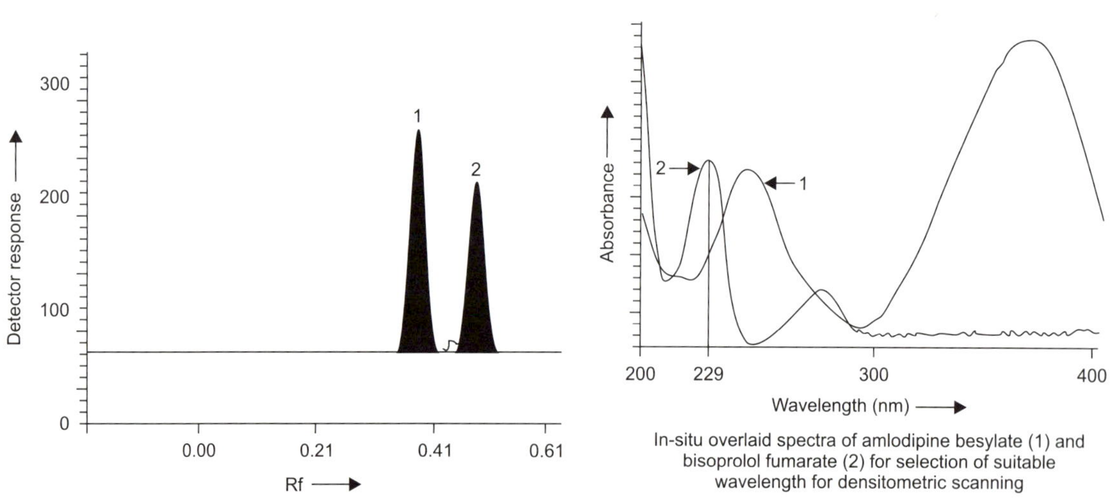

In-situ overlaid spectra of amlodipine besylate (1) and bisoprolol fumarate (2) for selection of suitable wavelength for densitometric scanning

Typical densitogram of the standard containing amlodipine besylate and bisoprolol fumarate. For detailed experimental and chromatographic conditions, refer to Protocol No. 20. Peaks identification: 1. Amlodipine besylate; 2. Bisoprolol fumarate.

PROTOCOL FOR HPTLC ANALYSIS OF PHARMACEUTICAL FORMULATION

Protocol No. 20

Formulation: Amlodipine besylate, Bisoprolol fumarate
Classification: Cardiovascular System **Dosage form:** Tablets
Standard preparation: Prepare 1 mg/ml solution of each compound in methanol. Further dilutions made with methanol to get 100 μg/ml of each for chromatographic application.
Sample preparation: Powdered sample equivalent to 5 mg of amlodipine suspended in 30 ml of methanol, shake for 30 min, dilute to 50 ml, filter and an aliquot of filtrate suitably diluted with methanol to get 100 μg/ml of each to use for chromatographic analysis.

Chromatographic equipments:
Sample applicator: Camag Linomat–IV
Development chamber: Camag twin-trough glass chamber, 10 × 10 cm
Densitometric scanner: Camag TLC Scanner–III

Chromatographic conditions:
1. Stationary phase: Silica gel $60F_{254}$ pre-coated HPTLC plates, 10 × 10 cm (200 μm) – Merck
2. Mobile phase (MP): Methanol–ethyl acetate–25% ammonia (0.5 : 6 : 0.5 v/v)
3. Standard/Sample application:
   Band length: 4 mm Volume applied: 6 μl Spacing: 5 mm
4. Chamber saturation: 20 min (MP)
5. RH (%): 55 ± 5
6. Temperature °C: 22 ± 2
7. Separation technique: Ascending
8. Quantity of mobile phase: 14 ml
9. Migration distance: 70 mm
10. Migration time: 25 min

Densitometric evaluation:
Wavelength: UV–229 nm Scanning mode: Reflectance/Absorbance
HRF: Amlodipine besylate—36; Bisoprolol fumarate—48
Linearity (ng/band): Amlodipine besylate and Bisoprolol fumarate—500–1000
Recovery (%): Amlodipine besylate—99.38–100.11; Bisoprolol fumarate—99.31–100.40

References: R.B. Kakde, V.H. Kotak and N.N. Bawane, *Pharma Review*, 168–170, Dec. 2008.

Comments:
- The method validated for accuracy, precision, linearity, LOD, LOQ, ruggedness and robustness.
- The method is stability indicating (acid, base, oxidative, thermal and photolytic, both the compounds being prone to oxidative degradation).

HPTLC : High Performance Thin Layer Chromatography
HPTLC Densitogram

No. 21

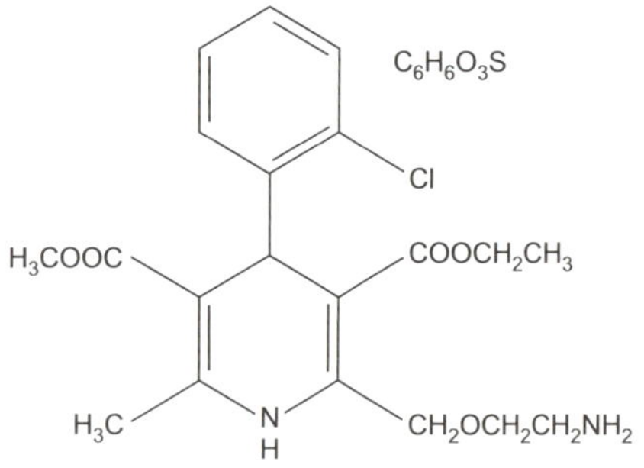

Amlodipine besylate

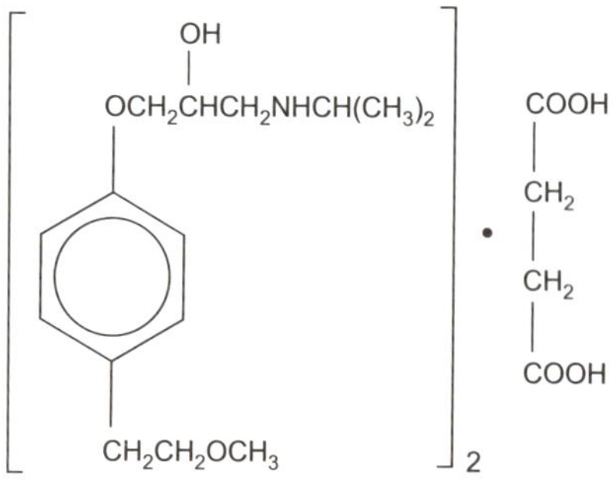

Metoprolol succinate

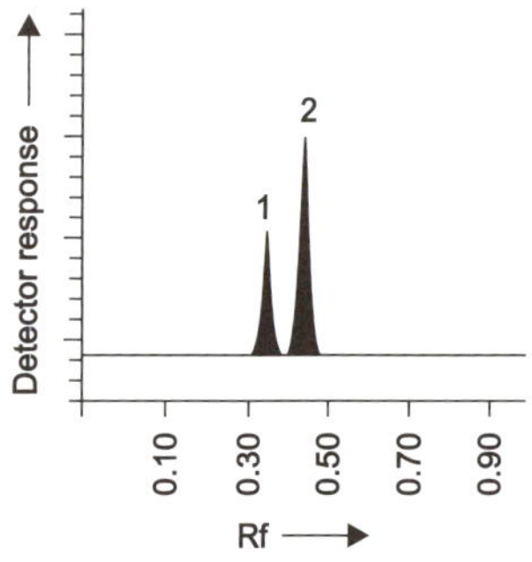

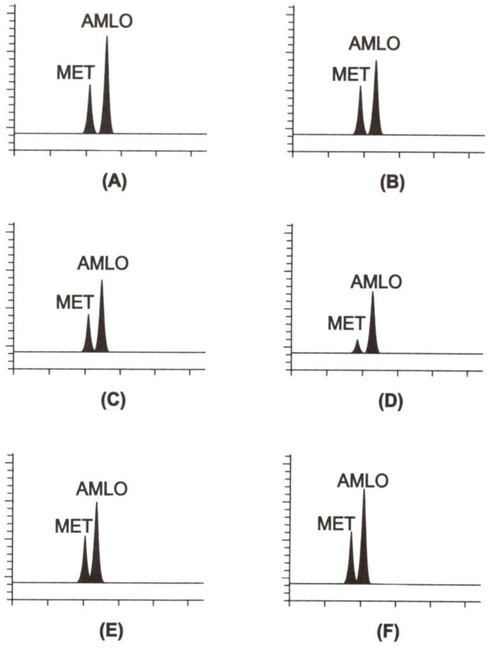

Densitograms obtained from: A, untreated tablet powder; B, acid hydrolysis-treated tablet powder; C, alkaline hydrolysis-treated tablet powder; D, H_2O_2-treated tablet powder; E, dry heat-treated tablet powder; F, UV light-treated tablet powder

Typical densitogram of the standard containing amlodipine besylate and metoprolol succinate. For detailed experimental and chromatographic conditions, refer to Protocol No. 21. Peaks identification: 1. Metoprolol succinate; 2. Amlodipine besylate.

PROTOCOL FOR HPTLC ANALYSIS OF PHARMACEUTICAL FORMULATION

Protocol No. 21

Formulation: **Amlodipine besylate, Metoprolol succinate**

Classification: Cardiovascular System **Dosage form:** Tablets

Standard preparation: Prepare 1 mg/ml solution of metoprolol succinate and 0.1 mg/ml solution of amlodipine (base), both in methanol. Further dilutions made to get 190 μg/ml of metoprolol and 28 μg/ml of amlodipine. Apply 10 μl of each solution for analysis.

Sample preparation: An appropriate quantity of the powdered sample suspended in 40 ml of methanol, sonicated for 15 min, then shaken for 30 min, diluted to 50 ml with methanol, filtered and an aliquot of filtrate suitably diluted to get 190 μg/ml (metoprolol) and 28 μg/ml (amlodipine). Apply 10 μl for assay.

Chromatographic equipments:

Sample applicator: Camag Linomat–IV

Development chamber: Camag twin-trough glass chamber, 10 × 10 cm

Densitometric scanner: Camag TLC Scanner–III

Chromatographic conditions:

1. Stationary phase: Silica gel $60F_{254}$ pre-coated HPTLC plates, 10 × 10 cm (200 μm) – Merck, pre-washed with methanol dried (115°C) for 30 min, prior to use
2. Mobile phase (MP): Methanol–ethyl acetate–water–toluene–25% ammonia (1.5 : 5 : 0.3 : 3 : 0.3 v/v)
3. Standard/Sample application:
   Band length: 4 mm Volume applied: 10 μl Spacing: 4 mm
4. Chamber saturation: 20 min (MP)
5. RH (%): —
6. Temperature °C: 25 ± 2
7. Separation technique: Ascending
8. Quantity of mobile phase: 10 ml
9. Migration distance: 70 mm
10. Migration time: —

Densitometric evaluation:

Wavelength: UV–236 nm Scanning mode: Reflectance/Absorbance

HRF: Metoprolol succinate—31; Amlodipine besylate—43

Linearity (ng/band): Amlodipine besylate—18–28; Metoprolol succinate—180–280

Recovery (%): Amlodipine besylate—98.87–99.63; Metoprolol succinate—99.40–100.08

References: Rajendra Kakde and Nilesh Bawane, *J. Planar Chromatogr.*, **22(2)**, 115–199, 2009.

Comments:

- The method validated for accuracy, precision, linearity, LOD, LOQ and specificity.
- The method is stability indicating (HCl, NaOH, thermal, oxidative and photolytic). No extra peak but decrease in peak height, indicating degradation under different stress conditions.

HPTLC : High Performance Thin Layer Chromatography
HPTLC Densitogram

No. 22

Amlodipine besylate

Benazepril hydrochloride

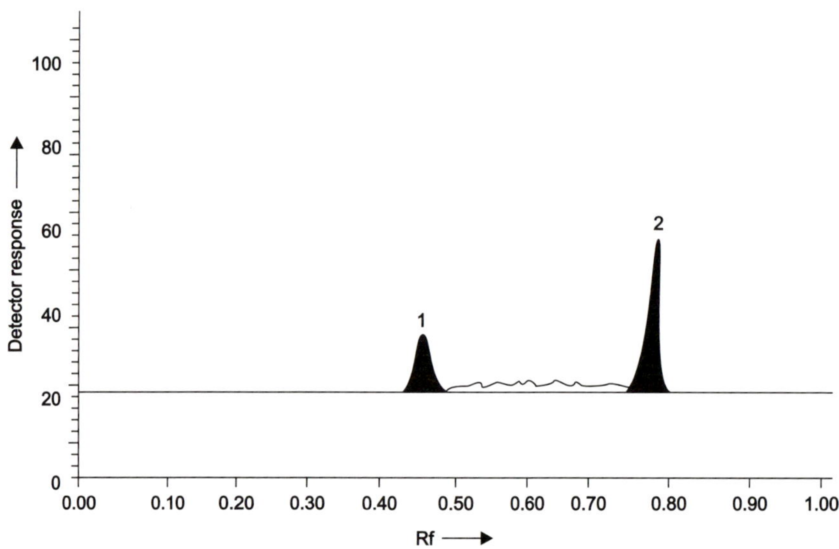

Typical densitogram of the sample containing amlodipine besylate and benazepril HCl. For detailed experimental and chromatographic conditions, refer to Protocol No. 22. Peaks identification: 1. Amlodipine besylate; 2. Benazepril HCl.

PROTOCOL FOR HPTLC ANALYSIS OF PHARMACEUTICAL FORMULATION

Protocol No. 22

Formulation: **Amlodipine besylate, Benazepril hydrochloride**

Classification: Cardiovascular System **Dosage form:** Tablets

Standard preparation: Prepare 250 μg/ml solution of each compound in methanol to use for application.

Sample preparation: Powdered sample equivalent to 10 mg of amlodipine or 20 mg of benazepril suspended in methanol, diluted to 10 ml, filtered through 0.2 μm nylon membrane filter, use for chromatographic application.

Chromatographic equipments:

Sample applicator: Camag Linomat–IV

Development chamber: Camag twin-trough glass chamber, 20 × 10 cm

Densitometric scanner: Camag TLC Scanner–III

Chromatographic conditions:

1. Stationary phase: Silica gel $60F_{254}$ pre-coated HPTLC plates, 20 × 10 cm (200 μm) – Merck
2. Mobile phase (MP): Ethyl acetate–methanol–chloroform–toluene (2.5 : 4 : 3 : 2 v/v)
3. Standard/Sample application:
   Band length: 4 mm Volume applied: 5 μl Spacing: 4 mm
4. Chamber saturation: 30 min (MP)
5. RH (%): 55 ± 5
6. Temperature °C: 25 ± 2
7. Separation technique: Ascending
8. Quantity of mobile phase: 23 ml
9. Migration distance: 70 mm
10. Migration time: 30 min

Densitometric evaluation:

Wavelength: UV–254 nm Scanning mode: Reflectance/Absorbance

HRF: Amlodipine besylate—45; Benazepril HCl—78

Linearity (ng/band): Amlodipine besylate—2–10; Benazepril hydrochloride—4–20

Recovery (%): Amlodipine besylate—99.08–101.1; Benazepril HCl—98.08–99.99

References: Gowri N, Vaidhyahugain V and Shnatha A, *Indian Drugs*, **40(1)**, 65–648, 2003.

Comments: The method validated for accuracy, precision, linearity, LOD, LOQ, specificity and ruggedness.

HPTLC : High Performance Thin Layer Chromatography
HPTLC Densitogram

No. 23

$C_6H_6O_3S$ Cl H_3COOC $COOCH_2CH_3$ H_3C N H $CH_2OCH_2CH_2NH_2$

Amlodipine besylate

H_3C O O O N COOH N H • HCl

Benazepril hydrochloride

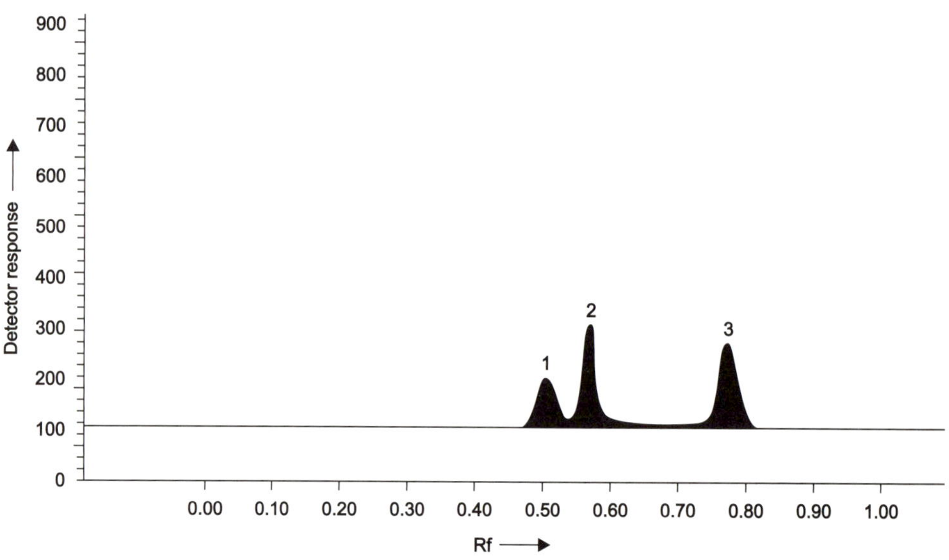

Typical densitogram of the standard containing amlodipine besylate and benazepril HCl. For detailed experimental and chromatographic conditions, refer to Protocol No. 23. Peaks identification: 1. Benazepril HCl; 2. Amlodipine besylate; 3. Zolpidem (IS).

PROTOCOL FOR HPTLC ANALYSIS OF PHARMACEUTICAL FORMULATION

Protocol No. 23

Formulation: Amlodipine besylate, Benazepril hydrochloride

Classification: Cardiovascular System **Dosage form:** Tablets

Standard preparation: Prepare 1 mg/ml solution of each compound in methanol. Further serial dilutions made with methanol to get 0.1–0.8 μg/ml of amlodipine and 0.2–2 μg/ml of benazepril. Apply 5 μl of each solution for analysis.

Sample preparation: An appropriate quantity of powdered sample suspended in methanol, sonicated, diluted, filtered. The final solution should contain 0.5 μg/ml of amlodipine and 1 μg/ml of benazepril. Apply 5 μl for assay.

Note: Each solution under analysis contained 0.8 μg of zolpidem as IS.

Chromatographic equipments:

Sample applicator: Camag Linomat–IV

Development chamber: Camag twin-trough glass chamber, 10 × 10 cm

Densitometric scanner: Camag TLC Scanner–III

Chromatographic conditions:

1. Stationary phasc: Silica gel $60F_{254}$ pre-coated HPTLC plates, 10 × 10 cm (200 μm) – Merck, pre-washed with methanol
2. Mobile phase (MP): Ethyl acetate–methanol–10% ammonia (8.5 : 2 : 1 v/v)
3. Standard/Sample application:
   Band length: 6 mm Volume applied: 5 μl Spacing: 5 mm
4. Chamber saturation: —
5. RH (%): 55 ± 5
6. Temperature °C: 25 ± 2
7. Separation technique: Ascending
8. Quantity of mobile phase: 10 ml
9. Migration distance: —
10. Migration time: —

Densitometric evaluation:

Wavelength: UV–254 nm Scanning mode: Reflectance/Absorbance

HRF: Benazepril hydrochloride—50; Amlodipine besylate—58; Zolpidem (IS)—78

Linearity (ng/band): Amlodipine—0.1–0.8; Benazepril—0.2–2

Recovery (%): 99.79–100.25 for both the drugs

References: S.N. Meyyanathan and B. Suresh, *J. Chromatogr. Sci.*, **43(2)**, 73–75, 2005.

Comments: The method validated for accuracy, precision, linearity, system suitability, LOD, LOQ, ruggedness and robustness.

HPTLC : High Performance Thin Layer Chromatography
HPTLC Densitogram

No. 24

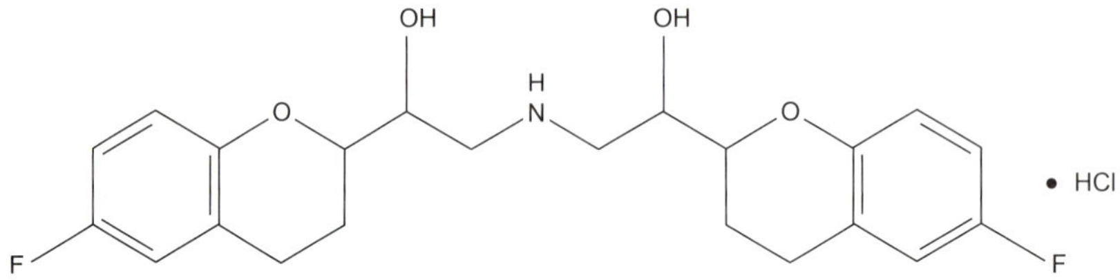

Nebivolol hydrochloride

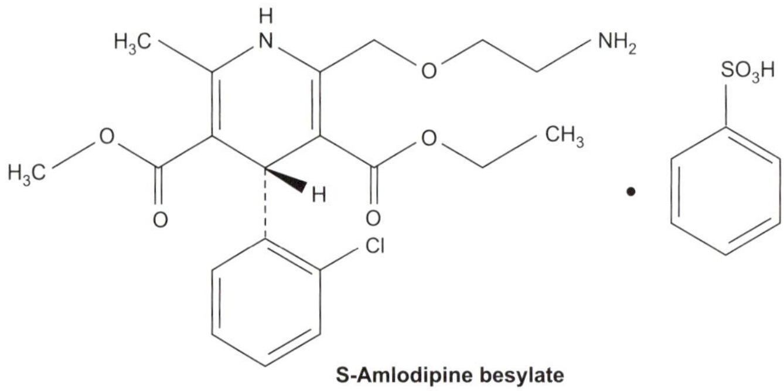

S-Amlodipine besylate

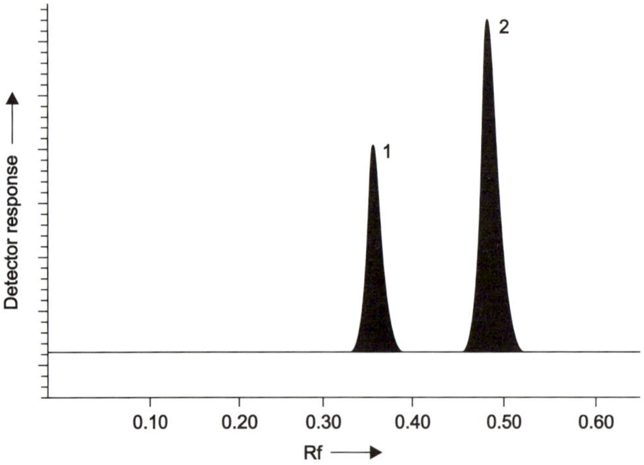

Typical densitogram of the standard containing S-amlodipine besylate and nebivolol hydrochloride. For detailed experimental and chromatographic conditions, refer to Protocol No. 24. Peaks identification: 1. S-amlodipine besylate; 2. Nebivolol HCl.

PROTOCOL FOR HPTLC ANALYSIS OF PHARMACEUTICAL FORMULATION

Protocol No. 24

Formulation: S-Amlodipine besylate, Nebivolol hydrochloride

Classification: Cardiovascular System **Dosage form:** Tablets

Standard preparation: Prepare solution of both the compounds in methanol to get 500 μg/ml of nebivolol hydrochloride and 250 μg/ml of S-amlodipine besylate. Apply varying volumes (1–5 μl) for linearity studies.

Sample preparation: Powdered sample equivalent to 5 mg of nebivolol or 2.5 mg of S-amlodipine besylate suspended in 5 ml of methanol, sonicated for 15 min, diluted to 10 ml and filtered. Apply 2 μl for assay.

Chromatographic equipments:

Sample applicator: Camag Linomat–IV

Development chamber: Camag twin-trough glass chamber, 20 × 10 cm

Densitometric scanner: Camag TLC Scanner–III

Chromatographic conditions:

1. Stationary phase: Silica gel 60F_{254} pre-coated HPTLC plates, 20 × 10 cm (200 μm) – Merck, pre-washed with methanol and dried at 50°C for 5 min, prior to use
2. Mobile phase (MP): Chloroform–toluene–methanol–glacial acetic acid (5 : 3 : 2 : 0.1 v/v)
3. Standard/Sample application:
   Band length: 6 mm Volume applied: 1–5 μl Spacing: 10 mm
4. Chamber saturation: 20 min (MP)
5. RH (%): 60 ± 5
6. Temperature °C: 25 ± 2
7. Separation technique: Ascending
8. Quantity of mobile phase: 20 ml
9. Migration distance: 80 mm
10. Migration time: 20 min

Densitometric evaluation:

Wavelength: UV–271 nm Scanning mode: Reflectance/Absorbance

HRF: S-amlodipine besylate—37; Nebivolol HCl—48

Linearity (ng/band): S-amlodipine besylate—250–1250; Nebivolol HCl—500–2500

Recovery (%): 99.35–99.89 for both the compounds

References: Anil Kumar Sharma, Bhavesh Patel and Rakshil Patel, *International J. Pharma and Biosciences*, **1(4)**, 339, 347, 2010.

Comments: The method validated for accuracy, precision, linearity, LOD, LOQ, ruggedness and robustness.

HPTLC : High Performance Thin Layer Chromatography
HPTLC Densitogram

No. 25

OH OH H N O O F F • HCl

Nebivolol hydrochloride

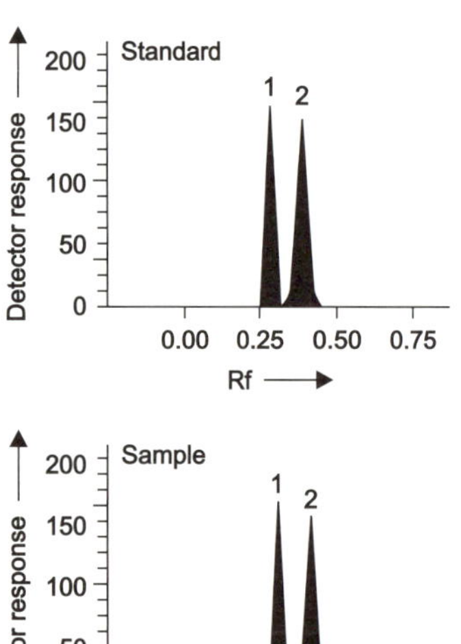

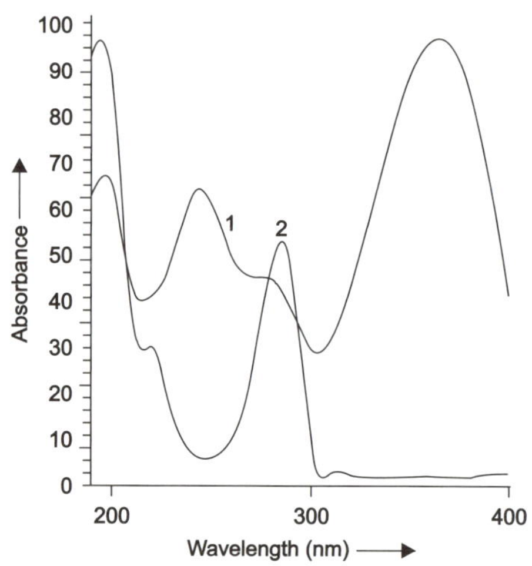

Overlaid UV-spectra of amlodipine (1) and nebivolol (2) for selection of suitable wavelength for densitometric scanning

Typical densitogram of the standard and the sample containing amlodipine besylate and nebivolol hydrochloride. For detailed experimental and chromatographic conditions, refer to Protocol No. 25. Peaks identification: 1. Amlodipine besylate; 2. Nebivolol HCl.

PROTOCOL FOR HPTLC ANALYSIS OF PHARMACEUTICAL FORMULATION

Protocol No. 25

Formulation: Amlodipine besylate, Nebivolol hydrochloride

Classification: Cardiovascular System **Dosage form:** Tablets

Standard preparation: Prepare 1 mg/ml solution of each compound in methanol separately. Carry out serial dilutions for linearity studies. Apply 10 μl of each solution for chromatographic analysis.

Sample preparation: Powdered sample equivalent to 5 mg of amlodipine is suspended in 8 ml of methanol, sonicated for 10 min, diluted to 10 ml, filtered and 1 ml of filtrate diluted to 10 ml. Apply 10 μl for chromatographic analysis.

Chromatographic equipments:

Sample applicator: Camag Linomat–V

Development chamber: Camag automatic development chamber (ADC-2), saturated with Camag saturation pad

Densitometric scanner: Camag TLC Scanner–III

Chromatographic conditions:

1. Stationary phase: Silica gel $60F_{254}$ pre-coated TLC glass plates, 20 × 10 cm (250 μm) – Merck
2. Mobile phase (MP): Ethyl acetate–methanol–25% ammonia (8.5 : 1 : 0.5 v/v)
3. Standard/Sample application:
   Band length: 8 mm Volume applied: 10 μl Spacing: 10 mm
4. Chamber saturation: 20 min (MP)
5. RH (%): 55 ± 5
6. Temperature °C: 25 ± 2
7. Separation technique: Ascending
8. Quantity of mobile phase: 20 ml
9. Migration distance: 70 mm
10. Migration time: 7 min

Densitometric evaluation:

Wavelength: UV–280 nm Scanning mode: Reflectance/Absorbance

HRF: Amlodipine besylate—27; Nebivolol HCl—36

Linearity: 200–1000 ng/band for both the compounds

Recovery (%): —

References: —

Comments: The method was optimized and analytical work carried out at **Anchrom's HPTLC Application Laboratory**, Mumbai, India.

HPTLC : High Performance Thin Layer Chromatography
HPTLC Densitogram

No. 26

d-nebivolol

l-nebivolol

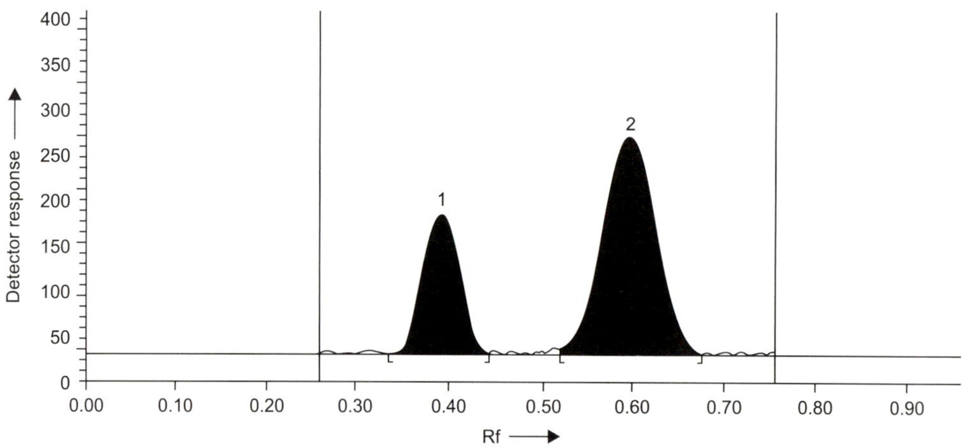

Typical densitogram of the standard containing amlodipine besylate (AB) and nebivolol HCl (NH). For detailed experimental and chromatographic conditions, refer to Protocol No. 26. Peaks identification: 1. Amlodipine besylate; 2. Nebivolol HCl.

PROTOCOL FOR HPTLC ANALYSIS OF PHARMACEUTICAL FORMULATION

Protocol No. 26

Formulation: Amlodipine besylate, Nebivolol hydrochloride

Classification: Cardiovascular System **Dosage form:** Tablets

Standard preparation: Prepare 500 μg/ml solution of each compound in methanol. Apply varying volumes of each solution for linearity profile.

Sample preparation: Powdered sample equivalent to 2.5 mg of amlodipine besylate was suspended in methanol, sonicated for 10 min, suitably diluted, filtered. The final concentration of the solution should contain 100 μg/ml of the drug. Apply 10 μl for chromatographic evaluation.

Chromatographic equipments:

Sample applicator: Camag Linomat–V

Development chamber: Camag twin-trough glass chamber, 10 × 10 cm

Densitometric scanner: Camag TLC Scanner–III

Chromatographic conditions:

1. Stationary phase: Silica gel $60F_{254}$ pre-coated TLC plates, 10 × 10 cm (250 μm) – Merck, pre-washed with methanol and activated at 110°C for 5 min prior to use
2. Mobile phase (MP): Ethyl acetate–methanol–diluted–ammonia (8.5 : 1 : 1 v/v)
3. Standard/Sample application:
   Band length: 6 mm Volume applied: 10 μl Spacing: 10 mm
4. Chamber saturation: 30 min (MP)
5. RH (%): 60 ± 5
6. Temperature °C: 25 ± 2
7. Separation technique: Ascending
8. Quantity of mobile phase: 10.5 ml
9. Migration distance: 80 mm
10. Migration time: 20 min

Densitometric evaluation:

Wavelength: UV–240 nm (AB) and 280 nm (NH)

Scanning mode: Reflectance/Absorbance

HRF: Amlodipine besylate—40; Nebivolol HCl—60

Linearity (ng/band): 500–200 for both the compounds

Recovery (%): Amlodipine besylate—98.50–99.10; Nebivolol HCl—99.50–100.10

References: Mahesh Dangi, Darshana Chaudhari, Mayur Sinker, Veena Racha and Mrinalini C. Damle, *Eurasian J. Anal Chem.*, **5(2)**, 161–169, 2010.

Comments:

- The method validated for accuracy, precision, linearity, LOD, LOQ, ruggedness and robustness.
- The method is stability indicating (acid, base, oxidative, thermolytic and photolytic).

HPTLC : High Performance Thin Layer Chromatography
HPTLC Densitogram

No. 27

Nebivolol hydrochloride

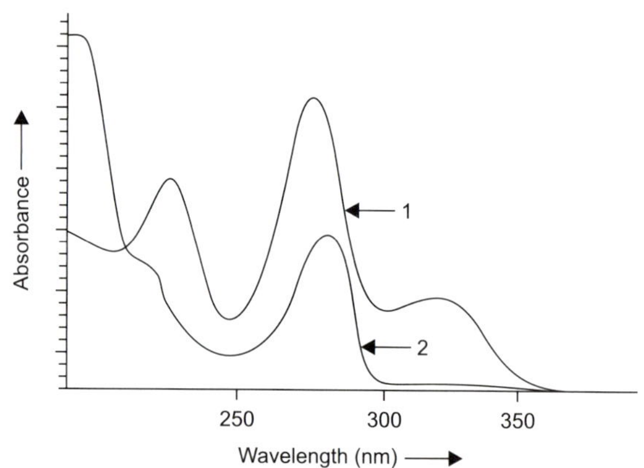

Overlaid UV-spectra of amlodipine besylate (1) and nebivolol HCl (2) for selection of suitable wavelength for densitometric scanning

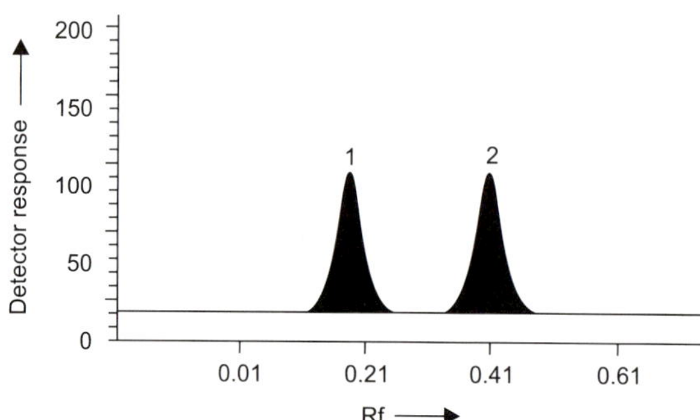

Typical densitogram of the sample containing amlodipine besylate and nebivolol HCl. For detailed experimental and chromatographic conditions, refer to Protocol No. 27. Peaks identification: 1. Amlodipine besylate; 2. Nebivolol HCl.

PROTOCOL FOR HPTLC ANALYSIS OF PHARMACEUTICAL FORMULATION

Protocol No. 27

Formulation: Amlodipine besylate, Nebivolol hydrochloride

Classification: Cardiovascular System **Dosage form:** Tablets

Standard preparation: Prepare 1 mg/ml solution of each compound in methanol. Further serial dilutions are made with methanol to get 100–500 μg/ml. Apply 2 μl of each dilution for linearity profile.

Sample preparation: Accurately weighed quantity of the powdered sample suspended in methanol, sonicated for 15 min, filtered and the filtrate suitably diluted to get 200 μg/ml of amlodipine. Apply 2 μl for chromatographic analysis.

Chromatographic equipments:

Sample applicator: Camag Linomat–V

Development chamber: Camag twin–trough glass chamber, 20 × 10 cm

Densitometric scanner: Camag TLC Scanner–III

Chromatographic conditions:

1. Stationary phase: Silica gel $60F_{254}$ pre-coated HPTLC plates, 10 × 10 cm (200 μm) – Merck, pre-washed with methanol and activated at 115°C for 10 min prior to use
2. Mobile phase (MP): Methylene chloride–methanol–25% ammonia (8.5 : 1 : 0.5 v/v)
3. Standard/Sample application:
   Band length: 8 mm Volume applied: 2 μl Spacing: 8 mm
4. Chamber saturation: 10 min (MP)
5. RH (%): 61 ± 5
6. Temperature °C: 26.4
7. Separation technique: Ascending
8. Quantity of mobile phase: 20 ml
9. Migration distance: 80 mm
10. Migration time: 20 min

Densitometric evaluation:

Wavelength: UV–285 nm Scanning mode: Reflectance/Absorbance

HRF: Amlodipine besylate—19; Nebivolol HCl—41

Linearity: 100–500 ng/band for both the compounds

Recovery (%): 99.96–102.11 for both the compounds

References: B. Dhandapani, S. Anjane Yulu, V. Venkateshwarhi, Shaik Harun Rasheed, *J. Pharmacy Research*, **3(2)**, 332–334, 2010.

Comments: The method validated for accuracy, precision, linearity, LOD, LOQ, specificity, robustness and ruggedness.

HPTLC : High Performance Thin Layer Chromatography
HPTLC Densitogram

No. 28

NH_2 COOH N H O N COOH • $2H_2O$

Lisinopril

$C_6H_6O_3S$ Cl H_3COOC $COOCH_2CH_3$ H_3C N H $CH_2OCH_2CH_2NH_2$

Amlodipine besylate

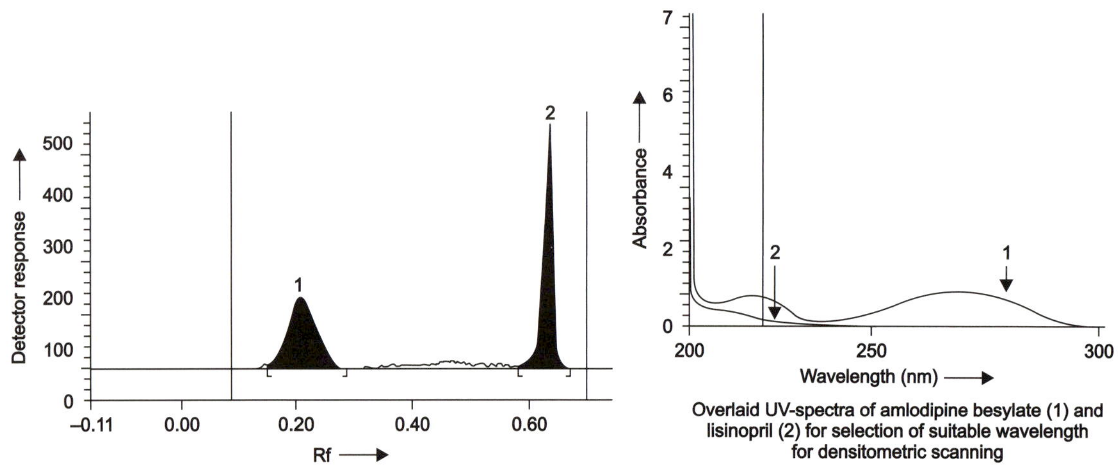

Overlaid UV-spectra of amlodipine besylate (1) and lisinopril (2) for selection of suitable wavelength for densitometric scanning

Typical densitogram of the sample containing amlodipine besylate and lisinopril. For detailed experimental and chromatographic conditions, refer to Protocol No. 28. Peaks identification: 1. Lisinopril; 2. Amlodipine besylate.

PROTOCOL FOR HPTLC ANALYSIS OF PHARMACEUTICAL FORMULATION

Protocol No. 28

Formulation: Amlodipine besylate, Lisinopril

Classification: Cardiovascular System **Dosage form:** Tablets

Standard preparation: Prepare 20 mg/ml solution of each compound in methanol. Carry out further serial dilutions for linearity studies. Apply 1 μl of each solution for chromatographic separation.

Sample preparation: Powdered sample equivalent to 5 mg of amlodipine suspended in 20 ml of methanol, sonicated for 15 min, diluted to 25 ml, filtered and apply 1 μl of the filtrate for analysis.

Chromatographic equipments:

Sample applicator: Camag Linomat–V

Development chamber: Camag twin–trough glass chamber, 20 × 10 cm

Densitometric scanner: Camag TLC Scanner–III

Chromatographic conditions:

1. Stationary phase: Silica gel $60F_{254}$ pre-coated TLC plates, 20 × 10 cm, pre-washed with methanol, activated at 110°C for 5 min prior to use
2. Mobile phase (MP): Methanol–ethyl acetate–0.2% amm. sulphate (3.0 : 6.0 : 4.0 v/v)
3. Standard/Sample application:
   Band length: 6 mm Volume applied: 1 μl Spacing: 6 mm
4. Chamber saturation: 30 min (MP)
5. RH (%): 60 ± 5
6. Temperature °C: 25 ± 2°C
7. Separation technique: Ascending
8. Quantity of mobile phase: 20 ml
9. Migration distance: 80 mm
10. Migration time: 18 min

Densitometric evaluation:

Wavelength: UV–218 nm Scanning mode: Reflectance/Absorbance

HRF: Lisinopril—22; Amlodipine besylate—65

Linearity (ng/band): 2000–10,000 for both the compounds

Recovery (%): 98.05–100.02 for both the compounds

References: K.H. Gopani, S.S. Havele and S.R. Dhaneshwar, *International J. Pharm and Tech.*, **3(2)**, 2353–2367, 2011.

Comments: The method validated for accuracy, precision, linearity, LOD, LOQ and specificity.

HPTLC : High Performance Thin Layer Chromatography
HPTLC Densitogram

No. 29

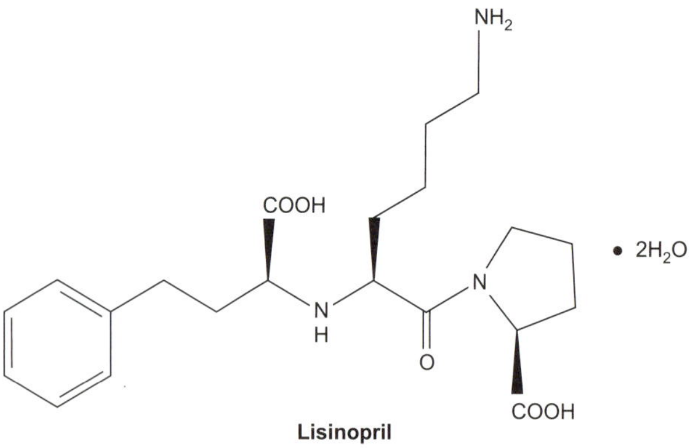

Lisinopril • $2H_2O$

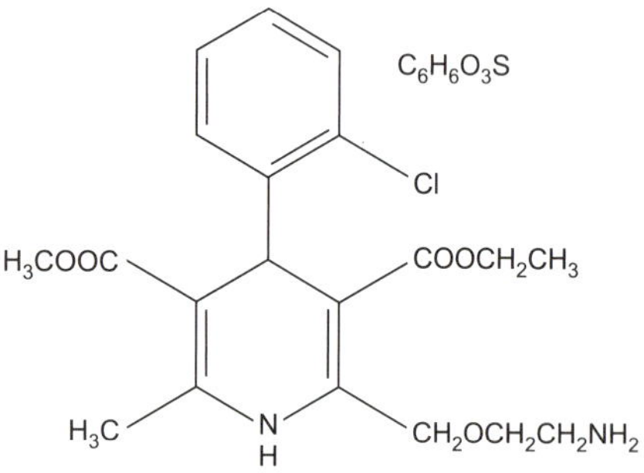

Amlodipine besylate ($C_6H_6O_3S$)

Standard

Sample

Detector response

Rf

Absorbance

Wavelength (nm)

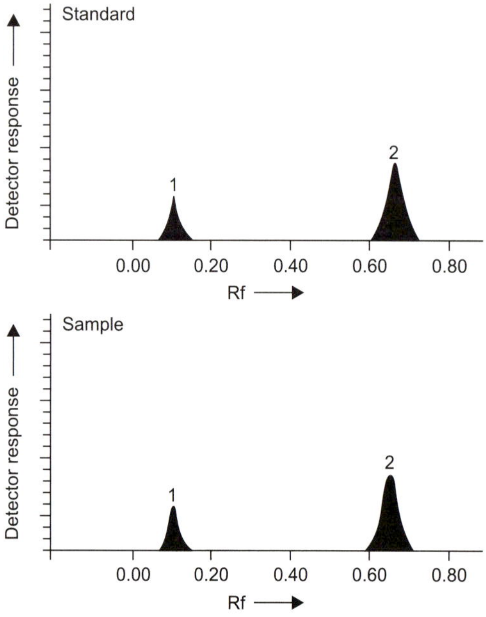

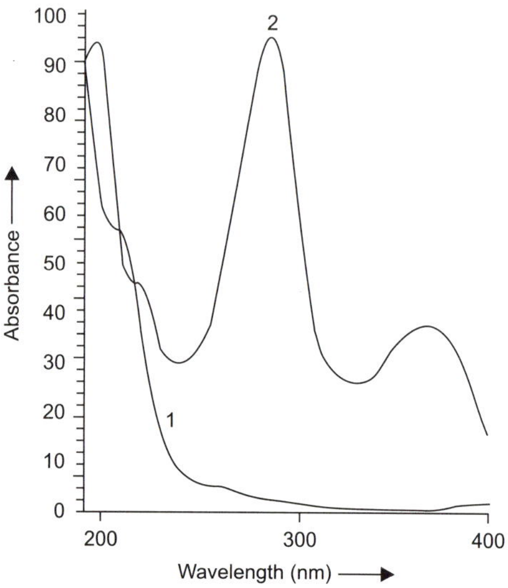

Overlaid UV-spectra of lisinopril (1) and amlodipine (2) for selection of suitable wavelength for densitometric scanning

Typical densitogram of the standard and the sample containing lisinopril and amlodipine. For detailed experimental and chromatographic conditions, refer to Protocol No. 29. Peaks identification: 1. Lisinopril; 2. Amlodipine.

PROTOCOL FOR HPTLC ANALYSIS OF PHARMACEUTICAL FORMULATION

Protocol No. 29

Formulation: Amlodipine besylate, Lisinopril

Classification: Cardiovascular System **Dosage form:** Tablets

Standard preparation: Prepare 1 mg/ml solution of each compound in methanol separately. Carry out serial dilutions for linearity studies. Apply 10 µl of each solution for chromatographic analysis.

Sample preparation: Powdered sample equivalent 5 mg of amlodipine is suspended in 8 ml of methanol, sonicated for 10 min, diluted to 10 ml, filtered, 1 ml of the filtrate diluted to 10 ml. Apply 10 µl for analysis.

Chromatographic equipments:

Sample applicator: Camag Linomat–V

Development chamber: Camag automatic development chamber saturated with Camag saturation pad

Densitometric scanner: Camag TLC Scanner–III

Chromatographic conditions:

1. Stationary phase: Silica gel $60F_{254}$ pre-coated TLC plate-glass, 20 × 10 cm (250 µm) – Merck
2. Mobile phase (MP): n-butanol–methanol–25% ammonia (3 : 1 : 1 v/v)
3. Standard/Sample application:
   Band length: 8 mm Volume applied: 10 µl Spacing: 10 mm
4. Chamber saturation: 20 min (MP)
5. RH (%): 55 ± 5
6. Temperature °C: 25 ± 2
7. Separation technique: Ascending
8. Quantity of mobile phase: 20 ml
9. Migration distance: 70 mm
10. Migration time: 30 min

Densitometric evaluation:

Wavelength: UV–200 nm Scanning mode: Reflectance/Absorbance

HRF: Lisinopril—10; Amlodipine besylate—68

Linearity: 200–1000 ng/band for both the compounds

Recovery (%): —

References: —

Comments: The method was optimized and analysis work carried out at **Anchrom's HPTLC Application Laboratory**, Mumbai, India.

HPTLC : High Performance Thin Layer Chromatography
HPTLC Densitogram

No. 30

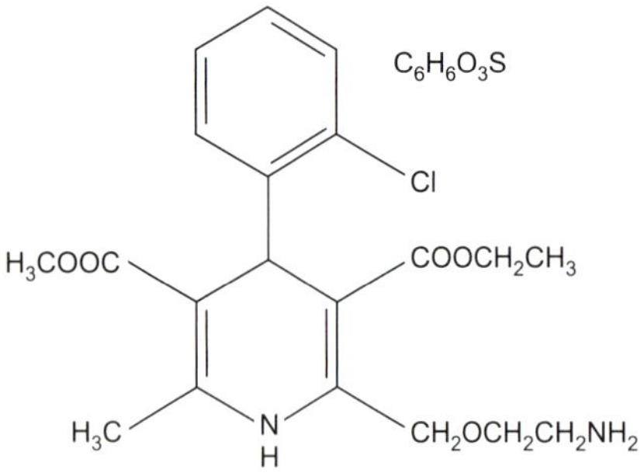
$C_6H_6O_3S$
Cl
H_3COOC
$COOCH_2CH_3$
H_3C
N
H
$CH_2OCH_2CH_2NH_2$

Amlodipine besylate

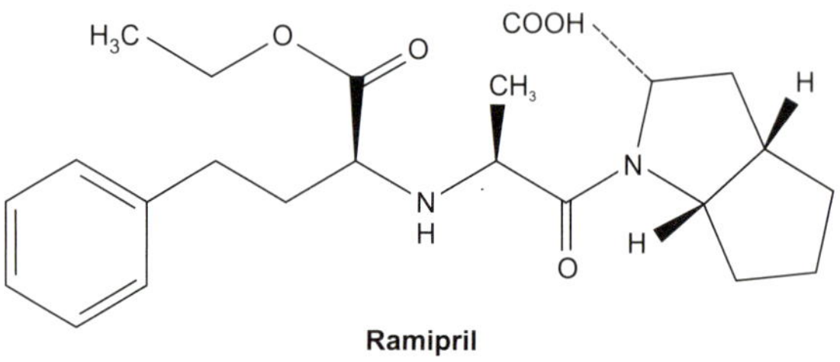
H_3C
O
O
COOH
CH_3
H
N
N
H
H
O

Ramipril

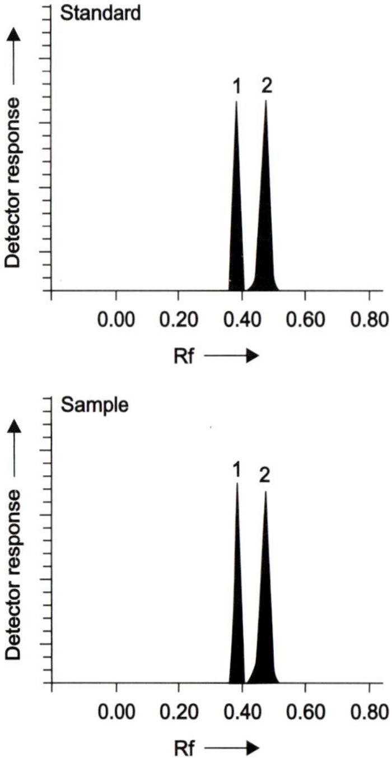
Standard
1
2
Detector response
0.00
0.20
0.40
0.60
0.80
Rf
Sample
1
2
Detector response
0.00
0.20
0.40
0.60
0.80
Rf

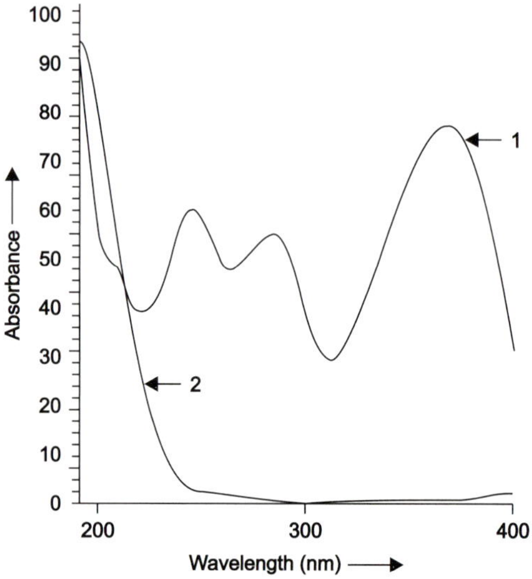
100
90
80
70
60
50
40
30
20
10
0
Absorbance
1
2
200
300
400
Wavelength (nm)

Overlaid UV-spectra of amlodipine (1) and ramipril (2) for selection of suitable wavelength for densitometric scanning

Typical densitogram of the standard and the sample containing amlodipine besylate and ramipril. For detailed experimental and chromatographic conditions, refer to Protocol No. 30. Peaks identification: 1. Amlodipine besylate; 2. Ramipril.

PROTOCOL FOR HPTLC ANALYSIS OF PHARMACEUTICAL FORMULATION

Protocol No. 30

Formulation: Amlodipine besylate, Ramipril

Classification: Cardiovascular System **Dosage form:** Tablets

Standard preparation: Prepare 1 mg/ml solution of each compound in methanol separately. Carry out serial dilutions for linearity studies. Apply 10 μl of each solution for chromatographic analysis.

Sample preparation: Powdered sample equivalent 5 mg of amlodipine is suspended in 8 ml of methanol, sonicated for 10 min, diluted to 10 ml, filtered, 1 ml of filtrate diluted to 10 ml. Apply 10 μl for analysis.

Chromatographic equipments:

Sample applicator: Camag Linomat–V

Development chamber: Camag automatic development chamber saturated with Camag saturation pad

Densitometric scanner: Camag TLC Scanner–III

Chromatographic conditions:

1. Stationary phase: Silica gel $60F_{254}$ pre-coated TLC plate-glass, 20 × 10 cm (250 μm) – Merck
2. Mobile phase (MP): Upper layer of mixture of glacial acetic acid–water–methylisobutyl ketone (25 : 25 : 50 v/v)
3. Standard/Sample application:
   Band length: 8 mm Volume applied: 10 μl Spacing: 10 mm
4. Chamber saturation: 20 min (MP)
5. RH (%): 55 ± 5
6. Temperature °C: 25 ± 2
7. Separation technique: Ascending
8. Quantity of mobile phase: 20 ml
9. Migration distance: 70 mm
10. Migration time: 24 min

Densitometric evaluation:

Wavelength: UV–210 nm Scanning mode: Reflectance/Absorbance

HRF: Amlodipine besylate—38; Ramipril—47

Linearity: 200–1000 ng/band for both the compounds

Recovery (%): —

References: —

Comments: The method was optimized and analysis work carried out at **Anchrom's HPTLC Application Laboratory**, Mumbai, India.

HPTLC : High Performance Thin Layer Chromatography
HPTLC Densitogram

No. 31

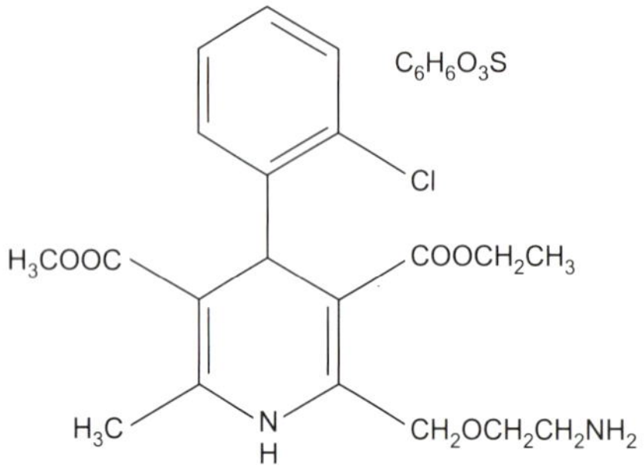

Amlodipine besylate

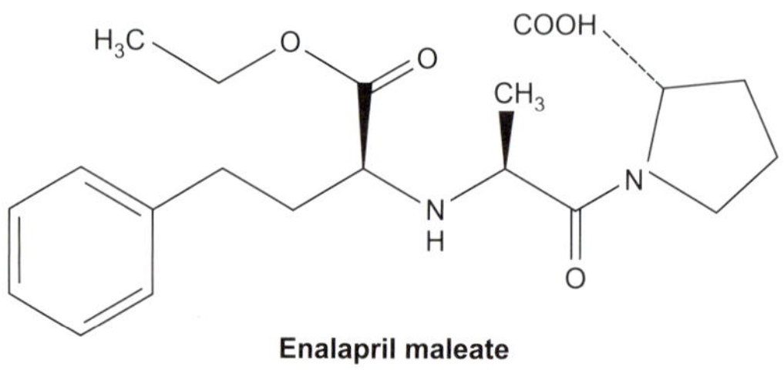

Enalapril maleate

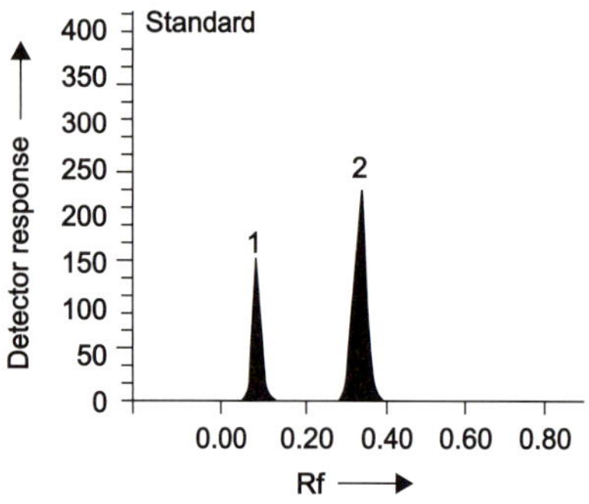

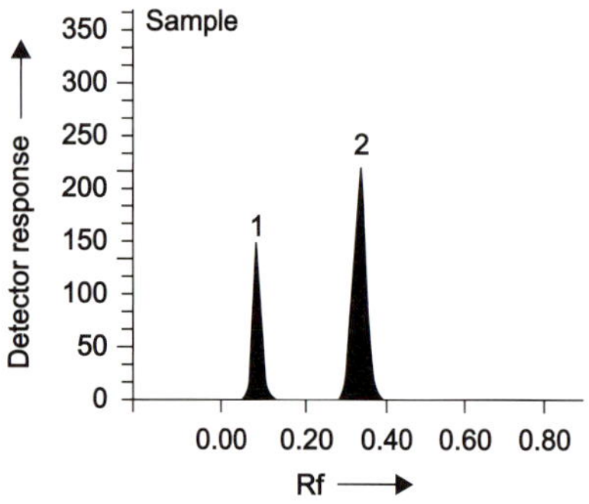

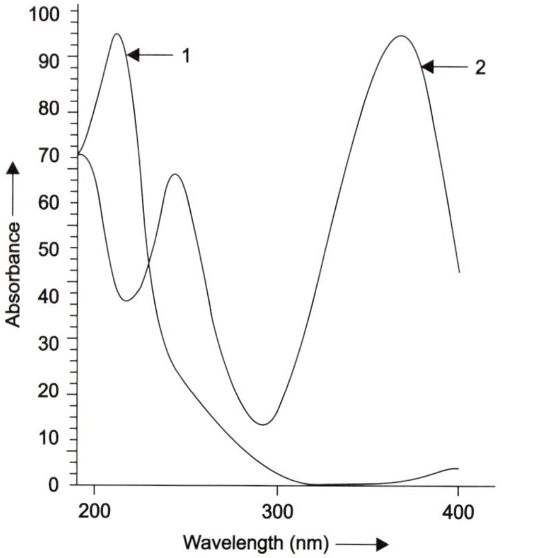

Overlaid UV-spectra of enalapril maleate (1) and amlodipine (2) for selection of suitable wavelength for densitometric scanning

Typical densitogram of the standard and the sample containing enalapril maleate and amlodipine. For detailed experimental and chromatographic conditions, refer to Protocol No. 31. Peaks identification: 1. Enalapril maleate; 2. Amlodipine besylate.

PROTOCOL FOR HPTLC ANALYSIS OF PHARMACEUTICAL FORMULATION

Protocol No. 31

Formulation: Amlodipine besylate, Enalapril maleate

Classification: Cardiovascular System **Dosage form:** Tablets

Standard preparation: Prepare 1 mg/ml solution of each compound in methanol separately. Carry out serial dilutions for linearity studies. Apply 10 μl of each solution for chromatographic analysis.

Sample preparation: Powdered sample equivalent to 5 mg of amlodipine is suspended in 8 ml of methanol, sonicated for 10 min, diluted to 10 ml, filtered, 1 ml of the filtrate diluted to 10 ml. Apply 10 μl for analysis.

Chromatographic equipments:

Sample applicator: Camag Linomat–V

Development chamber: Camag automatic development chamber saturated with Camag saturation pad

Densitometric scanner: Camag TLC Scanner–III

Chromatographic conditions:

1. Stationary phase: Silica gel $60F_{254}$ pre-coated TLC plate-glass, 20 × 10 cm (250 μm) – Merck
2. Mobile phase (MP): Chloroform–methanol–glacial acetic acid (8.5 : 1.5 : 1 v/v)
3. Standard/Sample application:

   Band length: 8 mm Volume applied: 10 μl Spacing: 10 mm
4. Chamber saturation: 20 min (MP)
5. RH (%): 55 ± 5
6. Temperature °C: 25 ± 2
7. Separation technique: Ascending
8. Quantity of mobile phase: 22 ml
9. Migration distance: 70 mm
10. Migration time: 8 min

Densitometric evaluation:

Wavelength: UV–230 nm Scanning mode: Reflectance/Absorbance

HRF: Enalapril maleate—10; Amlodipine besylate—37

Linearity: 200–1000 ng/band for both the compounds

Recovery (%): —

References: —

Comments: The method was optimized and analysis work carried out at **Anchrom's HPTLC Application Laboratory**, Mumbai, India.

HPTLC : High Performance Thin Layer Chromatography
HPTLC Densitogram

No. 32

$C_6H_6O_3S$

Amlodipine besylate

Telmisartan

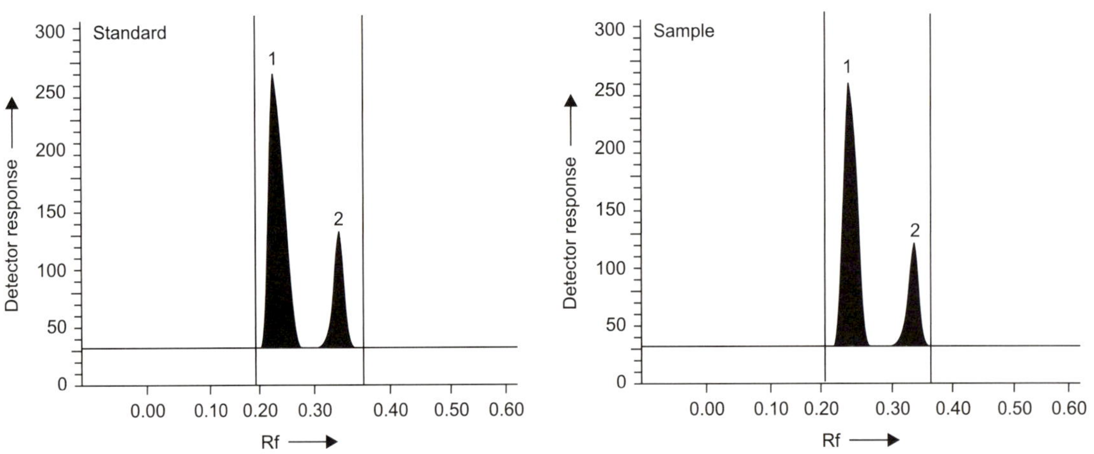

Typical densitogram of the sample and standard containing amlodipine besylate and telmisartan. For detailed experimental and chromatographic conditions, refer to Protocol No. 32. Peaks identification: 1. Telmisartan; 2. Amlodipine besylate.

PROTOCOL FOR HPTLC ANALYSIS OF PHARMACEUTICAL FORMULATION

Protocol No. 32

Formulation: Amlodipine besylate, Telmisartan

Classification: Cardiovascular System **Dosage form:** Tablets

Standard preparation: Prepare 1 mg/ml solution of each compound in solvent. Further serial dilutions made for linearity studies.

Solvent: Mixture of methanol–25% ammonia (8 : 2 v/v).

Sample preparation: Powdered sample equivalent to 100 mg of telmisartan suspended in solvent, sonicated for 10 min, diluted to 100 ml with solvent, filtered and an aliquot of filtrate suitably diluted with solvent to get 1000 μg/ml (telmisartan) to 250 μg/ml (amlodipine). Apply 2 μl for analysis.

Chromatographic equipments:

Sample applicator: Camag Linomat–IV

Development chamber: Camag twin-trough glass chamber, 20 × 10 cm

Densitometric scanner: Camag TLC Scanner–III

Chromatographic conditions:

1. Stationary phase: Silica gel $60F_{254}$ pre-coated HPTLC plates, 10 × 10 cm (200 μm) – Merck
2. Mobile phase (MP): Ethyl acetate–1,4-dioxane–methanol–25% ammonia (15 : 1.5 : 3 : 1.5 v/v)
3. Standard/Sample application:

   Band length: 80 mm Volume applied: 2 μl Spacing: 10 mm
4. Chamber saturation: 20 min (MP)
5. RH (%): 55 ± 5
6. Temperature °C: 25 ± 2
7. Separation technique: Ascending
8. Quantity of mobile phase: 21 ml
9. Migration distance: 80 mm
10. Migration time: 14 min

Densitometric evaluation:

Wavelength: UV–323 nm Scanning mode: Reflectance/Absorbance

HRF: Telmisartan—22; Amlodipine besylate—33

Linearity (ng/band): Telmisartan—500–2500; Amlodipine besylate—250–2000

Recovery (%): 100.24–100.38 for both the compounds

References: A.R. Chabukswar S.C. Jadgale, S.V. Kumbhar and R.D. Wavhale, Abstract No. PA–230; both IPC, 2008.

Comments: The method validated for accuracy, precision, linearity, LOD and LOQ.

HPTLC : High Performance Thin Layer Chromatography
HPTLC Densitogram

No. 33

Amlodipine besylate

Telmisartan

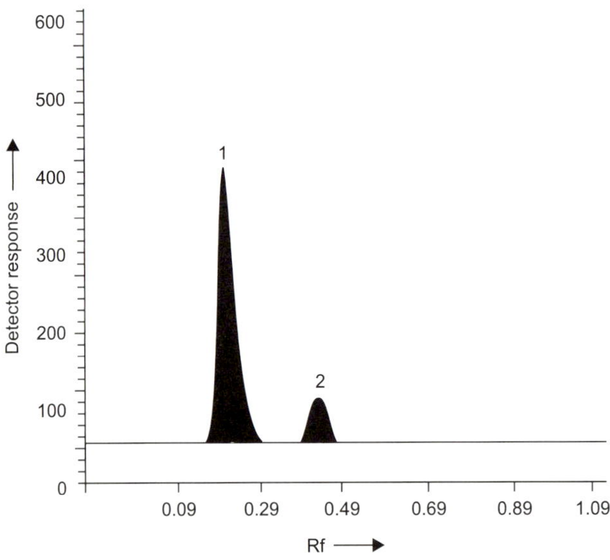

Typical densitogram of the sample containing amlodipine besylate and telmisartan. For detailed experimental and chromatographic conditions, refer to Protocol No. 33. Peaks identification: 1. Telmisartan; 2. Amlodipine besylate.

PROTOCOL FOR HPTLC ANALYSIS OF PHARMACEUTICAL FORMULATION

Protocol No. 33

Formulation: Amlodipine besylate, Telmisartan

Classification: Cardiovascular System **Dosage form:** Tablets

Standard preparation: Prepare 1 mg/ml solution of each compound separately in methanol. Further serial dilutions made for linearity profile. Apply 5 μl of each solution for analysis.

Sample preparation: Powdered sample equivalent to 5 mg of amlodipine besylate suspended in methanol, sonicated, diluted, filtered and filtrate suitably diluted. Apply 5 μl for chromatographic evaluation.

Chromatographic equipments:

Sample applicator: Camag Linomat–IV

Development chamber: Camag twin-trough glass chamber, 10 × 10 cm

Densitometric scanner: Camag TLC Scanner–III

Chromatographic conditions:

1. Stationary phase: Silica gel $60F_{254}$ pre-coated HPTLC plates, 10 × 10 cm (200 μm) – Merck
2. Mobile phase (MP): Tetrahydrofuran–dichloromethane–methanol–25% ammonia (6 : 2 : 1 : 0.4 v/v) or (6 : 2 : 1 : 0.2 v/v)
3. Standard/Sample application:
   Band length: 5 mm Volume applied: 5 μl Spacing: 10 mm
4. Chamber saturation: 30 min (MP)
5. RH (%): 55 ± 5
6. Temperature °C: 22 ± 2
7. Separation technique: Ascending
8. Quantity of mobile phase: 18 ml
9. Migration distance: 80 mm
10. Migration time: —

Densitometric evaluation:

Wavelength: UV–326 nm Scanning mode: Reflectance/Absorbance

HRF: Telmisartan—22; Amlodipine besylate—45

Linearity (ng/band): Amlodipine besylate—400–1400; Telmisartan—1200–7200

Recovery (%): 100.60–101.08 for both the compounds.

References: N.R. Vakariaya, M.B. Patel, G.F. Patel and R.B. Dholakiya, *J. Young Pharmacist*, **1(3)**, 260–263, 2009; *Int. J. Pharm. Tech. Res.*, **1(4)**, 1644–1649, 2009.

Comments: The method validated for accuracy, precision, linearity, LOD, LOQ, specificity and robustness.

HPTLC : High Performance Thin Layer Chromatography
HPTLC Densitogram

No. 34

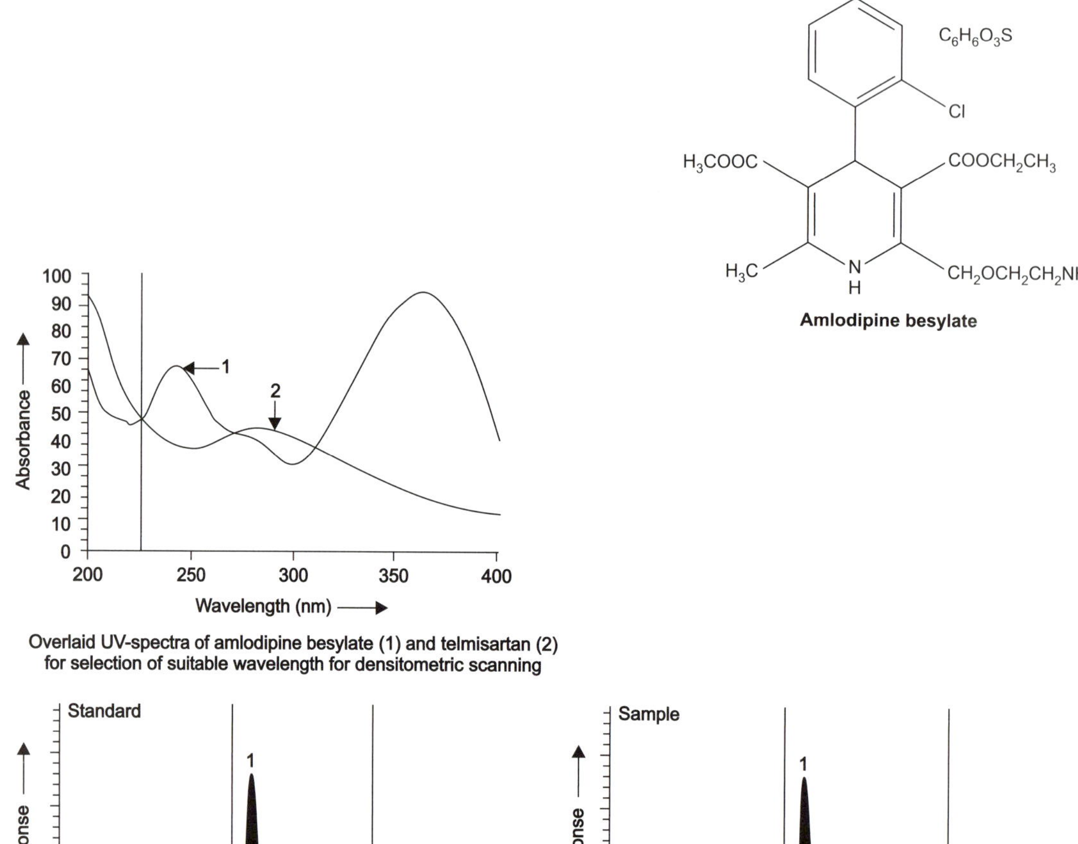

Overlaid UV-spectra of amlodipine besylate (1) and telmisartan (2) for selection of suitable wavelength for densitometric scanning

Typical densitogram of the sample and the standard containing amlodipine besylate and telmisartan. For detailed experimental and chromatographic conditions, refer to Protocol No. 34. Peaks identification: 1. Amlodipine besylate; 2. Telmisartan.

PROTOCOL FOR HPTLC ANALYSIS OF PHARMACEUTICAL FORMULATION

Protocol No. 34

Formulation: Amlodipine besylate, Telmisartan

Classification: Cardiovascular System **Dosage form:** Tablets

Standard preparation: Prepare 10 mg/ml solution of each compound separately in methanol. Further serial dilutions made to get 500–6000 μg/ml (amlodipine besylate) and 1000–8000 μg/ml (telmisartan). Apply 1 μl of each solution for linearity studies.

Sample preparation: Powdered sample equivalent to 100 mg of amlodipine suspended in methanol, sonicated for 10 min, diluted to 100 ml with methanol, filtered and used for application. Apply 0.5 μl (500 ng of AB) and (4000 ng of T) for analysis.

Chromatographic equipments:

Sample applicator: Camag Linomat–V
Development chamber: Camag twin-trough glass chamber, 10 × 10 cm
Densitometric scanner: Camag TLC Scanner–III

Chromatographic conditions:

1. Stationary phase: Silica gel $60F_{254}$ pre-coated TLC plates, 10 × 10 cm (250 μm) – Merck, pre-washed with methanol, dried at 110°C for 15 min, prior to use
2. Mobile phase (MP): Ethyl acetate–methanol–25% ammonia–glacial acetic acid (7.5 : 1.5 : 1 : 0.2 v/v)
3. Standard/Sample application:
   Band length: 6 mm Volume applied: 1 μl Spacing: 10 mm
4. Chamber saturation: 20 min (MP)
5. RH (%): 55 ± 5
6. Temperature °C: 25 ± 2
7. Separation technique: Ascending
8. Quantity of mobile phase: 10 ml
9. Migration distance: 80 mm
10. Migration time: 20 min

Densitometric evaluation:

Wavelength: UV–226 nm (iso-absorption point)
Scanning mode: Reflectance/Absorbance
HRF: Amlodipine besylate—34; Telmisartan—60
Linearity (ng/band): Amlodipine besylate—500–6000; Telmisartan—1000–8000
Recovery (%): 99.20–101.10 for both the compounds

References: A.B. Thomas, S.N. Jagdale, R.K. Nanda, L.P. Kothapalli and A.D. Deshpande, *J. Pharm. Res.*, **10(2)**, 66–72, 2011.

Comments:

- The method validated for accuracy, precision, linearity, LOD, LOQ, specificity and robustness.
- The method is stability indicating (acid, base, oxidative, thermal, photolytic). The degradation products were separated from main compounds.

HPTLC : High Performance Thin Layer Chromatography
HPTLC Densitogram

No. 35

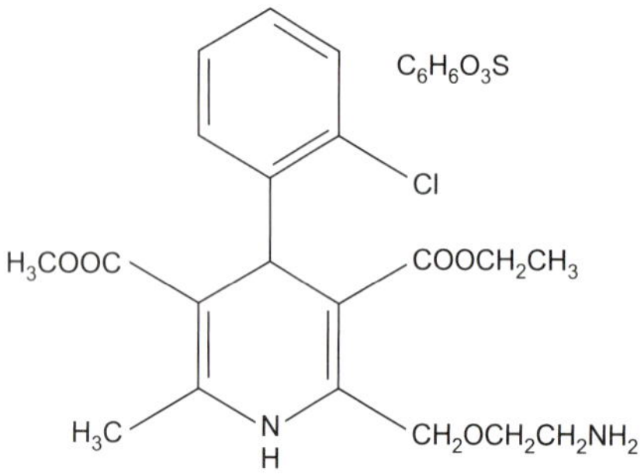

$C_6H_6O_3S$

Cl

H_3COOC

$COOCH_2CH_3$

H_3C

N
H

$CH_2OCH_2CH_2NH_2$

Amlodipine besylate

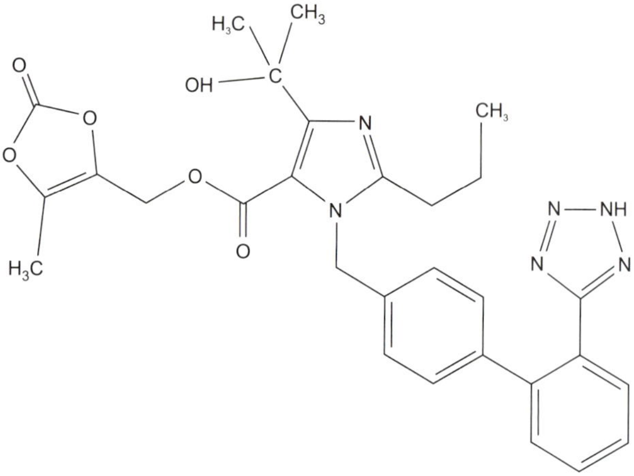

H_3C CH_3

OH C

O O O O N CH_3

N N—NH

H_3C O N N

Olmesartan medoxomil

Detector response ⟶

250
200
150
100
50
0

1
2

–0.20 0.00 0.20 0.40 0.60 0.80

Rf ⟶

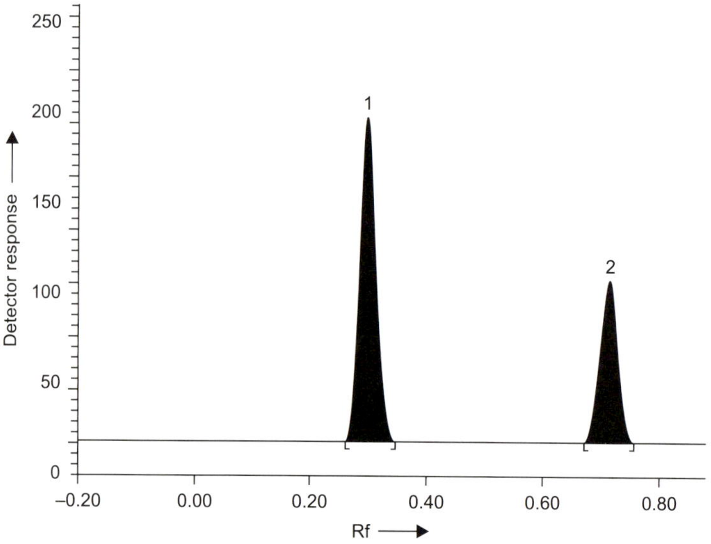

Typical densitogram of the sample containing amlodipine besylate and olmesartan medoxomil. For detailed experimental and chromatographic conditions, refer to Protocol No. 35. Peaks identification: 1. Amlodipine besylate; 2. Olmesartan medoxomil.

PROTOCOL FOR HPTLC ANALYSIS OF PHARMACEUTICAL FORMULATION

Protocol No. 35

Formulation: Amlodipine besylate, Olmesartan medoxomil

Classification: Cardiovascular System **Dosage form:** Tablets

Standard preparation: Prepare solution of both the drugs in methanol to get 1 mg/ml of amlodipine and 4 mg/ml of olmesartan. Dilute 1 ml to 10 ml with methanol and use for chromatographic analysis.

Sample preparation: Powdered sample equivalent to 10 mg of amlodipine suspended in 20 ml of methanol, sonicated for 30 min, diluted to 25 ml with methanol. Filtered and diluted to get 100 μg/ml and 400 μg/ml for amlodipine and olmesartan. Apply 2 μl for chromatographic analysis.

Chromatographic equipments:

Sample applicator: Camag Linomat–V
Development chamber: Camag twin-trough glass chamber, 10 × 10 cm
Densitometric scanner: Camag TLC Scanner–III

Chromatographic conditions:

1. Stationary phase: Silica gel 60F_{254} pre-coated TLC plates, 10 × 10 cm (250 μm) – Merck, pre-washed with methanol, dried at 110°C for 15 min prior to use
2. Mobile phase (MP): n-butanol–glacial acetic acid–water (5 : 1 : 0.1 v/v)
3. Standard/Sample application:
   Band length: 5 mm Volume applied: 2–10 μl Spacing: 5 mm
4. Chamber saturation: 30 min (MP)
5. RH (%): 60 ± 5
6. Temperature °C: 25 ± 2
7. Separation technique: Ascending
8. Quantity of mobile phase: 12 ml
9. Migration distance: 80 mm
10. Migration time: 20 min

Densitometric evaluation:

Wavelength: UV–254 nm Scanning mode: Reflectance/Absorbance
HRF: Amlodipine besylate—30; Olmesartan medoxomil—72
Linearity (ng/band): Amlodipine besylate—100–1000; Olmesartan medoxomil—400–4000
Recovery (%): 97.10–98.3 for both the drugs

References: Asmita Y. Kamble, Mahadev V. Mahadik, Laxam D. Khalat and Sunil R. Dhaneshwar, *Anal. Letters*, **43**, 251–258, 2010.

Comments:

- The method validated for accuracy, precision, linearity, LOD, LOQ, specificity, robustness and ruggedness.
- The sample was also analysed by validated RP-HPLC method. The results by both the methods were comparable.

HPTLC : High Performance Thin Layer Chromatography
HPTLC Densitogram

No. 36

Amlodipine besylate

Olmesartan medoxomil

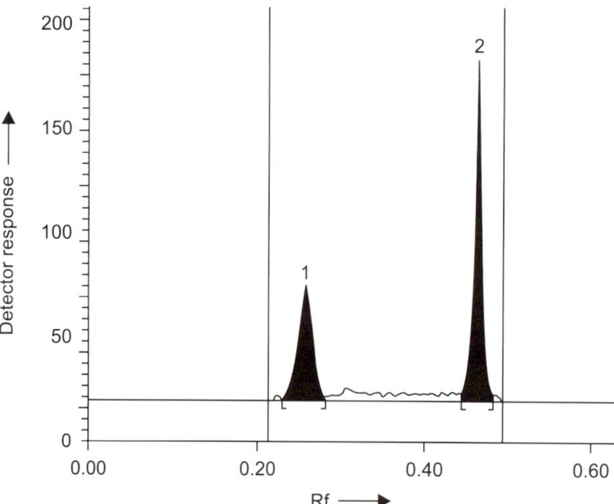

Typical densitogram of the sample containing amlodipine besylate and olmesartan medoxomil. For detailed experimental and chromatographic conditions, refer to Protocol No. 36. Peaks identification: 1. Amlodipine besylate; 2. Olmesartan medoxomil.

PROTOCOL FOR HPTLC ANALYSIS OF PHARMACEUTICAL FORMULATION

Protocol No. 36

Formulation: **Amlodipine besylate, Olmesartan medoxomil**

Classification: Cardiovascular System **Dosage form:** Tablets

Standard preparation: Prepare 1 mg/ml solution of each compound separately in methanol. Further serial dilutions are made for linearity profile. Apply 10 μl of each solution.

Sample preparation: Powdered sample equivalent to 5 mg of amlodipine suspended in methanol, sonicated for 5 min, diluted to 100 ml, filtered and filtrate used for chromatographic analysis.

Chromatographic equipments:

Sample applicator: Camag Linomat–V

Development chamber: Camag twin-trough glass chamber, 20 × 10 cm

Densitometric scanner: Camag TLC Scanner–III

Chromatographic conditions:

1. Stationary phase: Silica gel 60F_{254} pre-coated TLC plates, 20 × 10 cm (250 μm) – Merck, pre-washed with methanol, dried at 110°C for 5 min prior to use
2. Mobile phase (MP): Chloroform–methanol–toluene–acetic acid (8 : 1 : 1 : 0.1 v/v)
3. Standard/Sample application:
   Band length: 8 mm Volume applied: 10 μl Spacing: 10 mm
4. Chamber saturation: 20 min (MP)
5. RH (%): 60 ± 5
6. Temperature °C: 25 ± 2
7. Separation technique: Ascending
8. Quantity of mobile phase: 20 ml
9. Migration distance: —
10. Migration time: —

Densitometric evaluation:

Wavelength: UV–254 nm Scanning mode: Reflectance/Absorbance

HRF: Amlodipine besylate—25; Olmesartan medoxomil—45

Linearity (ng/band): Amlodipine besylate—200–1400; Olmesartan medoxomil—800–5600

Recovery (%): 98.0–102 for both the compounds

References: Dhanshri J. Desai, Archana S. More, Aniruddha R. Chabukswar, B.S. Kuchekar, Swati C. Jagdale and Pradeep D. Lokhande, *Der Pharma Chemica*, **2(4)**, 135–141, 2010.

Comments: The method validated for accuracy, precision, linearity, LOD, LOQ, specificity, robustness and ruggedness.

HPTLC : High Performance Thin Layer Chromatography
HPTLC Densitogram

No. 37

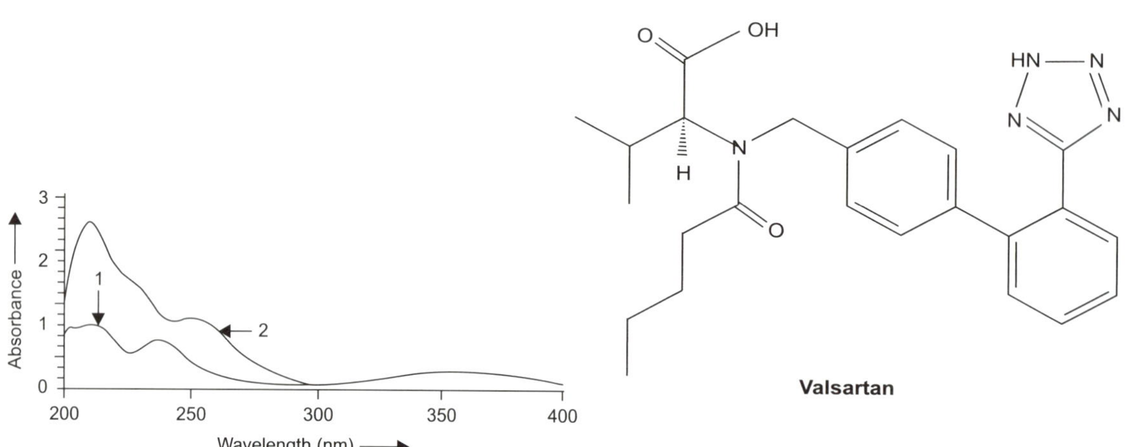

Overlaid UV-spectra of amlodipine (1) and valsartan (2) for selection of suitable wavelength for densitometric scanning

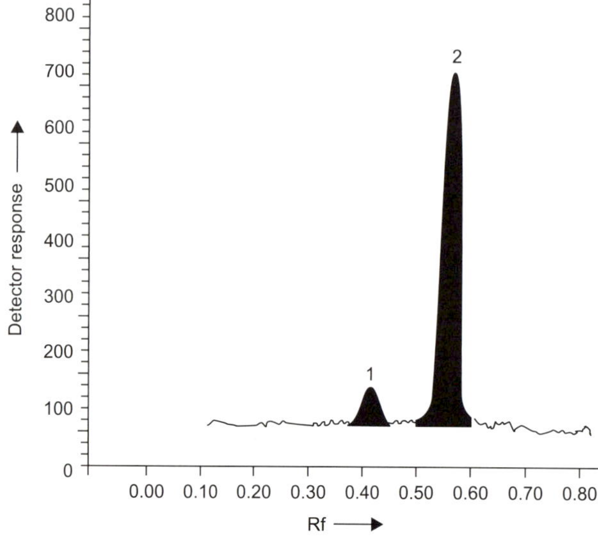

Typical densitogram of the sample containing amlodipine besylate and valsartan. For detailed experimental and chromatographic conditions, refer to Protocol No. 37. Peaks identification: 1. Amlodipine besylate; 2. Valsartan.

PROTOCOL FOR HPTLC ANALYSIS OF PHARMACEUTICAL FORMULATION

Protocol No. 37

Formulation: Amlodipine besylate, Valsartan

Classification: Cardiovascular System **Dosage form:** Tablets

Standard preparation: Prepare 1 mg/ml solution of amlodipine besylate and 16 mg/ml of valsartan, both in methanol. Further diluted to get 0.1 mg/ml (amlodipine besylate) and 1.6 mg/ml (valsartan). Apply 1–6 μl for linearity.

Sample preparation: Powdered sample equivalent to 10 mg of amlodipine suspended in 20 ml of methanol, sonicated for 30 min, diluted to 25 ml, centrifuged (3000 rpm) for 5 min. 2.5 ml of supernatant suitably diluted to get 100 μg/ml (amlodipine) and 1600 μg/ml (valsartan). Apply 2 μl for chromatographic analysis.

Chromatographic equipments:

Sample applicator: Camag Linomat–IV

Development chamber: Camag twin-trough glass chamber, 10 × 10 cm

Densitometric scanner: Camag TLC Scanner–III

Chromatographic conditions:

1. Stationary phase: Silica gel $60F_{254}$ pre-coated HPTLC plates, 10 × 10 cm (200 μm) – Merck
2. Mobile phase (MP): Toluene–methanol–acetic acid (7 : 3 : 0.1 v/v)
3. Standard/Sample application:
   Band length: 5 mm Volume applied: 2 μl Spacing: 7 mm
4. Chamber saturation: 30 min (MP)
5. RH (%): 60 ± 5
6. Temperature °C: 25 ± 2
7. Separation technique: Ascending
8. Quantity of mobile phase: 10 ml
9. Migration distance: 80 mm
10. Migration time: —

Densitometric evaluation:

Wavelength: UV–244 nm Scanning mode: Reflectance/Absorbance

HRF: Amlodipine besylate—41; Valsartan—54

Linearity (ng/band): Amlodipine besylate—100–600; Valsartan—1600–9600

Recovery (%): Amlodipine besylate—98.69–100.40; Valsartan—98.54–100.03

References: Sunil R. Dhaneshwar, Narendra G. Patre and Mahadeo V. Mahadek, *Chromatographia*, **69(1, 2)**, 157–161, 2009.

Comments: The method validated for accuracy, precision, linearity, LOD, LOQ, specificity and robustness.

HPTLC : High Performance Thin Layer Chromatography
HPTLC Densitogram

No. 38

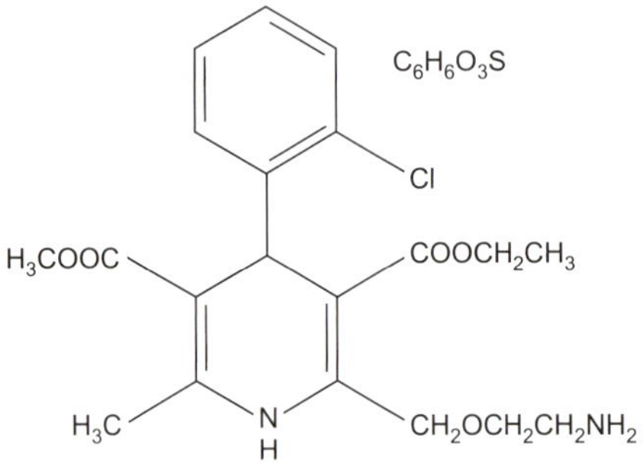

$C_6H_6O_3S$ Cl H_3COOC $COOCH_2CH_3$ H_3C N H $CH_2OCH_2CH_2NH_2$

Amlodipine besylate

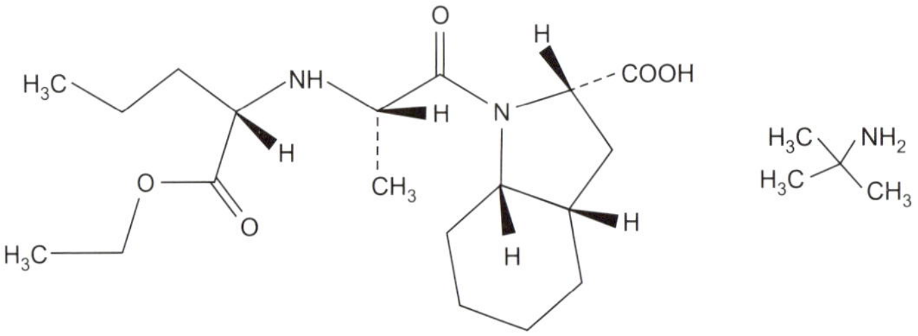

O H COOH H_3C NH H N H CH_3 O O H_3C H H H_3C NH_2 H_3C CH_3

Perindopril erbumine

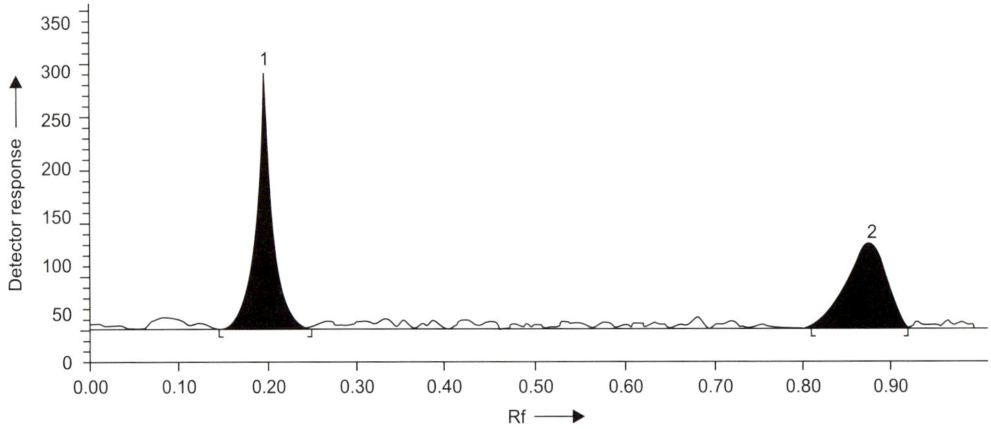

Detector response → 350 300 250 200 150 100 50 0 1 2 0.00 0.10 0.20 0.30 0.40 0.50 0.60 0.70 0.80 0.90 Rf →

Typical densitogram of the sample containing amlodipine besylate and perindopril erbumine. For detailed experimental and chromatographic conditions, refer to Protocol No. 38. Peaks identification: 1. Amlodipine besylate; 2. Perindopril erbumine.

PROTOCOL FOR HPTLC ANALYSIS OF PHARMACEUTICAL FORMULATION

Protocol No. 38

Formulation: Amlodipine besylate, Perindopril erbumine

Classification: Cardiovascular System **Dosage form:** Tablets

Standard preparation: Prepare 250 μg/ml solution of each compound separately in methanol. Further dilutions suitably made for linearity studies.

Sample preparation: Powdered sample equivalent to 10 mg of perindopril erbumine suspended in 5 ml of methanol, sonicated, diluted to 10 ml, filtered. Apply 9 μl of the solution for assay of amlodipine besylate. Dilute 2 ml of above solution to 10 ml and apply 6 μl for assay of perindopril.

Chromatographic equipments:

Sample applicator: Camag Linomat–V

Development chamber: Camag twin-trough glass chamber, 10 × 10 cm

Densitometric scanner: Camag TLC Scanner–III

Chromatographic conditions:

1. Stationary phase: Silica gel 60F_{254} pre-coated TLC plate, 10 × 10 cm (250 μm) – Merck, pre-washed with methanol and dried at 80°C for 5 min prior to use
2. Mobile phase (MP): Dichloromethane–methanol–glacial acetic acid (8.5 : 1.5 : 0.1 v/v)
3. Standard/Sample application:
   Band length: 4 mm Volume applied: 6 μl Spacing: 5 mm
4. Chamber saturation: 15 min (MP)
5. RH (%): 55 ± 5
6. Temperature °C: 22 ± 2
7. Separation technique: Ascending
8. Quantity of mobile phase: 10 ml
9. Migration distance: 90 mm
10. Migration time: 20 min

Densitometric evaluation:

Wavelength: UV–238 nm Scanning mode: Reflectance/Absorbance

HRF: Amlodipine besylate—20; Perindopril erbumine—89

Linearity (ng/band): Amlodipine besylate—6000–18000; Perindopril erbumine—500–2500

Recovery (%): 99.60–99.76 for both the compounds

References: T.C. Borole, S.P. Gandhi, A.V. Ladke and M.C. Damle, *The Pharma Review*, 113–116, 2011.

Comments: The method validated for accuracy, precision, linearity, LOD, LOQ, specificity and robustness.

HPTLC : High Performance Thin Layer Chromatography
HPTLC Densitogram

No. 39

$C_6H_6O_3S$

Amlodipine besylate

Losartan potassium

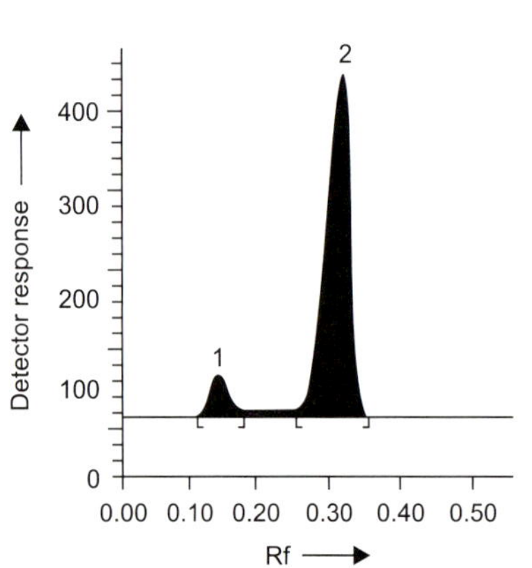

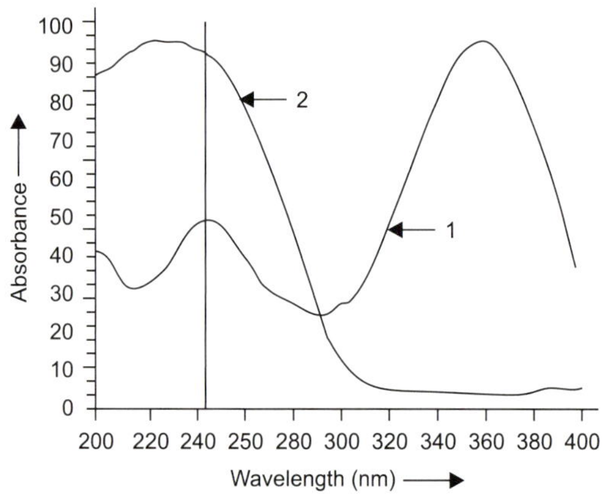

In-situ overlaid spectra of amlodipine besylate (1) and losartan (2) for selection of suitable wavelength for densitogram scanning

Typical densitogram of the standard containing amlodipine besylate and losartan K^+. For detailed experimental and chromatographic conditions, refer to Protocol No. 39. Peaks identification: 1. Amlodipine besylate; 2. Losartan K^+.

PROTOCOL FOR HPTLC ANALYSIS OF PHARMACEUTICAL FORMULATION

Protocol No. 39

Formulation: Amlodipine besylate, Losartan potassium

Classification: Cardiovascular System **Dosage form:** Tablets

Standard preparation: Prepare 100 μg/ml solution of amlodipine and 1000 μg/ml solution of losartan potassium in methanol to use for analysis.

Sample preparation: Powdered sample equivalent to 50 mg of atenolol or losartan potassium suspended in 40 ml of methanol, sonicated for 30 min, diluted to 50 ml with methanol, filtered through Whatman No. 41 filter paper. Filtrate to be used for analysis.

Chromatographic equipments:

Sample applicator: Camag Linomat–IV

Development chamber: Camag twin-trough glass chamber, 20 × 10 cm

Densitometric scanner: Camag TLC Scanner–III

Chromatographic conditions:

1. Stationary phase: Silica gel $60F_{254}$ pre-coated HPTLC plates, 20 × 10 cm (200 μm) – Merck, pre-washed with methanol, dried (110°C) for 30 min, prior to use
2. Mobile phase (MP): Toluene–methanol–chloroform (2 : 2.5 : 5.5 v/v)
3. Standard/Sample application:
   Band length: 4 mm Volume applied: 7 μl Spacing: 4 mm
4. Chamber saturation: 30 min (MP)
5. RH (%): 55 ± 5
6. Temperature °C: 25 ± 5
7. Separation technique: Ascending
8. Quantity of mobile phase: —
9. Migration distance: 80 mm
10. Migration time: —

Densitometric evaluation:

Wavelength: UV–254 nm

Scanning mode: Reflectance/Absorbance

HRF: Amlodipine besylate—14; Losartan K^+—32

Linearity (ng/band): Amlodipine besylate—250–1000; Losartan—500–2000

Recovery (%): 100.74–101.15 for both the compounds

References: K.R. Mahadik, H. Aggrawal and N. Kaul, *Indian Drugs*, **41(1)**, 32–35, 2004.

Comments: The method validated for accuracy, precision, linearity, LOD, LOQ and specificity.

HPTLC : High Performance Thin Layer Chromatography
HPTLC Densitogram

No. 40

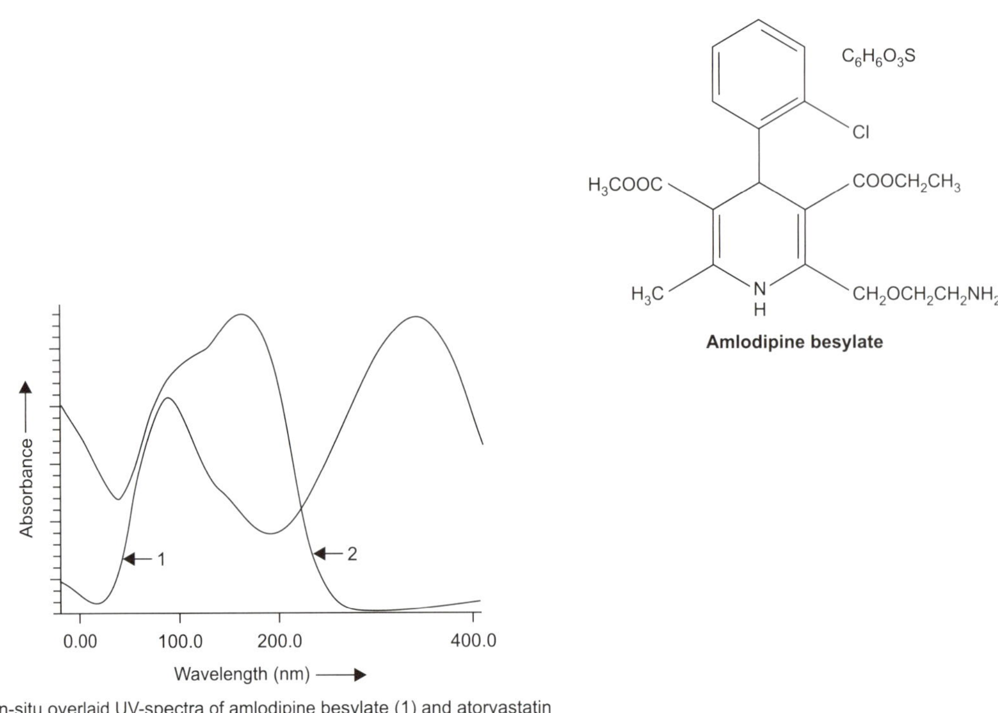

In-situ overlaid UV-spectra of amlodipine besylate (1) and atorvastatin calcium (2) for selection of suitable wavelength for densitogram scanning

Detector response
600.0
500.0
400.0
300.0
200.0
100.0
0.0
1
2
0.00 0.15 0.30 0.45 0.60 0.75
Rf

Typical densitogram of the sample containing amlodipine besylate and atorvastatin calcium. For detailed experimental and chromatographic conditions, refer to Protocol No. 40. Peaks identification: 1. Amlodipine besylate; 2. Atorvastatin Ca^{++}.

PROTOCOL FOR HPTLC ANALYSIS OF PHARMACEUTICAL FORMULATION

Protocol No. 40

Formulation: **Amlodipine besylate, Atorvastatin calcium**

Classification: Cardiovascular System **Dosage form:** Tablets

Standard preparation: Prepare 1 mg/ml solution of each compound in methanol. To prepare mixed standard solution, take 2 ml of amlodipine solution and 1 ml of atorvastatin solution, dilute to 10 ml with methanol to use for chromatographic application.

Sample preparation: Powdered sample equivalent to 5 mg of amlodipine besylate and 10 mg of atorvastatin calcium suspended in methanol, sonicated for 10 min, diluted, filtered, the filtrate containing 1 mg/ml of atorvastatin calcium and 500 μg/ml of amlodipine besylate suitably diluted for chromatographic analysis.

Chromatographic equipments:

Sample applicator: Camag Linomat–IV

Development chamber: Camag twin-trough glass chamber, 20 × 10 cm

Densitometric scanner: Camag TLC Scanner–III

Chromatographic conditions:

1. Stationary phase: Silica gel $60F_{254}$ pre-coated TLC plates, 10 × 10 cm (250 μm) – Merck
2. Mobile phase (MP): Ethyl acetate–1,4-dioxane–methanol–25% ammonia (10 : 1 : 2 : 1 v/v)
3. Standard/Sample application:
   Band length: 5 mm Volume applied: 5 μl Spacing: 10 mm
4. Chamber saturation: 30 min (MP)
5. RH (%): 60 ± 5
6. Temperature °C: 25 ± 2
7. Separation technique: Ascending
8. Quantity of mobile phase: 14 ml
9. Migration distance: 70 mm
10. Migration time: 25 min

Densitometric evaluation:

Wavelength: UV–254 nm Scanning mode: Reflectance/Absorbance

HRF: Amlodipine besylate—42; Atorvastatin Ca^{++}—68

Linearity (ng/band): Amlodipine besylate—400–2000; Atorvastatin—200–1000

Recovery (%): 100–104 for both the compounds

References: M.G. Pai, Swati Bhende and Rajashree Gude, Personal communication Dr. Rajashree Gude, Goa College of Pharmacy.

Comments: The method validated for accuracy, precision, linearity LOD, LOQ, specificity ruggedness and robustness.

HPTLC : High Performance Thin Layer Chromatography
HPTLC Densitogram

No. 41

Atorvastatin calcium

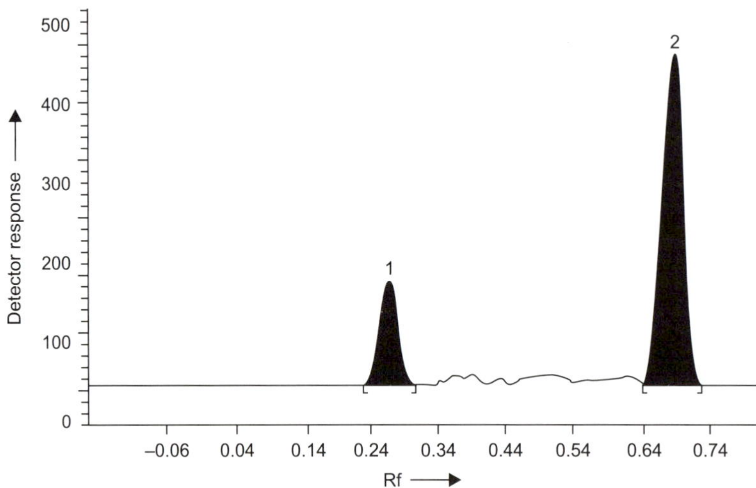

Typical densitogram of the standard containing amlodipine besylate and atorvastatin calcium. For detailed experimental and chromatographic conditions, refer to Protocol No. 41. Peaks identification: 1. Amlodipine besylate; 2. Atorvastatin Ca^{++}.

PROTOCOL FOR HPTLC ANALYSIS OF PHARMACEUTICAL FORMULATION

Protocol No. 41

Formulation: Amlodipine besylate, Atorvastatin calcium

Classification: Cardiovascular System **Dosage form:** Tablets

Standard preparation: Prepare 1 mg/ml solution of each compound in methanol. Further serial dilutions made with methanol to get different concentrations. Apply 10 μl of each solution for chromatographic analysis.

Sample preparation: Powdered sample equivalent to 10 mg of atorvastatin or 5 mg of amlodipine suspended in methanol, sonicated for 30 min, filtered, filtrate suitably diluted to get 500 μg/ml (atorvastatin) and 250 μg/ml (amlodipine) to use for assay.

Chromatographic equipments:

Sample applicator: Camag Linomat–V
Development chamber: Camag twin-trough glass chamber, 20 × 10 cm
Densitometric scanner: Camag TLC Scanner–III

Chromatographic conditions:

1. Stationary phase: Silica gel $60F_{254}$ pre-coated the plates, 10 × 10 cm (200 μm) – Merck, pre-washed with methanol to activated (60°C) for 5 min, prior to use
2. Mobile phase (MP): Chloroform–toluene–methanol–acetic acid (7 : 3 : 3 : 0.3 v/v)
3. Standard/Sample application:
   Band length: 7 mm Volume applied: 10 μl Spacing: 10 mm
4. Chamber saturation: 30 min (MP)
5. RH (%): 60 ± 5
6. Temperature °C: 25 ± 2
7. Separation technique: Ascending
8. Quantity of mobile phase: 26 ml
9. Migration distance: 75 mm
10. Migration time: 30 min

Densitometric evaluation:

Wavelength: UV–254 nm Scanning mode: Reflectance/Absorbance
HRF: Amlodipine besylate—28; Atorvastatin Ca^{++}—68
Linearity (ng/band): Amlodipine besylate—100–1500; Atorvastatin—100–1200
Recovery (%): Atorvastatin Ca^{++}—99.84–101.25; Amlodipine besylate—99.51–100.35

References: B.G. Chaudhari, N.M. Patel and P.B. Shah, *Indian Drugs*, **43(8)**, 649–654, 2006.

Comments:

- The method validated for accuracy, precision, linearity, LOD, LOQ, specificity and robustness.
- The method was suitable for impurity profile.

HPTLC : High Performance Thin Layer Chromatography
HPTLC Densitogram

No. 42

$C_6H_6O_3S$
Cl
H_3COOC
$COOCH_2CH_3$
H_3C
N
H
$CH_2OCH_2CH_2NH_2$

Amlodipine besylate

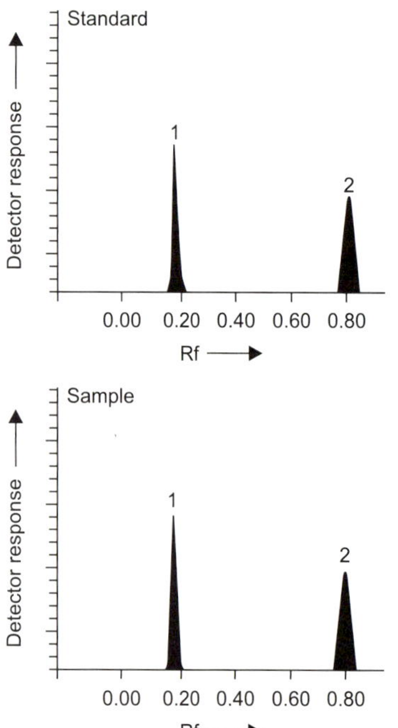

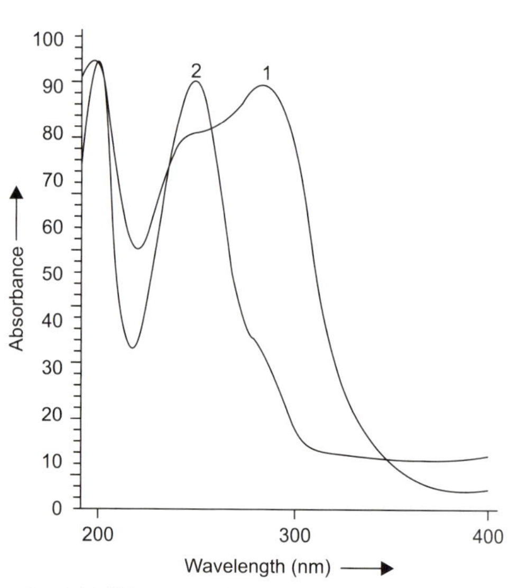

Overlaid UV-spectra of amlodipine (2) and atorvastatin (1) for selection of suitable wavelength for densitometric scanning

Typical densitogram of the standard and the sample containing atorvastatin and amlodipine besylate. For detailed experimental and chromatographic conditions, refer to Protocol No. 42. Peaks identification: 1. Atorvastatin Ca^{++}; 2. Amlodipine besylate.

PROTOCOL FOR HPTLC ANALYSIS OF PHARMACEUTICAL FORMULATION

Protocol No. 42

Formulation: Amlodipine besylate, Atorvastatin calcium

Classification: Cardiovascular System **Dosage form:** Tablets

Standard preparation: Prepare 1 mg/ml solution of each compound in methanol separately. Further serial dilutions are made with methanol for linearity studies. Apply 10 μl of each solution for analysis.

Sample preparation: Powdered sample equivalent to 5 mg of amlodipine is suspended in 8 ml of methanol, sonicated for 15 min, diluted to 10 ml, filtered and 1 ml of filtrate diluted to 10 ml with methanol and apply 10 μl for chromatographic analysis.

Chromatographic equipments:

Sample applicator: Camag Linomat–V

Development chamber: Camag automatic development chamber saturated with camag saturation pad

Densitometric scanner: Camag TLC Scanner–III

Chromatographic conditions:

1. Stationary phase: Silica gel $60F_{254}$ pre-coated TLC plate-glass, 20 × 10 cm (200 μm) – Merck
2. Mobile phase (MP): Chloroform–methanol–acetone–25% ammonia (18 : 6 : 10 : 3 v/v)
3. Standard/Sample application:
   Band length: 8 mm Volume applied: 10 μl Spacing: 10 mm
4. Chamber saturation: 20 min (MP)
5. RH (%): 55 ± 5
6. Temperature °C: 25 ± 2
7. Separation technique: Ascending
8. Quantity of mobile phase: 35 ml
9. Migration distance: 70 mm
10. Migration time: 8 min

Densitometric evaluation:

Wavelength: UV–240 nm Scanning mode: Reflectance/Absorbance

HRF: Atorvastatin—19; Amlodipine besylate—80

Linearity (ng/band): Amlodipine besylate—200–1000; Atorvastatin calcium—500–2000

Recovery (%): —

References: —

Comments: The method was optimized and analytical work carried out at **Anchrom's HPTLC Application Laboratory**, Mumbai, India.

HPTLC : High Performance Thin Layer Chromatography
HPTLC Densitogram

No. 43

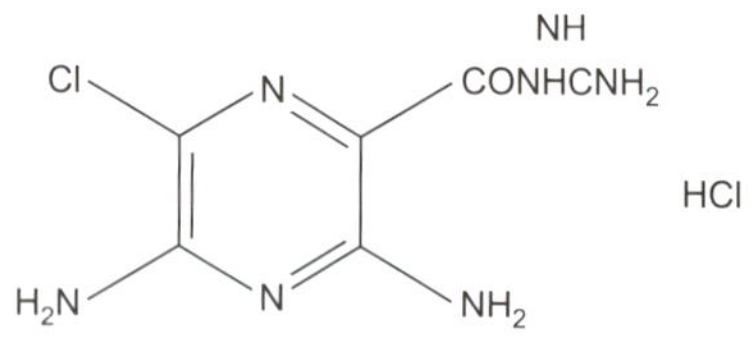

Amiloride hydrochloride

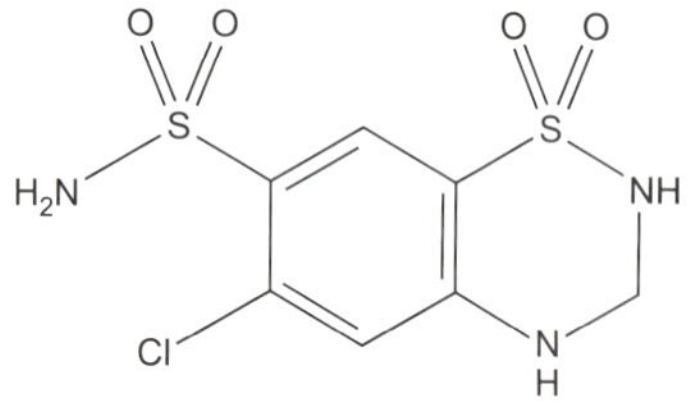

Hydrochlorothiazide

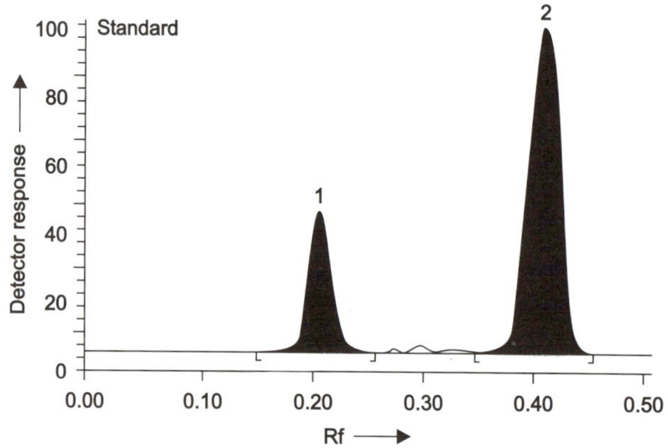

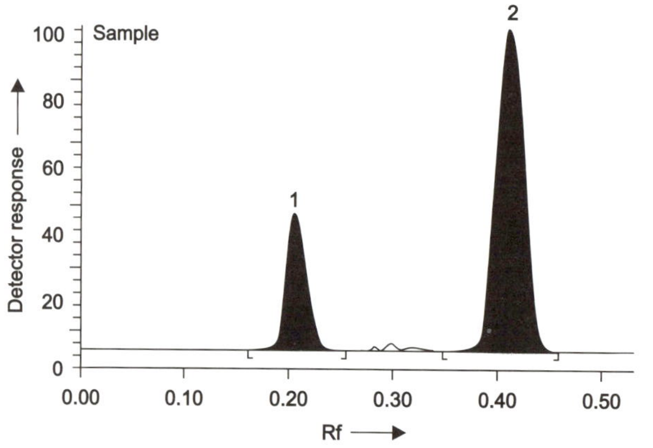

Typical densitogram of the sample and standard containing hydrochlorothiazide and amiloride hydrochloride. For detailed experimental and chromatographic conditions, refer to Protocol No. 43. Peaks identification: 1. Amiloride HCl; 2. Hydrochlorothiazide.

PROTOCOL FOR HPTLC ANALYSIS OF PHARMACEUTICAL FORMULATION

Protocol No. 43

Formulation: Hydrochlorothiazide, Amiloride hydrochloride

Classification: Cardiovascular System **Dosage form:** Tablets

Standard preparation: Dissolve 5 mg of amiloride hydrochloride and 50 mg of hydrochlorothiazide in 50 ml of methanol. Dilute 1 ml of the resulting solution to 10 ml with methanol and use for analysis.

Sample preparation: Powdered sample equivalent to 5 mg of amiloride HCl suspended in 30–35 ml of methanol, sonicate for 5 min, dilute to 50 ml with methanol, filter and dilute 1 ml of the filtrate to 10 ml with methanol to use for assay.

Chromatographic equipments:

Sample applicator: Camag Linomat–IV

Development chamber: Camag twin-trough glass chamber, 10 × 10 cm

Densitometric scanner: Camag TLC Scanner–II

Chromatographic conditions:

1. Stationary phase: Silica gel 60F_{254} pre-coated HPTLC plates, 5 × 10 cm (200 μm) – Merck
2. Mobile phase (MP): Chloroform–methanol–25% ammonia (8 : 2.6 : 0.2 v/v)
3. Standard/Sample application:
   Band length: 8 mm Volume applied: 4 μl Spacing: 10 mm
4. Chamber saturation: 20 min (MP)
5. RH (%): 55 ± 5
6. Temperature °C: 22 ± 2
7. Separation technique: Ascending
8. Quantity of mobile phase: 10.8 ml
9. Migration distance: 50 mm
10. Migration time: 12 min

Densitometric evaluation:

Wavelength: UV–290 nm Scanning mode: Reflectance/Absorbance

HRF: Amiloride HCl—22; Hydrochlorothiazide—42

Linearity (ng/band): Amiloride HCl—10–100; Hydrochlorothiazide—50–500

Recovery (%): 99.68–103.60 for both the compounds

References: —

Comments:

- The method was optimized and analytical work carried out at **Anchrom's HPTLC Application Laboratory**, Mumbai, India.
- The MP consisting of ethyl acetate–methanol–25% ammonia (7.5 : 1.0 : 0.8 v/v) also gave good resolution.

HPTLC : High Performance Thin Layer Chromatography
HPTLC Densitogram

No. 44

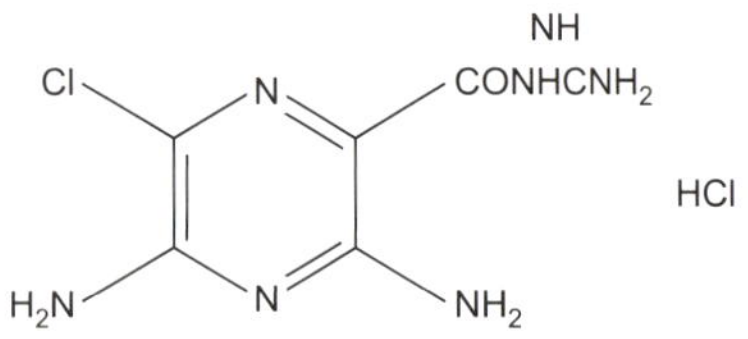

Amiloride hydrochloride

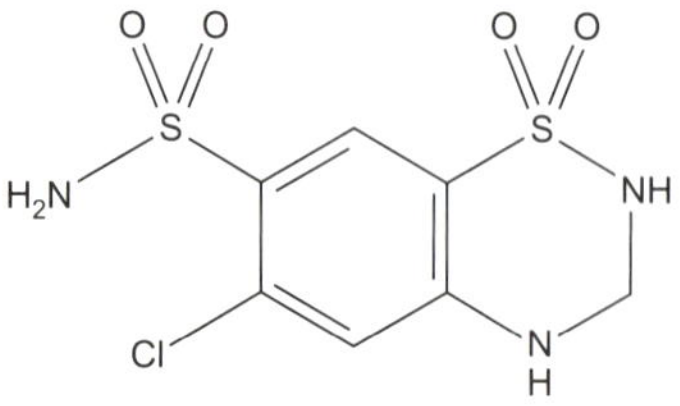

Hydrochlorothiazide

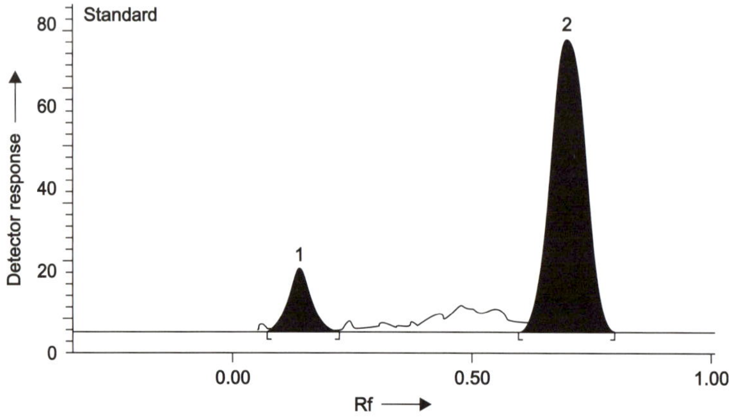

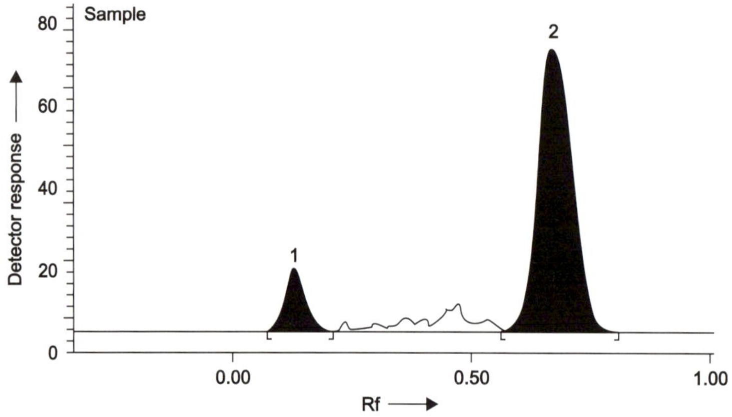

Typical densitogram of the sample and standard containing hydrochlorothiazide and amiloride hydrochloride. For detailed experimental and chromatographic conditions, refer to Protocol No. 44. Peaks identification: 1. Amiloride HCl; 2. Hydrochlorothiazide.

PROTOCOL FOR HPTLC ANALYSIS OF PHARMACEUTICAL FORMULATION

Protocol No. 44

Formulation: Hydrochlorothiazide, Amiloride hydrochloride

Classification: Cardiovascular System **Dosage form:** Tablets

Standard preparation: Dissolve 5 mg of amiloride hydrochloride and 50 mg of hydrochlorothiazide in 50 ml of methanol. Dilute 1 ml of the resulting solution to 10 ml with methanol and use for analysis.

Sample preparation: Powdered sample equivalent to 5 mg of amiloride HCl suspended in 30–35 ml of methanol, sonicated for 5 min, diluted to 50 ml, filtered and 1 ml of filtrate diluted to 10 ml with methanol for assay.

Chromatographic equipments:

Sample applicator: Camag Linomat–IV

Development chamber: Camag twin-trough glass chamber, 10 × 10 cm

Densitometric scanner: Camag TLC Scanner–II

Chromatographic conditions:

1. Stationary phase: Silica gel 60 RP–18F_{254s} pre-coated HPTLC plates, 10 × 10 cm (200 μm) – Mcrck
2. Mobile phase (MP): 0.5 M sodium chloride–methanol–glacial acetic acid (12 : 8 : 0.01 v/v)
3. Standard/Sample application:
   Band length: 50 mm Volume applied: 4 μl Spacing: 80 mm
4. Chamber saturation: 30 min (MP)
5. RH (%): 55 ± 5
6. Temperature °C: 22 ± 2
7. Separation technique: Ascending
8. Quantity of mobile phase: 20 ml
9. Migration distance: 50 mm
10. Migration time: 40 min

Densitometric evaluation:

Wavelength: UV–290 nm Scanning mode: Reflectance/Absorbance

HRF: Amiloride HCl—14; Hydrochlorothiazide—70

Linearity (ng/band): Amiloride HCl—10–100; Hydrochlorothiazide—50–500

Recovery (%): 98.70–102.5 for both the compounds

References: —

Comments:

- The method was optimized and analytical work carried out at **Anchrom's HPTLC Application Laboratory**, Mumbai, India.
- The RP-HPTLC analysis carried out on silicon oil impregnated (5% silicon oil in pet. ether). HPTLC pre-coated RP-18 plates gave equally good separation for quantitative analysis.
- No reversal of retention order was observed in RP-HPTLC.

HPTLC : High Performance Thin Layer Chromatography
HPTLC Densitogram

No. 45

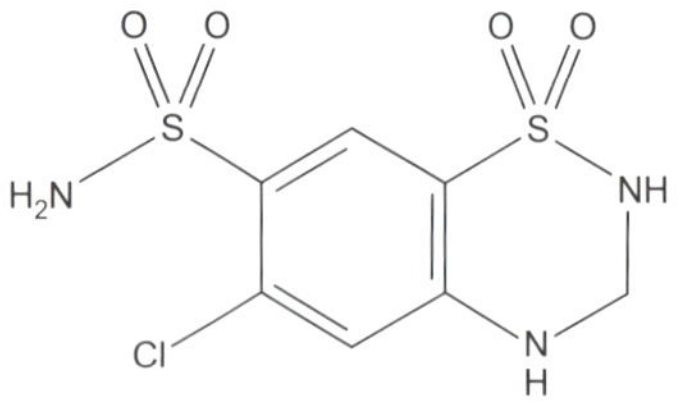

Hydrochlorothiazide

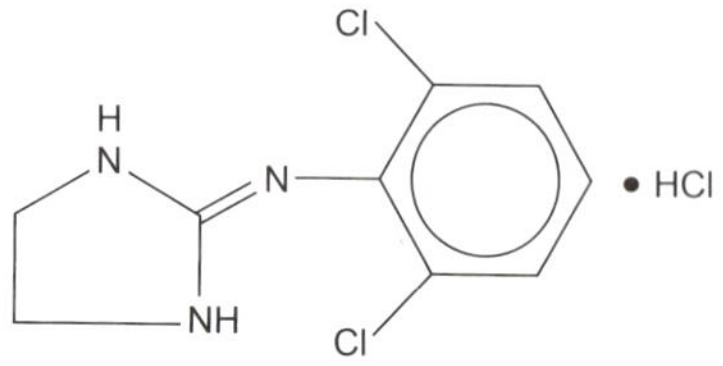

Clonidine hydrochloride

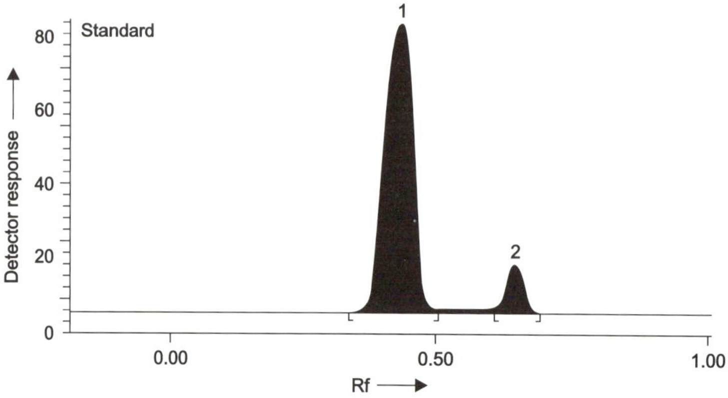

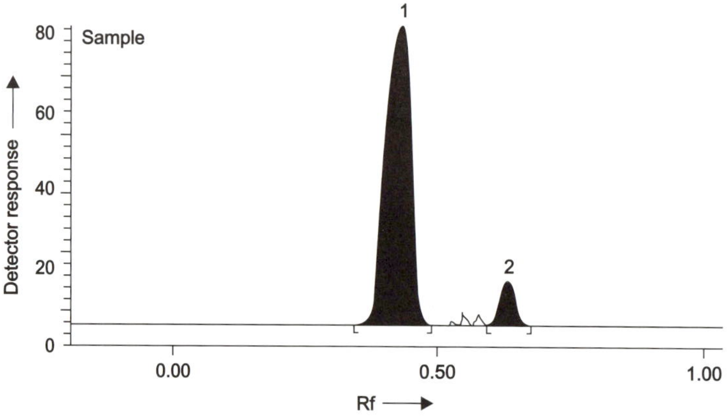

Typical densitogram of the sample and standard containing hydrochlorothiazide and clonidine hydrochloride. For detailed experimental and chromatographic conditions, refer to Protocol No. 45. Peaks identification: 1. Hydrochlorothiazide; 2. Clonidine HCl.

PROTOCOL FOR HPTLC ANALYSIS OF PHARMACEUTICAL FORMULATION

Protocol No. 45

Formulation: Hydrochlorothiazide, Clonidine hydrochloride
Classification: Cardiovascular System **Dosage form:** Tablets
Standard preparation: (1) Prepare 1 mg/ml solution of clonidine in methanol; (2) prepare 1 mg/ml solution of hydrochlorothiazide in methanol; (3) dilute 0.5 ml of solution-1 to 10 ml; (4) mix 0.5 ml of solution-2 and 0.1 ml of solution-3 and dilute to 10 ml with methanol and use for analysis.
Sample preparation: Powdered sample equivalent to 10 mg of hydrochlorothiazide suspended in 6–7 ml of methanol, sonicate, dilute to 10 ml. Filter and dilute 0.5 ml of filtrate to 10 ml with methanol for application.
Chromatographic equipments:
Sample applicator: Camag Linomat–IV
Development chamber: Camag twin-trough glass chamber, 10 × 10 cm
Densitometric scanner: Camag TLC Scanner–II
Chromatographic conditions:

1. Stationary phase: Silica gel $60F_{254}$ pre-coated HPTLC plates, 10 × 10 cm (200 μm) – Merck
2. Mobile phase (MP): Toluene–acetone–25% ammonia (5 : 5 : 0.1 v/v)
3. Standard/Sample application:
   Band length: 7 mm Volume applied: 5 μl Spacing: 10 mm
4. Chamber saturation: 20 min (MP)
5. RH (%): 55 ± 5
6. Temperature °C: 22 ± 2
7. Separation technique: Ascending
8. Quantity of mobile phase: 10 ml
9. Migration distance: 55 mm
10. Migration time: 15 min

Densitometric evaluation:
Wavelength: UV–202 nm, Vis-430 nm Scanning mode: Reflectance/Absorbance
HRF: Hydrochlorothiazide—43; Clonidine—63
Linearity (ng/band): Hydrochlorothiazide—50–500; Clonidine HCl—1–10
Recovery (%): 98.0–99.5 for both the drugs
References: —
Comments:

- The method was optimized and analytical work carried out at **Anchrom's HPTLC Application Laboratory**, Mumbai, India.
- The developed plate was first scanned at 202 nm and then dipped in Dragondorff's reagent (1 s). The orange spot corresponding to clonidine scanned at 430 nm.

HPTLC : High Performance Thin Layer Chromatography
HPTLC Densitogram

No. 46

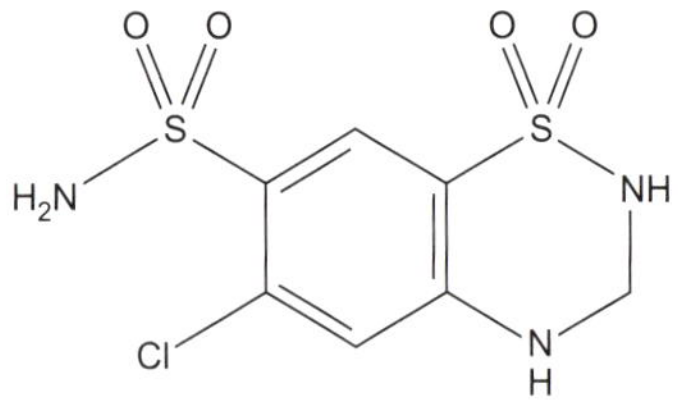

Hydrochlorothiazide

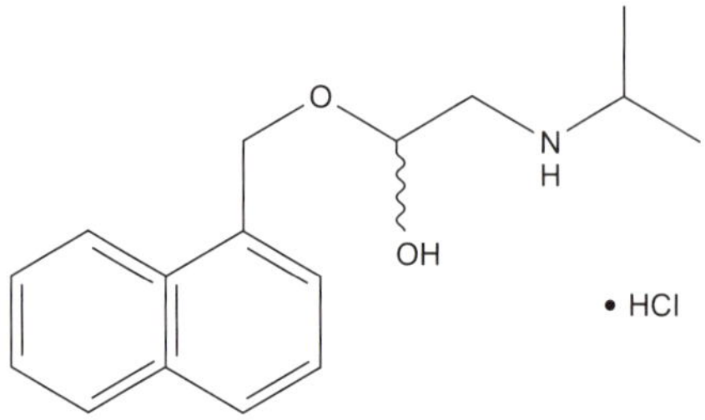

Propranolol HCl

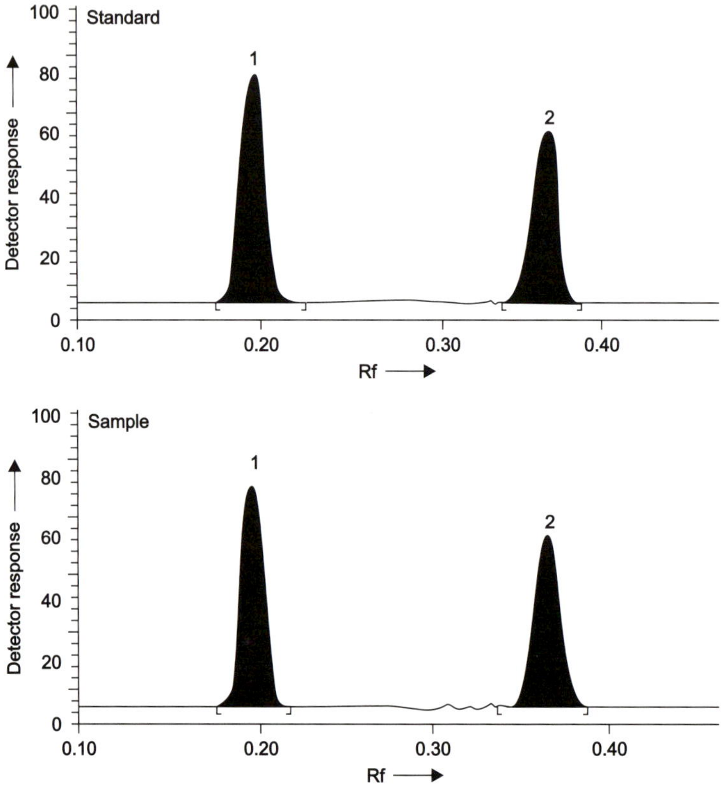

Standard

Detector response →

Rf →

Sample

Detector response →

Rf →

Typical densitogram of the sample and standard containing propranolol HCl and hydrochlorothiazide. For detailed experimental and chromatographic conditions, refer to Protocol No. 46. Peaks identification: 1. Hydrochlorothiazide; 2. Propranolol HCl.

PROTOCOL FOR HPTLC ANALYSIS OF PHARMACEUTICAL FORMULATION

Protocol No. 46

Formulation: **Hydrochlorothiazide, Propranolol hydrochloride**

Classification: Cardiovascular System **Dosage form:** Tablets

Standard preparation: Weigh accurately about 25 mg of hydrochlorothiazide and 40 mg of propranolol hydrochloride, dissolve in methanol to produce 25 ml. Further dilutions made with methanol for analysis.

Sample preparation: Powdered sample equivalent to 25 mg of hydrochlorothiazide suspended in 20 ml of methanol, sonicated for 5 min, dilute to 15 ml with methanol. Filter and dilute 1 ml of the filtrate to 10 ml with methanol for analysis.

Chromatographic equipments:

Sample applicator: Camag Linomat–IV

Development chamber: Camag twin-trough glass chamber, 10 × 10 cm

Densitometric scanner: Camag TLC Scanner–II

Chromatographic conditions:

1. Stationary phase: Silica gel 60F_{254} pre-coated HPTLC plates, 5 × 10 cm (200 μm) – Merck (pre-washed with methanol and dried)
2. Mobile phase (MP): Chloroform–methanol–ammonia (9 : 1 : 0.04 v/v)
3. Standard/Sample application:
   Band length: 80 mm Volume applied: 4 μl Spacing: 10 mm
4. Chamber saturation: 10 min (MP)
5. RH (%): 55 ± 5
6. Temperature °C: 22 ± 2
7. Separation technique: Ascending
8. Quantity of mobile phase: 10.04 ml
9. Migration distance: 50 mm
10. Migration time: 16 min

Densitometric evaluation:

Wavelength: UV–254 nm Scanning mode: Reflectance/Absorbance

HRF: Hydrochlorothiazide—20; Propranolol HCl—37

Linearity (ng/band): Hydrochlorothiazide—200–500; Propranolol HCl—200–750

Recovery (%): 96.75–98.70 for both the compounds

References: —

Comments:

- The method was optimized and analytical work carried out at **Anchrom's HPTLC Application Laboratory**, Mumbai, India.
- The method developed in the laboratory routinely used with good reproducibility.

HPTLC : High Performance Thin Layer Chromatography
HPTLC Densitogram

No. 47

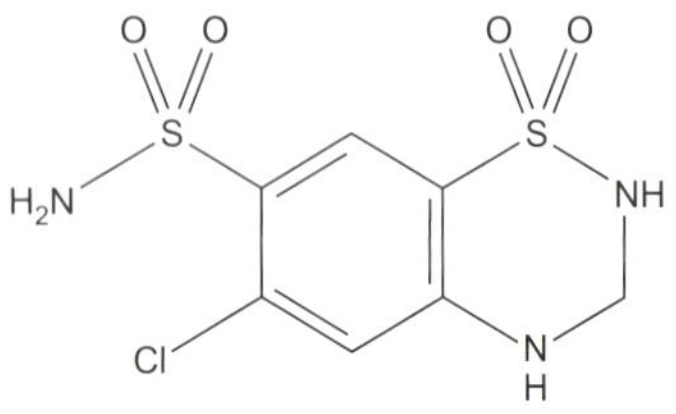

Hydrochlorothiazide

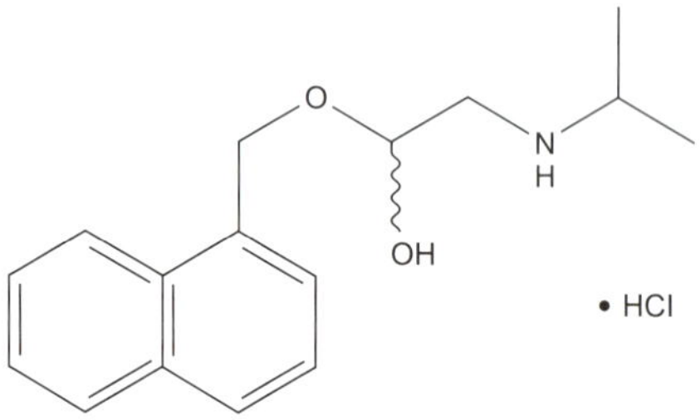

Propranolol HCl

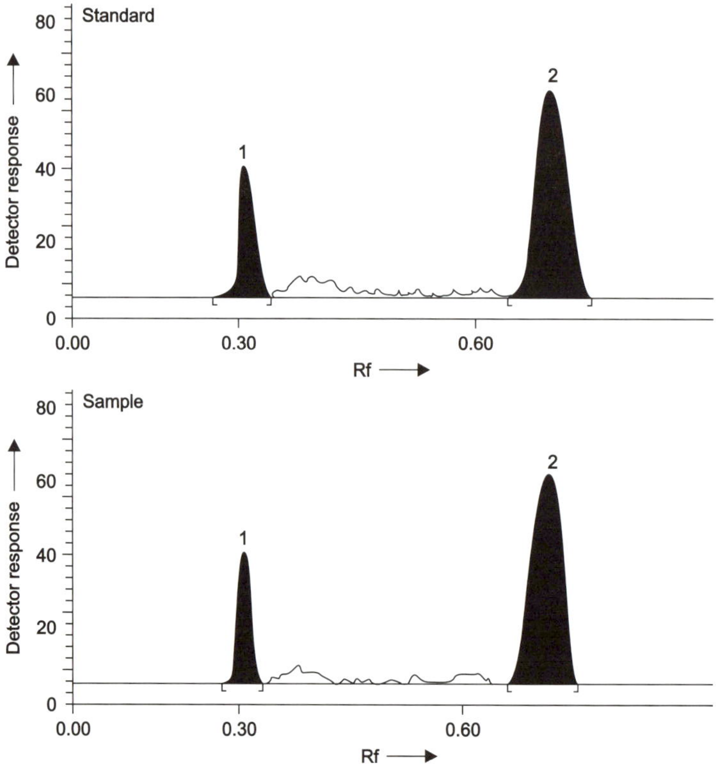

Typical densitogram of the sample and standard containing propranolol HCl and hydrochlorothiazide. For detailed experimental and chromatographic conditions, refer to Protocol No. 47. Peaks identification: 1. Propranolol HCl; 2. Hydrochlorothiazide.

PROTOCOL FOR HPTLC ANALYSIS OF PHARMACEUTICAL FORMULATION

Protocol No. 47

Formulation: Hydrochlorothiazide, Propranolol hydrochloride

Classification: Cardiovascular System **Dosage form:** Tablets

Standard preparation: Prepare 1 mg/ml solution of hydrochlorothiazide and 1.6 mg/ml solution of propranolol hydrochloride, both in methanol. Further dilutions made with methanol for analysis.

Sample preparation: Powdered sample equivalent to 40 mg of propranolol hydrochloride suspended in 20 ml of methanol, sonicated for 5 min, diluted to 25 ml with methanol, filtered and dilute 1 ml of the filtrate to 10 ml with methanol for assay.

Chromatographic equipments:

Sample applicator: Camag Linomat–IV
Development chamber: Camag twin-trough glass chamber, 10 × 10 cm
Densitometric scanner: Camag TLC Scanner–II

Chromatographic conditions:

1. Stationary phase: Silica gel 60 RP–18F_{254s} pre-coated HPTLC plates, 5 × 7.5 cm (200 μm) – Merck
2. Mobile phase (MP): 0.5 M Sodium chloride–methanol–glacial acetic acid (12 : 8 : 0.01 v/v)
3. Standard/Sample application:
   Band length: 8 mm Volume applied: 4 μl Spacing: 10 mm
4. Chamber saturation: 30 min (MP)
5. RH (%): 55 ± 5
6. Temperature °C: 22 ± 2
7. Separation technique: Ascending
8. Quantity of mobile phase: 20 ml
9. Migration distance: 50 mm
10. Migration time: 40 min

Densitometric evaluation:

Wavelength: UV–254 nm Scanning mode: Reflectance/Absorbance
HRF: Propranolol HCl—32; Hydrochlorothiazide—69
Linearity (ng/band): Hydrochlorothiazide—200–500; Propranolol HCl—200–750
Recovery (%): 101.92–103.95 for both the compounds

References: —

Comments:

- The method was optimized and analytical work carried out at **Anchrom's HPTLC Application Laboratory**, Mumbai, India.
- Reversed–phased chromatography resulted in reversal of retention order as compared to NP-HPTLC.
- RP-HPTLC carried out on silicon oil impregnated plates prepared in the laboratory gave equally good separation results.

HPTLC : High Performance Thin Layer Chromatography
HPTLC Densitogram

No. 48

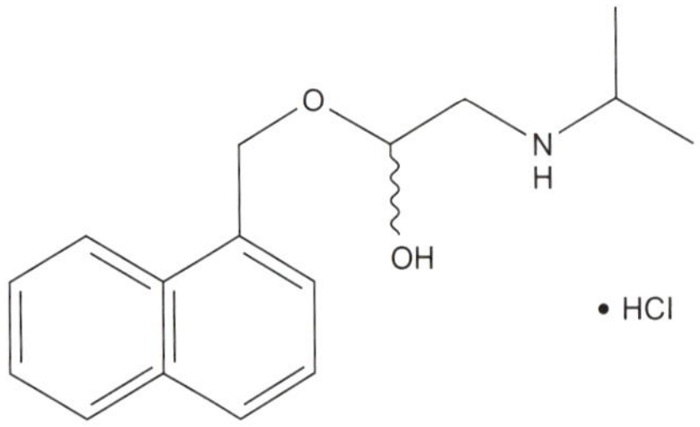

• HCl

Propranolol HCl

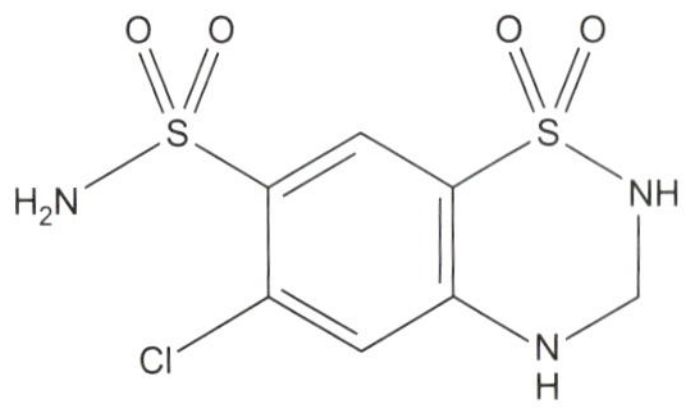

Hydrochlorothiazide

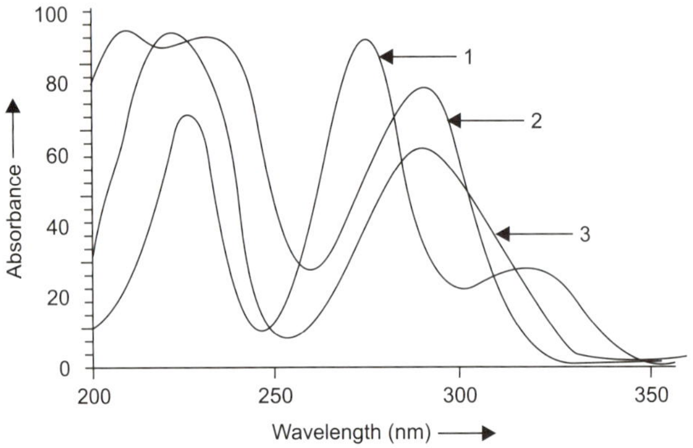

In-situ overlaid UV-spectra of propranolol HCl (1), trimethoprim-IS (2) and hydrochlorothiazide(3) for selection of suitable wavelength for densitometric scanning

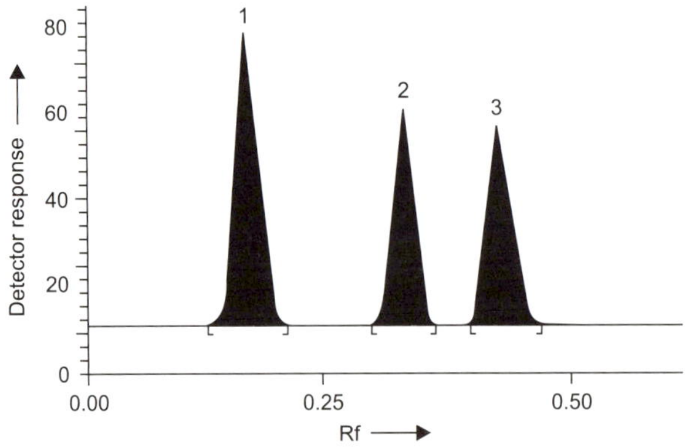

Typical densitogram of the sample containing propranolol HCl and hydrochlorothiazide. For detailed experimental and chromatographic conditions, refer to Protocol No. 48. Peaks identification: 1. Propranolol HCl; 2. Trimethoprim (IS); 3. Hydrochlorothiazide.

PROTOCOL FOR HPTLC ANALYSIS OF PHARMACEUTICAL FORMULATION

Protocol No. 48

Formulation: Hydrochlorothiazide, Propranolol hydrochloride

Classification: Cardiovascular System **Dosage form:** Tablets

Standard preparation: Prepare solution of both the compounds as well as IS in methanol to get 4 μg/ml (propranolol HCl); 2 μg/ml (hydrochlorothiazide) and 8 μg/ml (trimethoprim – IS). Apply 10 μl of each solution for analysis.

Sample preparation: Powdered sample equivalent to 40 mg of propranolol hydrochloride suspended in 20 ml of methanol, sonicated for 5 min, diluted to 25 ml with methanol, filtered and dilute 1 ml of the filtrate to 10 ml with methanol for assay.

Chromatographic equipments:

Sample applicator: Camag Linomat–IV

Development chamber: Camag twin-trough glass chamber, 10 × 10 cm

Densitometric scanner: Camag TLC Scanner–II

Chromatographic conditions:

1. Stationary phase: Silica gel $60F_{254}$ pre-coated HPTLC plates, 10 × 10 cm (200 μm) – Merck
2. Mobile phase (MP): Toluene–methanol–ethyl acetate–ammonia (8 : 2 : 1 : 0.2 v/v)
3. Standard/Sample application:
   Band length: 8 mm Volume applied: 10 μl Spacing: 10 mm
4. Chamber saturation: 20 min (MP)
5. RH (%): 50 ± 5
6. Temperature °C: 25 ± 2
7. Separation technique: Ascending
8. Quantity of mobile phase: 11.2 ml
9. Migration distance: 70 mm
10. Migration time: 36

Densitometric evaluation:

Wavelength: UV–280 nm Scanning mode: Reflectance/Absorbance

HRF: Propranolol HCl—16; Trimethoprim (IS)—31; Hydrochlorothiazide—42

Linearity (ng/band): Propranolol HCl—40–200; Hydrochlorothiazide—20–100

Recovery (%): Propranolol HCl—98.5–102; Hydrochlorothiazide—97–101

References: V.M. Shinde, B.S. Desai, N.M. Tendulkar, *Indian Drugs*, **31(5)**, 192–195, 1993.

Comments: The method validated for accurasy, precision, linearity, LOD, LOQ and specificity.

HPTLC : High Performance Thin Layer Chromatography
HPTLC Densitogram

No. 49

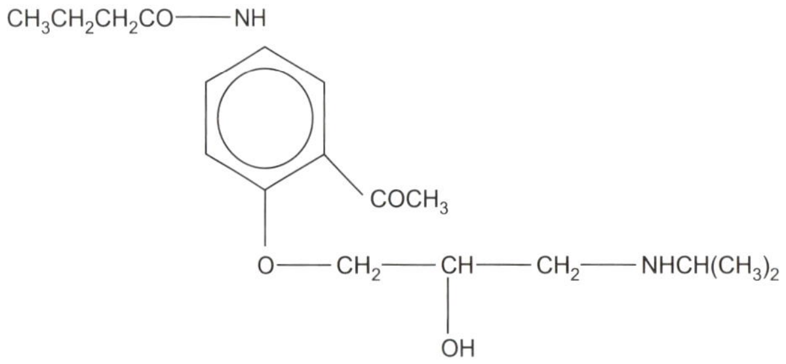

Acebutalol hydrochloride

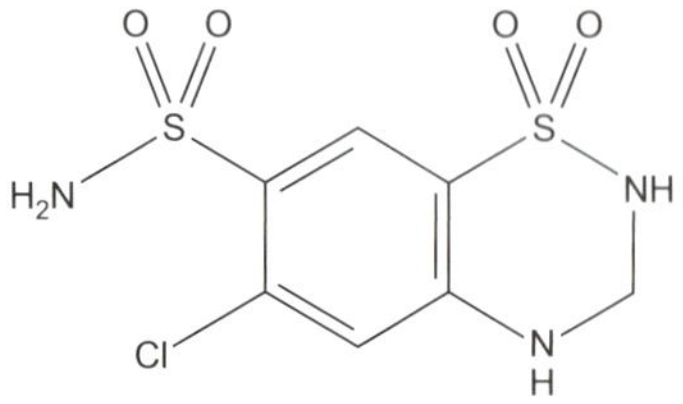

Hydrochlorothiazide

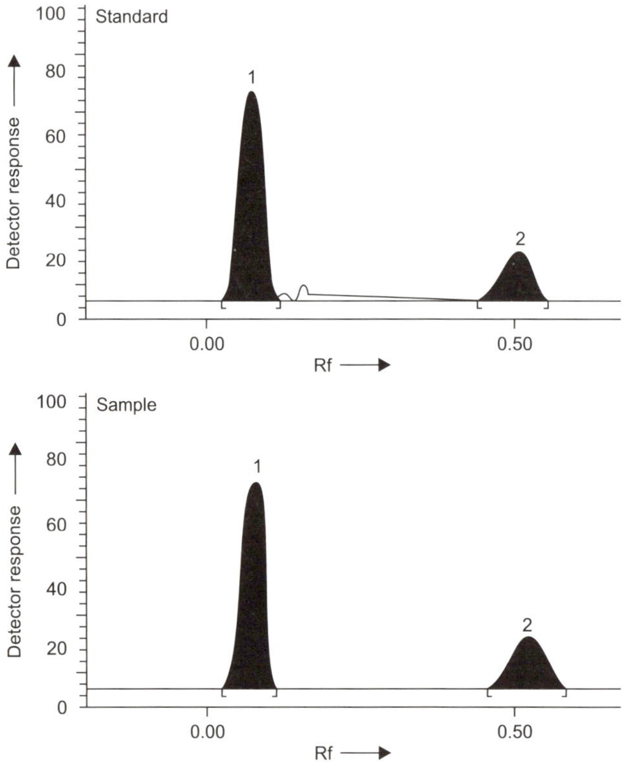

Typical densitogram of the sample and standard containing hydrochlorothiazide and acebutalol hydrochloride. For detailed experimental and chromatographic conditions, refer to Protocol No. 49. Peaks identification: 1. Acebutalol HCl; 2. Hydrochlorothiazide.

PROTOCOL FOR HPTLC ANALYSIS OF PHARMACEUTICAL FORMULATION

Protocol No. 49

Formulation: Hydrochlorothiazide, Acebutalol hydrochloride

Classification: Cardiovascular System **Dosage form:** Tablets

Standard preparation: Dissolve 12.5 mg of hydrochlorothiazide and 20 mg of acebutalol hydrochloride in 50 ml of methanol. Further dilute 4 ml to 10 ml with methanol and use for chromatographic analysis.

Sample preparation: Powdered sample equivalent to 12.5 mg of hydrochlorothiazide suspended in 40 ml of methanol, sonicate, dilute to 50 ml. Filter and dilute 4 ml of the filtrate to 10 ml with methanol and use for assay.

Chromatographic equipments:

Sample applicator: Camag Linomat–IV

Development chamber: Camag twin-trough glass chamber, 10 × 10 cm

Densitometric scanner: Camag TLC Scanner–II

Chromatographic conditions:

1. Stationary phase: Silica gel 60F_{254} pre-coated HPTLC plates, 10 × 10 cm (200 μm) – Merck
2. Mobile phase (MP): Toluene–n-propanol–25% ammonia (6 : 4 : 0.05 v/v)
3. Standard/Sample application:
   Band length: 8 mm Volume applied: 5 μl Spacing: 8 mm
4. Chamber saturation: 20 min (MP)
5. RH (%): 50 ± 5
6. Temperature °C: 22 ± 2
7. Separation technique: Ascending
8. Quantity of mobile phase: 10 ml
9. Migration distance: —
10. Migration time: 14 min

Densitometric evaluation:

Wavelength: UV–254 nm Scanning mode: Reflectance/Absorbance

HRF: Acebutalol HCl—10; Hydrochlorothiazide—52

Linearity (ng/band): Hydrochlorothiazide—100–500; Acetbutalol HCl—200–2000

Recovery (%): 97.68–98.76 for both the compounds

References: —

Comments: The method was optimized and analytical work carried out at **Anchrom's HPTLC Application Laboratory**, Mumbai, India.

HPTLC : High Performance Thin Layer Chromatography
HPTLC Densitogram

No. 50

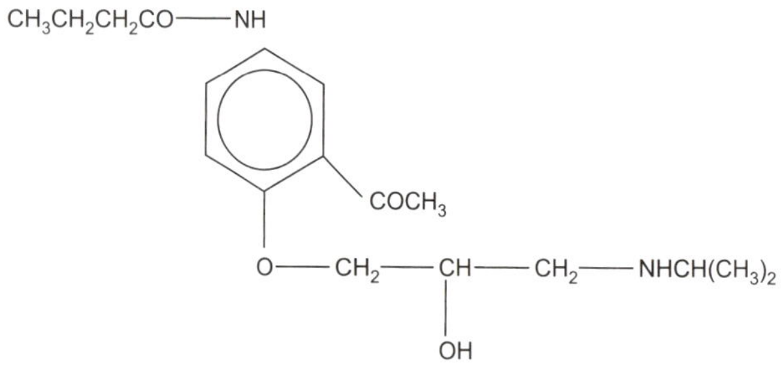

$CH_3CH_2CH_2CO$—NH

$COCH_3$

O—CH_2—CH—CH_2—$NHCH(CH_3)_2$

OH

Acebutalol hydrochloride

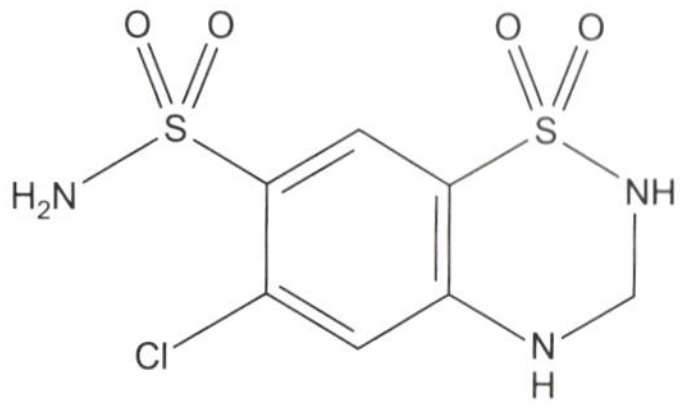

O O O O S S H_2N NH Cl N H

Hydrochlorothiazide

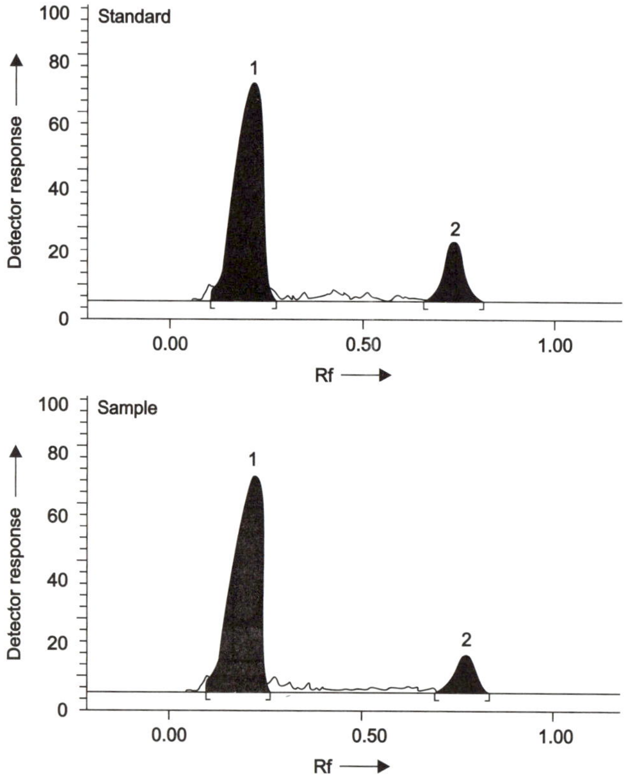

Standard

Detector response

100 80 60 40 20 0

1 2

0.00 0.50 1.00

Rf

Sample

Detector response

100 80 60 40 20 0

1 2

0.00 0.50 1.00

Rf

Typical densitogram of the sample and standard containing hydrochlorothiazide and acebutalol hydrochloride. For detailed experimental and chromatographic conditions, refer to Protocol No. 50. Peaks identification: 1. Acebutalol HCl; 2. Hydrochlorothiazide.

PROTOCOL FOR HPTLC ANALYSIS OF PHARMACEUTICAL FORMULATION

Protocol No. 50

Formulation: Hydrochlorothiazide, Acebutalol hydrochloride

Classification: Cardiovascular System **Dosage form:** Tablets

Standard preparation: Dissolve 25 mg of hydrochlorothiazide and 40 mg of acebutalol hydrochloride in 100 ml of methanol. Further dilute 4 ml to 10 ml with methanol and use for analysis.

Sample preparation: Powdered sample equivalent to 12.5 mg of hydrochlorothiazide suspended in 30–40 ml of methanol, sonicate, dilute to 50 ml. Filter and dilute 4 ml of the filtrate to 10 ml with methanol and use for assay.

Chromatographic equipments:

Sample applicator: Camag Linomat–IV

Development chamber: Camag twin-trough glass chamber, 10 × 10 cm

Densitometric scanner: Camag TLC Scanner–II

Chromatographic conditions:

1. Stationary phase: Silica gel 60 RP–18F_{254s} 5 × 7.5 cm (200 μm) – Merck
2. Mobile phase (MP): 0.5 M sodium chloride–methanol–acetonitrile–glacial acetic acid (5 : 2 : 3 : 0.1 v/v)
3. Standard/Sample application:
   Band length: 8 mm Volume applied: 5 μl Spacing: 10 mm
4. Chamber saturation: 30 min (MP)
5. RH (%): 50 ± 5
6. Temperature °C: 22 ± 2
7. Separation technique: Ascending
8. Quantity of mobile phase: 10 ml
9. Migration distance: 50 mm
10. Migration time: 25 min

Densitometric evaluation:

Wavelength: UV–254 nm Scanning mode: Reflectance/Absorbance

HRF: Acebutalol HCl—23; Hydrochlorothiazide—77

Linearity: —

Recovery (%): 100.38–104.57 for both the compounds

References: —

Comments:

- The method was optimized and analytical work carried out at **Anchrom's HPTLC Application Laboratory**, Mumbai, India. The reversed-phase chromatographic separation gave better resolution.
- RP-HPTLC carried out on silicon oil-impregnated plates (5% silicon oil in pet. ether) prepared in the laboratory gave good results.

HPTLC : High Performance Thin Layer Chromatography
HPTLC Densitogram

No. 51

Bisoprolol fumarate

Hydrochlorothiazide

In-vitro overlaid UV-spectra of hydrochlorothiazide (2) and bisoprolol fumarate (1) for selection of suitable wavelength for densitometric scanning

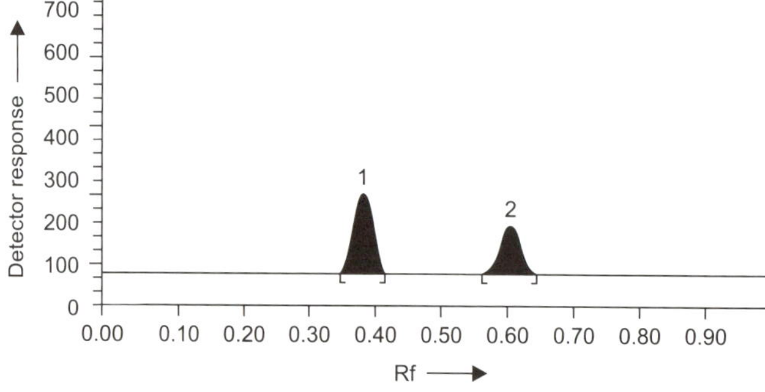

Typical densitogram of the sample containing hydrochlorothiazide and bisoprolol fumarate. For detailed experimental and chromatographic conditions, refer to Protocol No. 51. Peaks identification: 1. Hydrochlorothiazide; 2. Bisoprolol fumarate.

PROTOCOL FOR HPTLC ANALYSIS OF PHARMACEUTICAL FORMULATION

Protocol No. 51

Formulation: Hydrochlorothiazide, Bisoprolol fumarate

Classification: Cardiovascular System **Dosage form:** Tablets

Standard preparation: Prepare 1 mg/ml solution of each compound in methanol. Further dilutions made to get 100 μg/ml and use for application.

Sample preparation: Powdered sample equivalent to 25 mg of bisoprolol fumarate suspended in 20 ml of methanol, sonicated for 15 min, diluted to 35 ml, filtered through Whatman No. 40 filter paper, 1 ml of aliquot was further diluted to 10 ml with methanol to be used for chromatographic analysis.

Chromatographic equipments:

Sample applicator: Camag Linomat–V

Development chamber: Camag twin-trough glass chamber, 10 × 10 cm

Densitometric scanner: Camag TLC Scanner–III

Chromatographic conditions:

1. Stationary phase: Silica gel $60F_{254}$ pre-coated TLC plates, 10 × 10 cm (250 μm) – Merck, pre-washed with methanol, dried at 50°C for 5 min
2. Mobile phase (MP): Chloroform–methanol–25% ammonia (7 : 2 : 0.1 v/v)
3. Standard/Sample application:
   Band length: 8 mm Volume applied: 5 μl Spacing: 10 mm
4. Chamber saturation: 30 min (MP)
5. RH (%): 55 ± 5
6. Temperature °C: 25 ± 2
7. Separation technique: Ascending
8. Quantity of mobile phase: 18 ml
9. Migration distance: 80 mm
10. Migration time: 40 min

Densitometric evaluation:

Wavelength: UV–225 nm Scanning mode: Reflectance/Absorbance

HRF: Hydrochlorothiazide—39; Bisoprolol fumarate—62

Linearity (ng/band): Hydrochlorothiazide—50–800; Bisoprolol fumarate—200–1000

Recovery (%): Hydrochlorothiazide—99.89–102.32; Bisoprolol fumarate—99.68–102.09

References: L.J. Patel, B.N. Suhagia and P.B. Shah, *Indian Drugs*, **43(8)**, 630–635, 2006.

Comments: The method validated for accuracy, precision, linearity, LOD and LOQ.

HPTLC : High Performance Thin Layer Chromatography
HPTLC Densitogram

No. 52

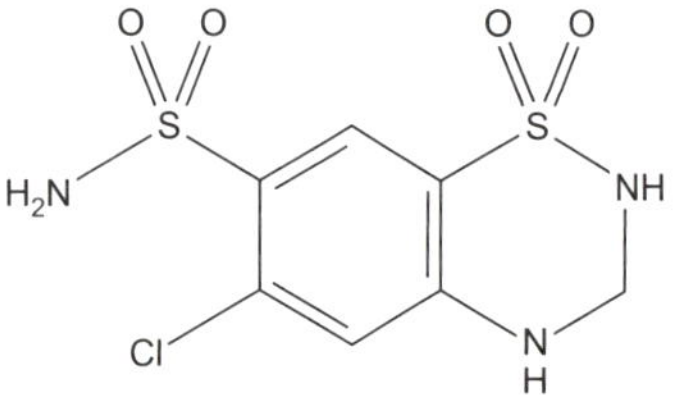

Hydrochlorothiazide

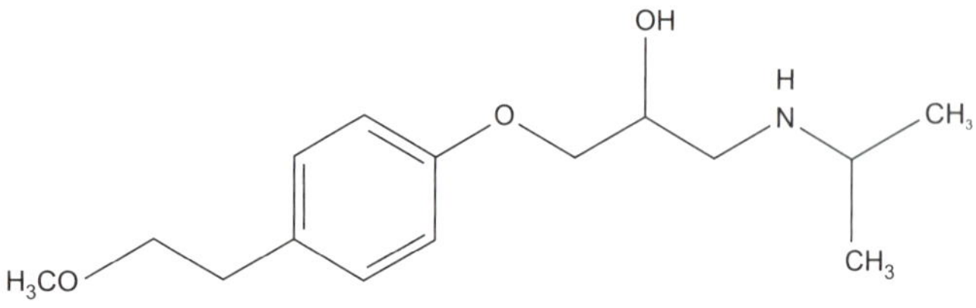

Metoprolol tartrate

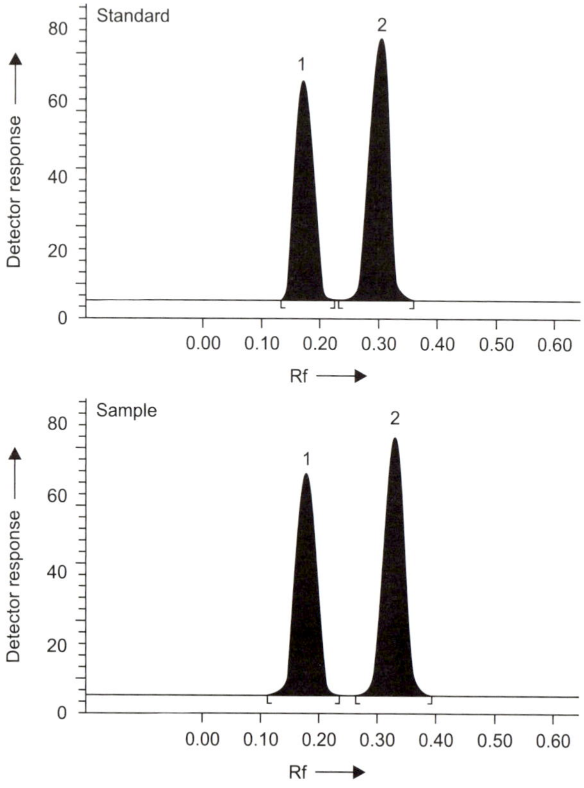

Typical densitogram of the sample and standard containing hydrochlorothiazide and metoprolol tartrate. For detailed experimental and chromatographic conditions, refer to Protocol No. 52. Peaks identification: 1. Hydrochlorothiazide; 2. Metoprolol tartrate.

PROTOCOL FOR HPTLC ANALYSIS OF PHARMACEUTICAL FORMULATION

Protocol No. 52

Formulation: Hydrochlorothiazide, Metoprolol tartrate

Classification: Cardiovascular System **Dosage form:** Tablets

Standard preparation: Prepare 1 mg/ml solution of hydrochlorothiazide in methanol (A). Weigh 10 mg of metoprolol tartrate, add 0.8 ml of solution–A and dilute to 10 ml with methanol and use for analysis.

Sample preparation: Weigh powdered sample equivalent to 100 mg of metoprolol tartrate, suspend in 70 ml of methanol, sonicate for 5 min, dilute to 100 ml with methanol, filter and use for assay.

Chromatographic equipments:

Sample applicator: Camag Linomat–IV

Development chamber: Camag twin-trough glass chamber, 10 × 10 cm

Densitometric scanner: Camag TLC Scanner–II

Chromatographic conditions:

1. Stationary phase: Silica gel $60F_{254}$ pre-coated TLC plates, 10 × 10 cm (250 μm) – Merck
2. Mobile phase (MP): Chloroform–methanol–25% ammonia (9 : 1 : 0.05 v/v)
3. Standard/Sample application:
   Band length: 7 mm Volume applied: 4 μl Spacing: 10 mm
4. Chamber saturation: 20 min (MP)
5. RH (%): 55 ± 5
6. Temperature °C: 22 ± 2
7. Separation technique: Ascending
8. Quantity of mobile phase: 10 ml
9. Migration distance: 50 mm
10. Migration time: 16 min

Densitometric evaluation:

Wavelength: UV–225 nm Scanning mode: Reflectance/Absorbance

HRF: Hydrochlorothiazide—17; Metoprolol tartrate—32

Linearity (ng/band): Hydrochlorothiazide—10–100 μg/ml; Metoprolol tartrate—25–250 μg/ml

Recovery (%): 98.65–99.70 for both the compounds.

References: —

Comments: The method was optimized and analytical work carried out at **Anchrom's HPTLC Application Laboratory**, Mumbai, India.

HPTLC : High Performance Thin Layer Chromatography
HPTLC Densitogram

No. 53

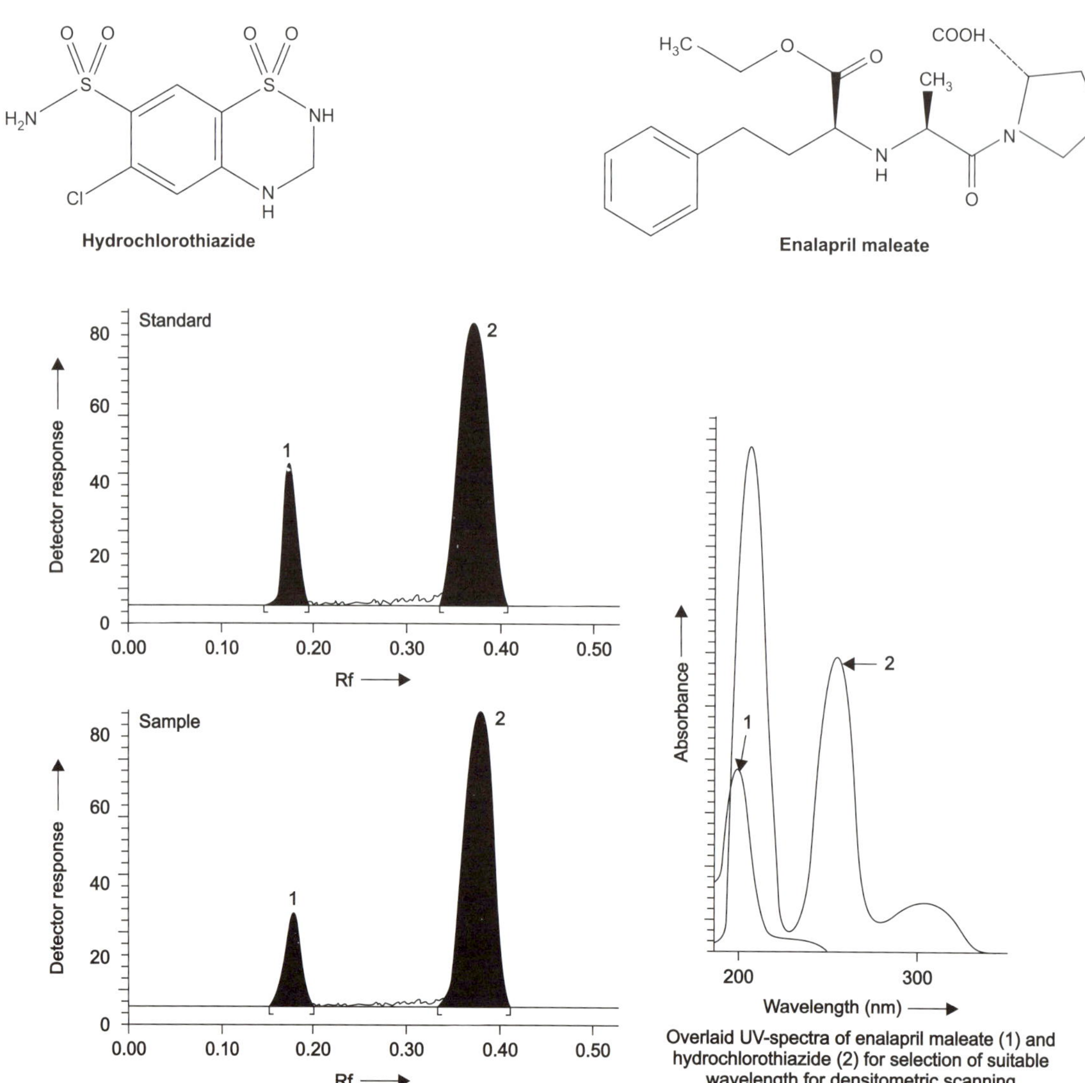

Overlaid UV-spectra of enalapril maleate (1) and hydrochlorothiazide (2) for selection of suitable wavelength for densitometric scanning

Typical densitogram of the sample and standard containing hydrochlorothiazide and enalapril maleate. For detailed experimental and chromatographic conditions, refer to Protocol No. 53. Peaks identification: 1. Enalapril maleate; 2. Hydrochlorothiazide.

PROTOCOL FOR HPTLC ANALYSIS OF PHARMACEUTICAL FORMULATION

Protocol No. 53

Formulation: Hydrochlorothiazide, Enalapril maleate

Classification: Cardiovascular System **Dosage form:** Tablets

Standard preparation: Prepare 400 μg/ml solution of enalapril maleate and 1 mg/ml solution of hydrochlorothiazide, both in methanol. Dilute 1 ml of the resulting solution to 10 ml with methanol for application.

Sample preparation: Powdered sample equivalent to 10 mg of enalapril maleate suspended in 20 ml of methanol, sonicate for 5 min, dilute to 25 ml, filter and dilute 1 ml of the filtrate to 10 ml with methanol for application.

Chromatographic equipments:

Sample applicator: Camag Linomat–IV

Development chamber: Camag twin-trough glass chamber, 10 × 10 cm

Densitometric scanner: Camag TLC Scanner–II

Chromatographic conditions:

1. Stationary phase: Silica gel $60F_{254}$ pre-coated HPTLC plates, 10 × 10 cm (200 μm) – Merck
2. Mobile phase (MP): Chloroform–methanol–glacial acetic acid (8.5 : 1.5 : 0.1 v/v)
3. Standard/Sample application:
   Band length: 7 mm Volume applied: 5 μl Spacing: 10 mm
4. Chamber saturation: 20 min (MP)
5. RH (%): 55 ± 5
6. Temperature °C: 22 ± 2
7. Separation technique: Ascending
8. Quantity of mobile phase: 10 ml
9. Migration distance: 50 mm
10. Migration time: 15 min

Densitometric evaluation:

Wavelength: UV–215 nm or 258 nm Scanning mode: Reflectance/Absorbance

HRF: Enalapril maleate—17; Hydrochlorothiazide—37

Linearity (ng/band): Hydrochlorothiazide—200–800; Enalapril maleate—50–200

Recovery (%): 97.75–101.50 for both the compounds.

References: —

Comments: The method was optimized and analytical work carried out at **Anchrom's HPTLC Application Laboratory**, Mumbai, India.

HPTLC : High Performance Thin Layer Chromatography
HPTLC Densitogram

No. 54

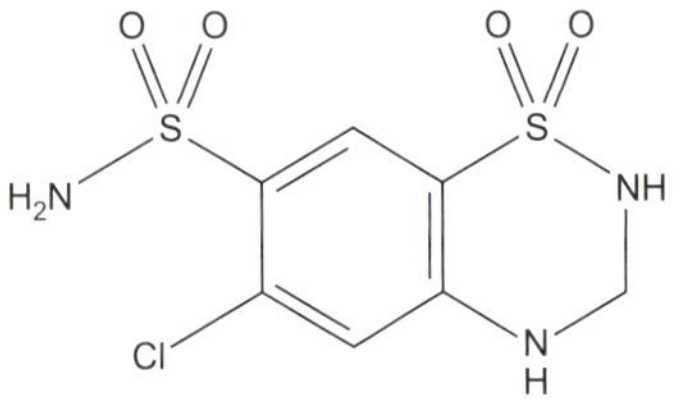

Hydrochlorothiazide

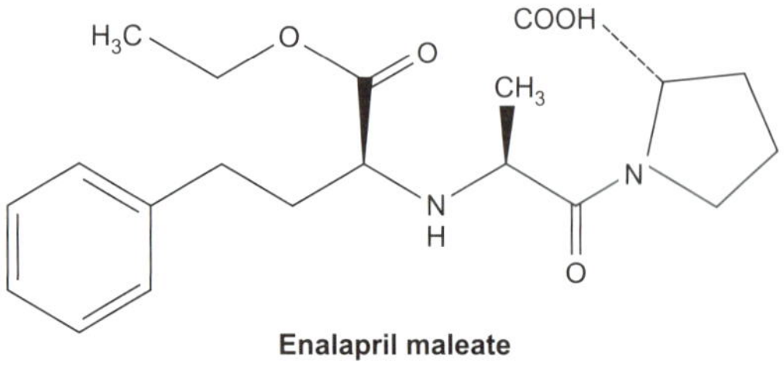

Enalapril maleate

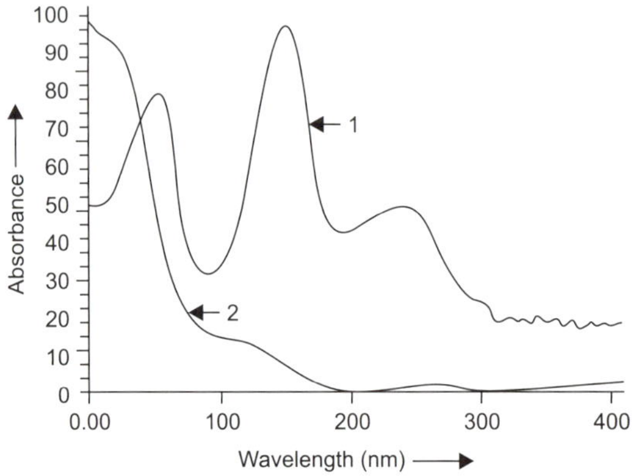

In-situ overlaid spectra of hydrochlorothiazide (1) and enalapril maleate (2) for selection of suitable wavelength for densitometric scanning

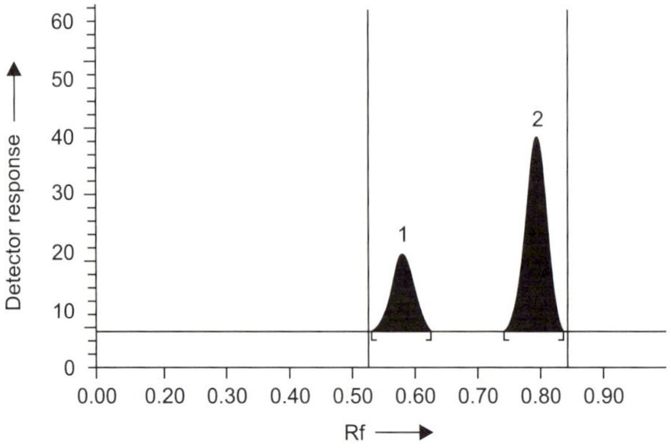

Typical densitogram of the sample containing hydrochlorothiazide and enalapril maleate. For detailed experimental and chromatographic conditions, refer to Protocol No. 54. Peaks identification: 1. Enalapril maleate; 2. Hydrochlorothiazide.

PROTOCOL FOR HPTLC ANALYSIS OF PHARMACEUTICAL FORMULATION

Protocol No. 54

Formulation: Hydrochlorothiazide (H), Enalapril maleate (E)

Classification: Cardiovascular System **Dosage form:** Tablets

Standard preparation: Standard solution of each compound prepared in methanol to get 200 μg/ml of enalapril and 625 μg/ml of hydrochlorothiazide and used for analysis.

Sample preparation: An appropriate quantity of the powdered sample shaken with 10 ml of methanol for 15 min, centrifuged and the supernatant used for determination. The solution contained 200 μg/ml of enalapril and 625 μg/ml of hydrochlorothiazide.

Chromatographic equipments:

Sample applicator: Camag Linomat–IV

Development chamber: Sigma Aldrich glass chamber, 18 × 9 × 10 cm

Densitometric scanner: Camag TLC Scanner–II

Chromatographic conditions:

1. Stationary phase: Silica gel $60F_{254}$ pre-coated HPTLC plates, 10 × 10 cm (200 μm) – Merck
2. Mobile phase (MP): n-butanol–glacial acetic acid–water (12 : 3 : 5 v/v)
3. Standard/Sample application:
   Band length: 10 mm Volume applied: 5 μl Spacing: 10 mm
4. Chamber saturation: 30 min (MP)
5. RH (%): 55 ± 5
6. Temperature °C: 22 ± 2
7. Separation technique: Ascending
8. Quantity of mobile phase: 20 ml
9. Migration distance: 95 mm
10. Migration time: 35 min

Densitometric evaluation:

Wavelength: UV–208 nm (E); UV–274 nm (H)

Scanning mode: Reflectance/Absorbance

HRF: Enalapril maleate—58; Hydrochlorothiazide—80

Linearity (ng/band): Enalapril—300–5000; Hydrochlorothiazide—100–1600

Recovery (%): Enalapril—97.8–102.2; Hydrochlorothiazide—98.3–102.0

References: Mariusz Stolareczyk, Maslanaka Anna and Jankrzek, *J. Liq. Chromatogr. and Related Technol.*, **31**, 1892–1902, 2008.

Comments: The method validated for accuracy, precision, linearity, LOD and LOQ.

HPTLC : High Performance Thin Layer Chromatography
HPTLC Densitogram

No. 55

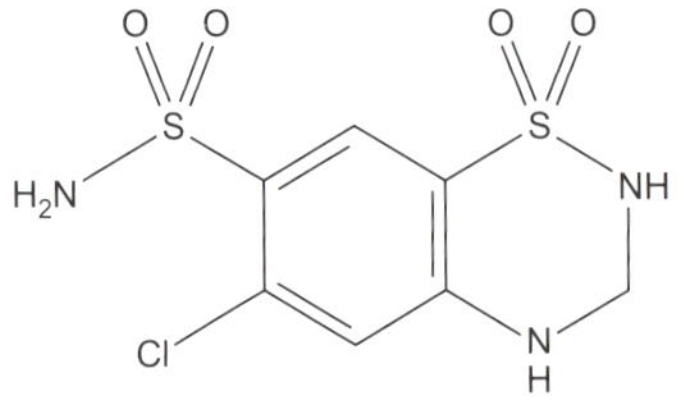

Hydrochlorothiazide

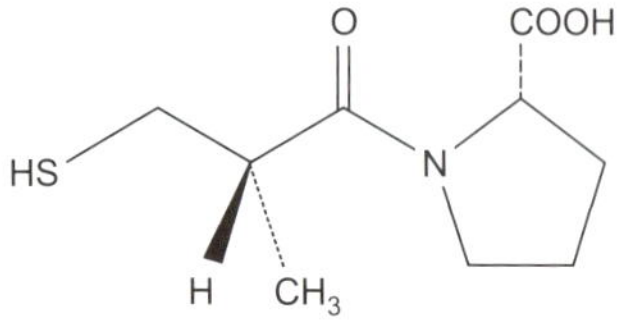

Captopril

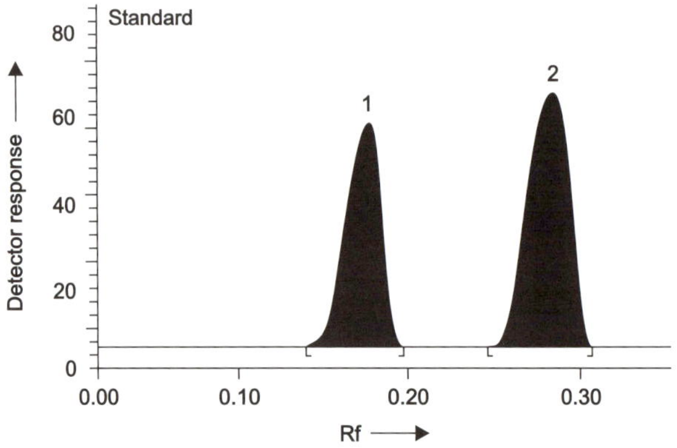

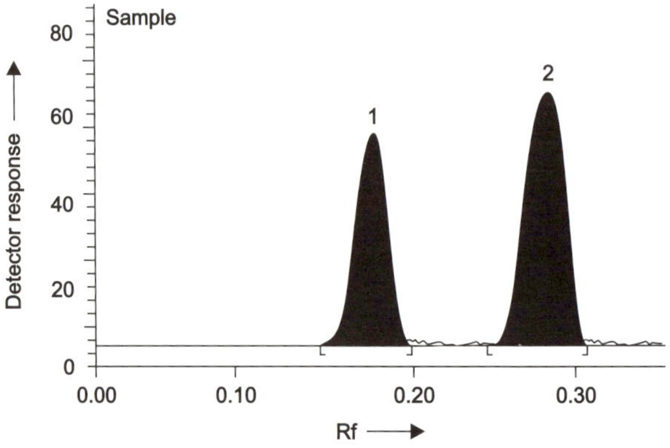

Standard

Sample

Typical densitogram of the sample and standard containing hydrochlorothiazide and captopril. For detailed experimental and chromatographic conditions, refer to Protocol No. 55. Peaks identification: 1. Captopril; 2. Hydrochlorothiazide.

PROTOCOL FOR HPTLC ANALYSIS OF PHARMACEUTICAL FORMULATION

Protocol No. 55

Formulation: Hydrochlorothiazide, Captopril

Classification: Cardiovascular System **Dosage form:** Tablets

Standard preparation: Prepare 400 μg/ml solution of each compound in methanol. Dilute 1 ml to 10 ml for application.

Sample preparation: Powdered sample equivalent to 10 mg of captorpil suspended in 20 ml of methanol, sonicate for 5 min, dilute to 25 ml, filter and dilute 1 ml of filtrate to 10 ml with methanol and use for application.

Chromatographic equipments:

Sample applicator: Camag Linomat–IV

Development chamber: Camag twin-trough glass chamber, 10 × 10 cm

Densitometric scanner: Camag TLC Scanner–II

Chromatographic conditions:

1. Stationary phase: Silica gel 60F_{254} pre-coated HPTLC plates, 5 × 10 cm (200 μm) – Merck
2. Mobile phase (MP): Chloroform–methanol–25% ammonia (8 : 2 : 0.2 v/v)
3. Standard/Sample application:

   Band length: 5 mm Volume applied: 5 μl Spacing: 5 mm
4. Chamber saturation: 20 min (MP)
5. RH (%): 55 ± 5
6. Temperature °C: 22 ± 2
7. Separation technique: Ascending
8. Quantity of mobile phase: 10 ml
9. Migration distance: 50 mm
10. Migration time: 15 min

Densitometric evaluation:

Wavelength: UV–210 nm or 238 nm Scanning mode: Reflectance/Absorbance

HRF: Captopril—17; Hydrochlorothiazide—28

Linearity: 100–750 ng for both the compounds

Recovery (%): 98.75–101.28 for both the compounds

References: —

Comments: The method was optimized and analytical work carried out at **Anchrom's HPTLC Application Laboratory**, Mumbai, India.

HPTLC : High Performance Thin Layer Chromatography
HPTLC Densitogram

No. 56

Hydrochlorothiazide

Captopril

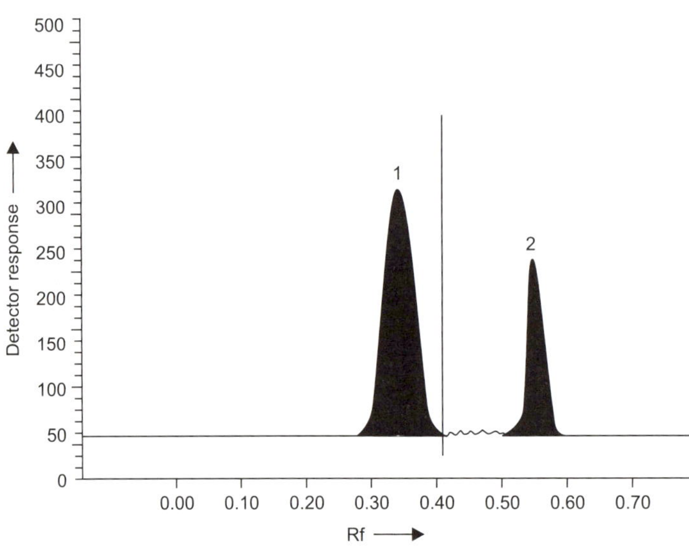

Typical densitogram of the standard containing hydrochlorothiazide and captopril. For detailed experimental and chromatographic conditions, refer to Protocol No. 56. Peaks identification: 1. Hydrochlorothiazide; 2. Captopril.

PROTOCOL FOR HPTLC ANALYSIS OF PHARMACEUTICAL FORMULATION

Protocol No. 56

Formulation: Hydrochlorothiazide, Captopril

Classification: Cardiovascular System **Dosage form:** Tablets

Standard preparation: 10 μg/ml of each compound prepared in methanol. Apply 2–14 μl of each solution for linearity.

Sample preparation: Powdered sample equivalent to 50 mg of captopril suspended in 40 ml of methanol, shaken for 15 min, diluted to 50 ml, filtered and filtrate suitably diluted for assay.

Chromatographic equipments:

Sample applicator: Camag Linomat–IV

Development chamber: Camag twin-trough glass chamber, 10 × 10 cm

Densitometric scanner: Camag TLC Scanner–III

Chromatographic conditions:

1. Stationary phase: Silica gel 60F_{254} pre-coated HPTLC plates, 5 × 10 cm (200 μm) – Merck
2. Mobile phase (MP): Methanol–toleuene–ethyl acetate–glacial acetic acid (1 : 6 : 3 : 0.5 v/v)
3. Standard/Sample application:
   Band length: 6 mm Volume applied: 6 μl Spacing: 10 mm
4. Chamber saturation: 15 Min (MP)
5. RH (%): 55 ± 5
6. Temperature °C: 22 ± 2
7. Separation technique: Ascending
8. Quantity of mobile phase: 10 ml
9. Migration distance: 70 mm
10. Migration time: 30 min

Densitometric evaluation:

Wavelength: UV–219 nm Scanning mode: Reflectance/Absorbance

HRF: Hydrochlorothiazide—34; Captopril—55

Linearity: 20–140 ng for both the drugs

Recovery (%): Hydrochlorothiazide 99.99–100.25; Captopril—100.02–100.2

References: S.G. Walode, M.S. Charde, M.R. Tajne and A.V. Kasture, *Indian Drugs*, **47(6)**, 340–344, 2005.

Comments: The method validated for different parameters as per ICH guidelines.

HPTLC : High Performance Thin Layer Chromatography
HPTLC Densitogram

No. 57

Captopril

Hydrochlorothiazide

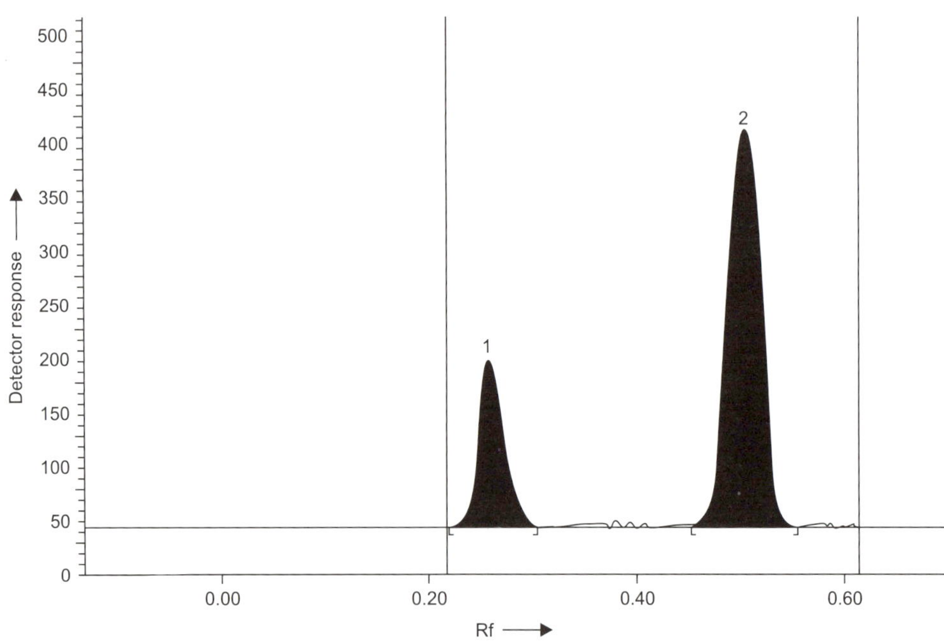

Typical densitogram of the standard containing hydrochlorothiazide and captopril. For detailed experimental and chromatographic conditions, refer to Protocol No. 57. Peaks identification: 1. Captopril; 2. Hydrochlorothiazide.

PROTOCOL FOR HPTLC ANALYSIS OF PHARMACEUTICAL FORMULATION

Protocol No. 57

Formulation: Hydrochlorothiazide, Captopril

Classification: Cardiovascular System **Dosage form:** Tablets

Standard preparation: Prepare 100 μg/ml solution of each compound separately in methanol. Apply varying volumes of each solution for linearity profile.

Sample preparation: An appropriate quantity of powdered sample suspended in methanol, sonicated, diluted, filtered and filtrate suitably diluted to get 100 ng/μl. Apply 5 μl of the resulting solution for assay.

Chromatographic equipments:

Sample applicator: Camag Linomat–V

Development chamber: Camag twin-trough glass chamber, 10 × 10 cm

Denistometric scanner: Camag TLC Scanner–III

Chromatographic conditions:

1. Stationary phase: Silica gel $60F_{254}$ pre-coated TLC plates, 10 × 10 cm (250 μm) – Merck, pre-washed with methanol and dried prior to use
2. Mobile phase (MP): Toluene–methanol (6 : 4 v/v)
3. Standard/Sample application:
   Band length: 5 mm Volume applied: 3–5 μl Spacing: 10 mm
4. Chamber saturation: 15 min (MP)
5. RH (%): 55 ± 5
6. Temperature °C: Ambient
7. Separation technique: Ascending
8. Quantity of mobile phase: 10 ml
9. Migration distance: 80 mm
10. Migration time: 15 min

Densitometric evaluation:

Wavelength: UV–210 nm Scanning mode: Reflectance/Absorbance

HRF: Captipril—24; Hydrochlorothiazide—50

Linearity: 300–550 ng/band for both the drugs

Recovery (%): 99.60–100.5 for both the drugs

References: Tushar Koyani, Kashyap N. Thumar and Navin R. Sheth, Manuscript submitted for Dr. P.D. Sethi Award, 2011. Data courtesy Prof. Kashyap.

Comments: The method validated for accuracy, precision, linearity, LOD, LOQ, specificity and robustness.

HPTLC : High Performance Thin Layer Chromatography
HPTLC Densitogram

No. 58

Hydrochlorothiazide

Quinapril hydrochloride

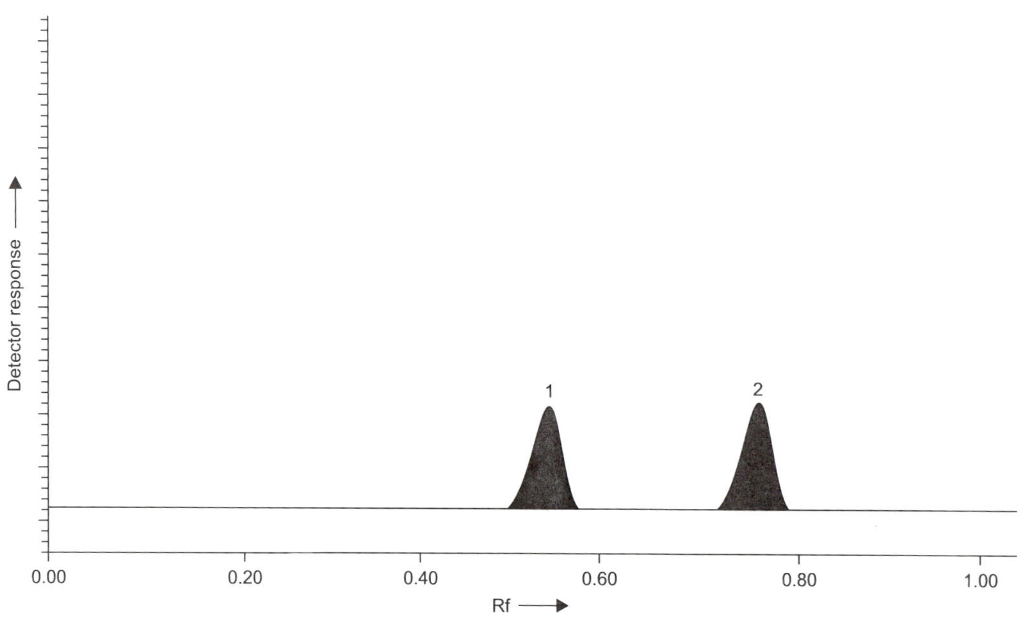

Typical densitogram of the sample containing hydrochlorothiazide and quinapril HCl. For detailed experimental and chromatographic conditions, refer to Protocol No. 58. Peaks identification: 1. Quinapril HCl; 2. Hydrochlorothiazide.

PROTOCOL FOR HPTLC ANALYSIS OF PHARMACEUTICAL FORMULATION

Protocol No. 58

Formulation: Hydrochlorothiazide, Quinapril hydrochloride

Classification: Cardiovascular System **Dosage form:** Tablets

Standard preparation: Prepare 125 μg/ml solution of hydrochlorothiazide and 100 μg/ml solution of quinapril hydrochloride, both in methanol and use for chromatographic analysis.

Sample preparation: Powdered sample equivalent to 10 mg of quinapril HCl or 12.5 mg of hydrochlorothiazide suspended in 70 ml of methanol, sonicated for 20 min, diluted to 100 ml, filtered and used for analysis.

Chromatographic equipments:

Sample applicator: Camag Linomat–V

Development chamber: Camag twin-trough glass chamber, 20 × 10 cm

Densitometric scanner: Camag TLC Scanner–III

Chromatographic conditions:

1. Stationary phase: Silica gel $60F_{254}$ pre-coated TLC plates, 20 × 10 cm (250 μm) – Merck
2. Mobile phase (MP): Ethyl acetate–acetone–acetic acid (6.5 : 3 : 0.5 v/v)
3. Standard/Sample application:

   Band length: 6 mm Volume applied: 2 μl Spacing: 10 mm
4. Chamber saturation: 15 min (MP)
5. RH (%): 55 ± 5
6. Temperature °C: 25 ± 2
7. Separation technique: Ascending
8. Quantity of mobile phase: 20 ml
9. Migration distance: 70 mm
10. Migration time: 25 min

Densitometric evaluation:

Wavelength: UV–208 nm Scanning mode: Reflectance/Absorbance

HRF: Quinapril HCl—53; Hydrochlorothiazide—76

Linearity (ng/band): Quinapril HCl—400–2800 ; Hydrochlorothiazide—500–3500

Recovery (%): Quinapril HCl—99.37–100.79; Hydrochlorothiazide—99.33–100.53

References: Girija B. Bhavar, V.A. Chatpalliwar, D.D. Patil and S.J. Surana. *Ind. J. Pharm. Sci.*, **71**, 529, 2008.

Comments: The method validated for accuracy, precision, linearity, LOD, LOQ and specificity as per ICH guidelines.

HPTLC : High Performance Thin Layer Chromatography
HPTLC Densitogram

No. 59

Hydrochlorothiazide

Quinapril hydrochloride

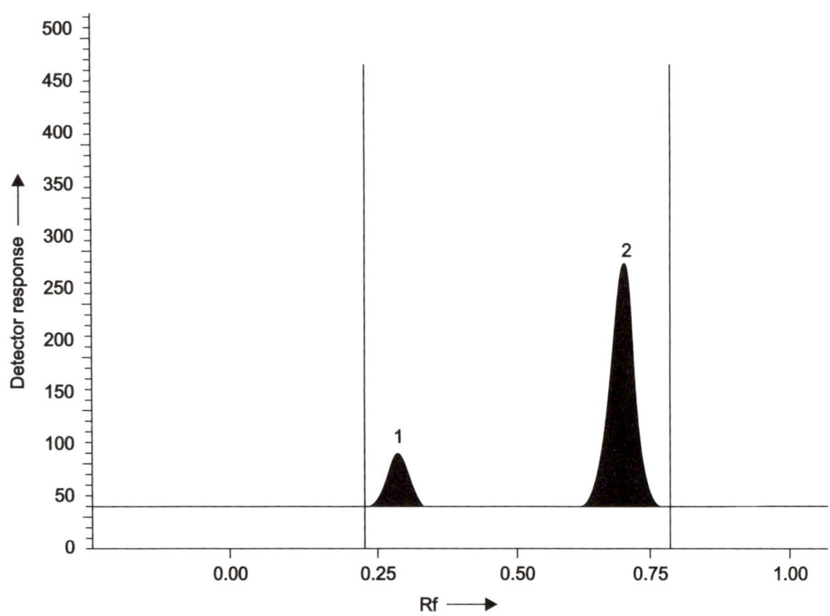

Typical densitogram of the sample containing hydrochlorothiazide and quinapril HCl. For detailed experimental and chromatographic conditions, refer to Protocol No. 59. Peaks identification: 1. Quinapril HCl; 2. Hydrochlorothiazide.

PROTOCOL FOR HPTLC ANALYSIS OF PHARMACEUTICAL FORMULATION

Protocol No. 59

Formulation: Hydrochlorothiazide, Quinapril hydrochloride

Classification: Cardiovascular System **Dosage form:** Tablets

Standard preparation: Dissolve 10 mg of quinapril and 12.5 mg of hydrochlorothiazide in 10 ml of methanol. Further dilute 1 ml to 10 ml with methanol and use the resulting solution for analysis.

Sample preparation: Powdered sample equivalent to 10 mg of quinapril suspended in 7–8 ml of methanol, sonicated for 5 min, diluted to 10 ml, filtered and 1 ml of filtrate diluted to 10 ml with methanol and used for assay.

Chromatographic equipments:

Sample applicator: Camag Linomat–V

Development chamber: Camag twin-trough glass chamber, 20 × 10 cm

Densitometric scanner: Camag TLC Scanner–III

Chromatographic conditions:

1. Stationary phase: Silica gel $60F_{254}$ pre-coated TLC plates, 20 × 10 cm (250 μm) – Merck, pre-washed with methanol, activated at 60°C for 5 min prior to use
2. Mobile phase (MP): Toluene–ethyl acetate–glacial acetic acid (1 : 6 : 0.5 v/v)
3. Standard/Sample application:
   Band length: 6 mm Volume applied: 7 μl Spacing: 5 mm
4. Chamber saturation: 30 min (MP)
5. RH (%): 55 ± 5
6. Temperature °C: 25 ± 2
7. Separation technique: Ascending
8. Quantity of mobile phase: 15 ml
9. Migration distance: 75 mm
10. Migration time: 25 min

Densitometric evaluation:

Wavelength: UV–273 nm Scanning mode: Reflectance/Absorbance

HRF: Quinapril HCl—30; Hydrochlorothiazide—68

Linearity (ng/band): Hydrochlorothiazide—480–960; Quinapril HCl—400–800

Recovery (%): 100.98–101.34 for both the compounds.

References: M. Gandhimati and T.K. Ravi, *Indian Drugs*, **46(2)**, 150–153, 2009.

Comments: The method validated for accuracy, precision, linearity, LOD, LOQ and robustness.

HPTLC : High Performance Thin Layer Chromatography
HPTLC Densitogram

No. 60

Hydrochlorothiazide

Benazepril hydrochloride

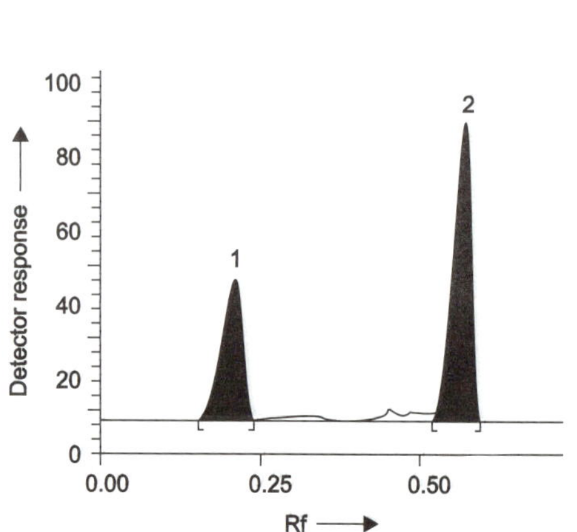

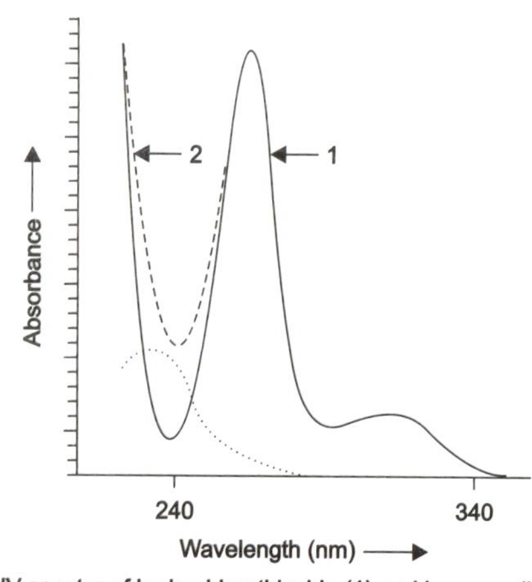

Overlaid UV-spectra of hydrochlorothiazide (1) and benazepril hydrochloride (2) for selection of suitable wavelength for densitometric scanning

Typical densitogram of the sample containing hydrochlorothiazide and benazepril HCl. For detailed experimental and chromatographic conditions, refer to Protocol No. 60. Peaks identification: 1. Benazepril HCl; 2. Hydrochlorothiazide.

PROTOCOL FOR HPTLC ANALYSIS OF PHARMACEUTICAL FORMULATION

Protocol No. 60

Formulation: Hydrochlorothiazide, Benazepril hydrochloride

Classification: Cardiovascular System **Dosage form:** Tablets

Standard preparation: Dissolve 100 mg of benazepril HCl and 12.5 mg of hydrochlorothiazide in methanol to produce 50 ml. Further dilute with methanol to get 0.2–2 mg/ml (benazepril HCl) and 0.25–2.5 mg/ml (hydrochlorothiazide). Apply 10 μl of each solution for linearity.

Sample preparation: Powdered sample equivalent to 50 mg of benazepril HCl suspeneded in methanol, shaken for 15 min, diluted to 50 ml, filtered and aliquot of filtrate suitably diluted for assay. Apply 10 μl final solution for analysis.

Chromatographic equipments:

Sample applicator: 10 μl Hamilton–micrisyringe

Development chamber: Flat bottom, glass chamber, 20 × 20 cm

Densitometric scanner: Shimadzu dual wavelength flying spot densitometer CS–9000

Chromatographic conditions:

1. Stationary phase: —
2. Mobile phase (MP): Ethyl acetate–methanol–chloroform (10 : 3 : 2 v/v)
3. Standard/Sample application:
   Band length: 5 mm Volume applied: 10 μl Spacing: 15 mm
4. Chamber saturation: 20 min (MP)
5. RH (%): 55 ± 5
6. Temperature °C: 22 ± 2
7. Separation technique: Ascending
8. Quantity of mobile phase: 30 ml
9. Migration distance: 80 mm
10. Migration time: 25 min

Densitometric evaluation:

Wavelength: UV–238 nm (benazepril HCl); 275 nm (hydrochlorothiazide)

Scanning mode: Reflectance/Absorbance

HRF: Benazepril HCl—22; Hydrochlorothiazide—60

Linearity (μg/band): Hydrochlorothiazide—2.5–25; Benazepril HCl—2–20

Recovery (%): Hydrochlorothiazide—99.0—100.6; Benazepril HCl—99.0–100.8

References: AlaaEl-Gindy, Ahmed Ashour, Laila Abdel-Fattah and Marwan M. Shabana, *J. Pharm. Biomed. Anal.*, **25**, 171–179, 2001.

Comments: The method validated for accuracy, precision, linearity, LOD, LOQ, selectivity, specificity, robustness and ruggedness.

HPTLC : High Performance Thin Layer Chromatography
HPTLC Densitogram

No. 61

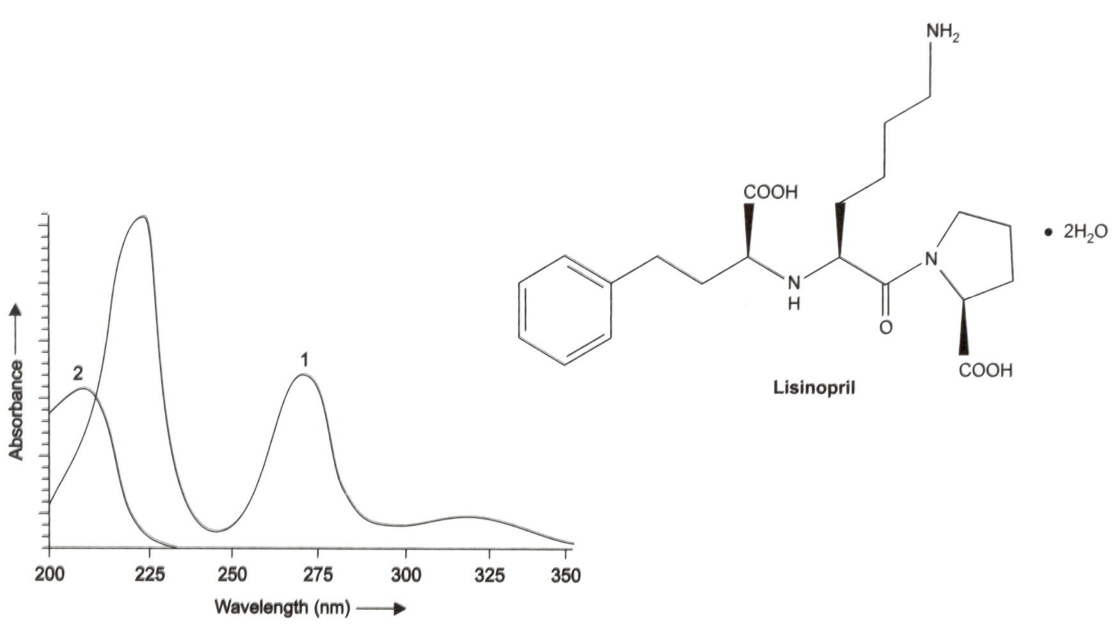

In-situ over-laid UV-spectra of hydrochlorothiazide (1) and lisinopril (2) for selection of suitable wavelength for densitometric scanning

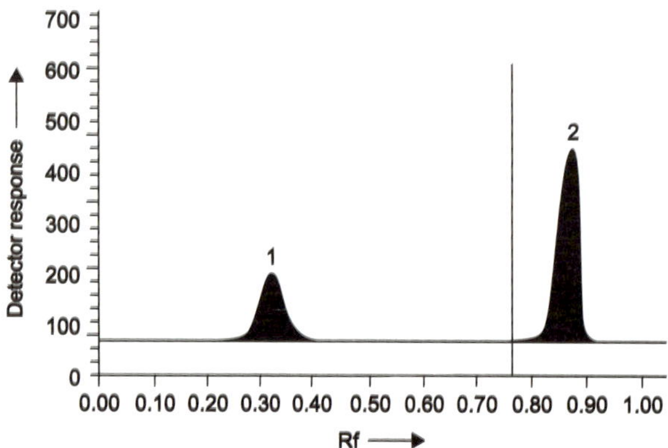

Typical densitogram of the sample containing hydrochlorothiazide and lisinopril. For detailed experimental and chromatographic conditions, refer to Protocol No. 61. Peaks identification: 1. Lisinopril; 2. Hydrochlorothiazide.

PROTOCOL FOR HPTLC ANALYSIS OF PHARMACEUTICAL FORMULATION

Protocol No. 61

Formulation: Hydrochlorothiazide, Lisinopril

Classification: Cardiovascular System **Dosage form:** Tablets

Standard preparation: Prepare solution of both the compounds in methanol to get 2 mg/ml (lisinopril) and 250 μg/ml (hydrochlorothiazide). Further serial dilutions made with methanol for linearity studies. Apply 10 μl of each solution for chromatographic analysis.

Sample preparation: Powdered sample equivalent to 25 mg of hydrochlorothiazide suspended in methanol, sonicated, diluted to 50 ml, filtered and the filtrate further diluted for assay. Apply 10 μl for analysis.

Chromatographic equipments:

Sample applicator: 10 μl Hamilton microsyringe

Development chamber: Flat bottom glass chamber, 20 × 20 cm

Densitometric scanner: Shimadzu dual wavelength flying spot, densitometer CS–9000

Chromatographic conditions:

1. Stationary phase: Silica gel $60F_{254}$ pre-coated HPTLC plates, 20 × 10 cm
2. Mobile phase (MP): Chloroform–ethyl acetate–acetic acid (10 : 3 : 2 v/v)
3. Standard/Sample application:
   Band length: 5 mm Volume applied: 10 μl Spacing: 15 mm
4. Chamber saturation: 20 min (MP)
5. RH (%): 55 ± 5
6. Temperature °C: 25 ± 2
7. Separation technique: Ascending
8. Quantity of mobile phase: 30 ml
9. Migration distance: 80 mm
10. Migration time: 25 min

Densitometric evaluation:

Wavelength: UV–210 nm (Lisinopril); 275 nm (Hydrochlorothiazide)

Scanning mode: Reflectance/Absorbance

HRF: Lisinopril—31; Hydrochlorothiazide—88

Linearity (μg/band): Lisinopril—4–20; Hydrochlorothiazide—2.5–25

Recovery (%): 99.8–100.6 for both the compounds

References: Alaa El-Gindy, Ahmed Ashour, Laila Abdel–Fattah and Marwan M. Shabana, *J. Pharm. Biomed. Anal.*, **25**, 923–931, 2001.

Comments: The method was validated for accuracy, precision, linearity, LOD, LOQ, selectivity, specificity, robustness and ruggedness.

HPTLC : High Performance Thin Layer Chromatography
HPTLC Densitogram

No. 62

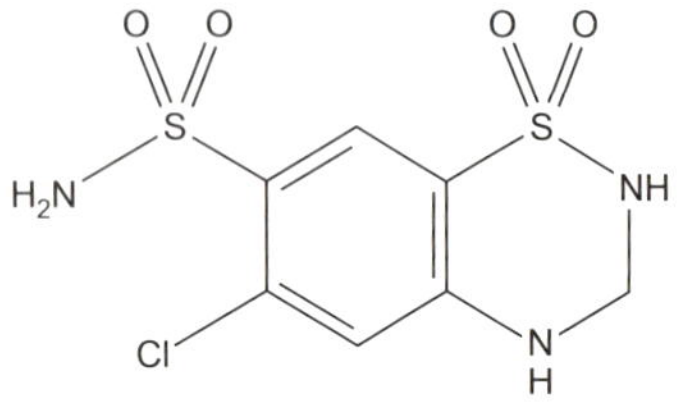

Hydrochlorothiazide

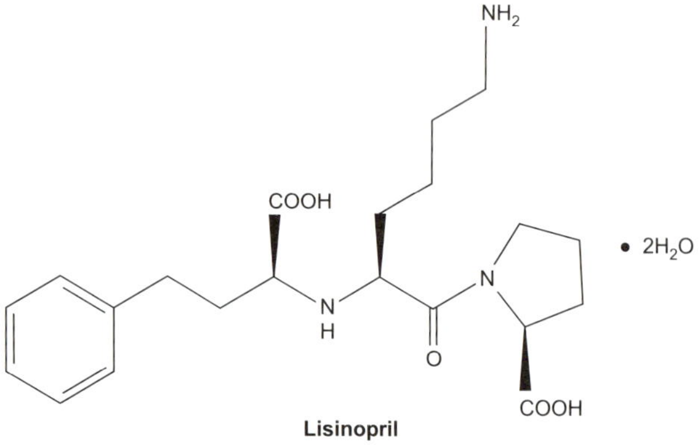

Lisinopril

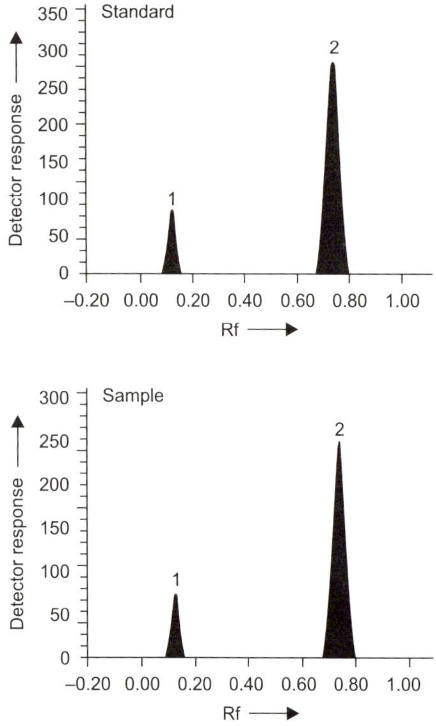

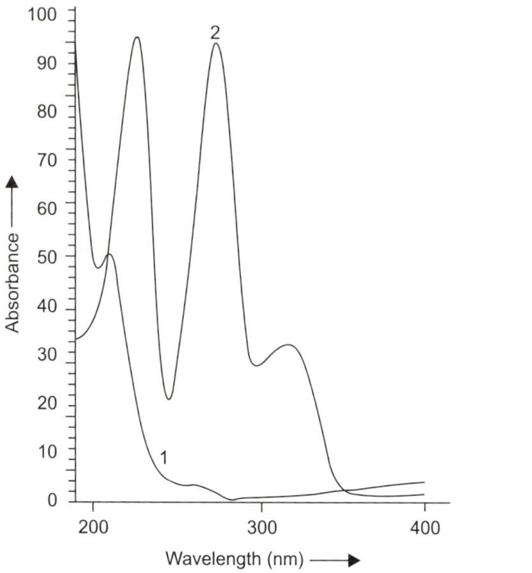

Overlaid UV-spectra of lisinopril (1) and hydrochlorothiazide (2) for selection of suitable wavelength for densitometric scanning

Typical densitogram of the standard and the sample containing lisinopril and hydrochlorothiazide. For detailed experimental and chromatographic conditions, refer to Protocol No. 62. Peaks identification: 1. Lisinopril; 2. Hydrochlorothiazide.

PROTOCOL FOR HPTLC ANALYSIS OF PHARMACEUTICAL FORMULATION

Protocol No. 62

Formulation: Hydrochlorothiazide, Lisinopril

Classification: Cardiovascular System **Dosage form:** Tablets

Standard preparation: Prepare 1 mg/ml solution of each compound in methanol separately. Further serial dilutions made with methanol for linearity profile. Apply 10 μl of each solution for chromatographic analysis.

Sample preparation: Powdered sample equivalent to 12.5 mg of hydrochlorothiazide is suspended in 7 ml of methanol, sonicated, diluted to 10 ml with methanol. Filtered and 1 ml of filtrate diluted to 10 ml with methanol for chromatographic analysis.

Chromatographic equipments:

Sample applicator: Camag Linomat–V

Development chamber: Camag automatic development chamber saturated with camag saturation pad

Densitometric scanner: Camag TLC Scanner–III

Chromatographic conditions:

1. Stationary phase: Silica gel $60F_{254}$ pre-coated TLC plates glass, 20 × 10 cm (250 μm) – Merck
2. Mobile phase (MP): n-Butanol–methanol–water (3 : 1 : 1 v/v)
3. Standard/Sample application:
   Band length: 8 mm Volume applied: 10 μl Spacing: 10 mm
4. Chamber saturation: 20 min (MP)
5. RH (%): 55 ± 5
6. Temperature °C: 25 ± 2
7. Separation technique: Ascending
8. Quantity of mobile phase: 20 ml
9. Migration distance: 70 mm
10. Migration time: 46 min

Densitometric evaluation:

Wavelength: UV–200 nm Scanning mode: Reflectance/Absorbance

HRF: Lisinopril—12; Hydrochlorothiazide—73

Linearity: 500–2000 ng/band for both the compounds

Recovery (%): —

References: —

Comments: The method was optimized and analytical work carried out at **Anchrom's HPTLC Application Laboratory**, Mumbai, India.

HPTLC : High Performance Thin Layer Chromatography
HPTLC Densitogram

No. 63

Ramipril

Hydrochlorothiazide

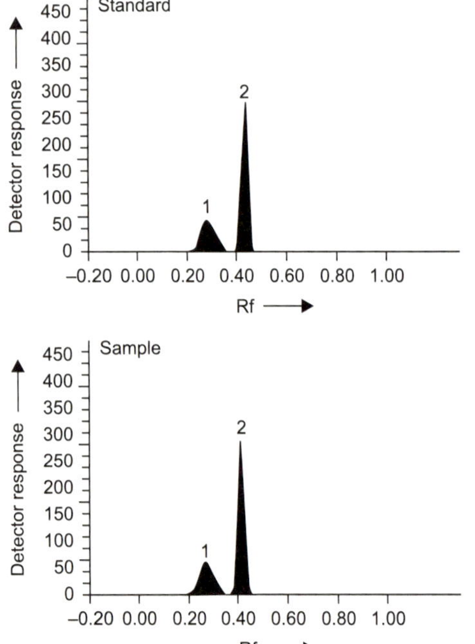

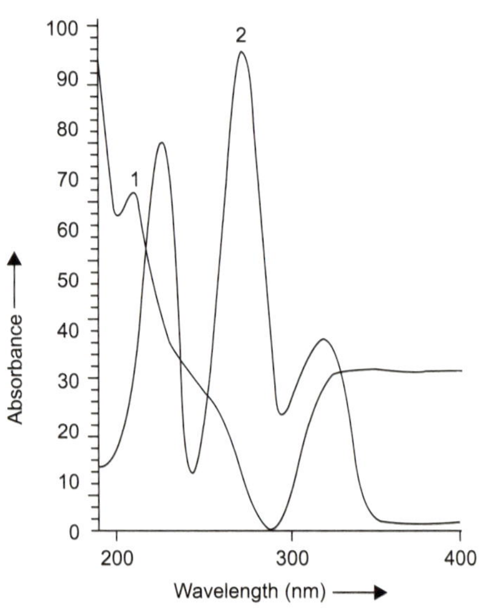

Overlaid UV-spectra of ramipril (1) and hydrochlorothiazide (2) for selection of suitable wavelength for densitometric scanning

Typical densitogram of the standard and the sample containing hydrochlorothiazide and ramipril. For detailed experimental and chromatographic conditions, refer to Protocol No. 63. Peaks identification: 1. Ramipril; 2. Hydrochlorothiazide.

PROTOCOL FOR HPTLC ANALYSIS OF PHARMACEUTICAL FORMULATION

Protocol No. 63

Formulation: **Hydrochlorothiazide, Ramipril**

Classification: Cardiovascular System **Dosage form:** Tablets

Standard preparation: Prepare 1 mg/ml solution of each compound in methanol separately. Further serial dilutions made with methanol for linearity profile. Apply 10 μl of each solution for chromatographic analysis.

Sample preparation: Powdered sample equivalent to 12.5 mg of hydrochlorothiazide suspended in 7 ml of methanol, sonicated, diluted to 10 ml with methanol. Filtered and 1 ml of filtrate diluted to 10 ml with methanol for chromatographic analysis.

Chromatographic equipments:

Sample applicator: Camag Linomat–V

Development chamber: Camag automatic development chamber saturated with camag saturation pad

Densitometric scanner: Camag TLC Scanner–III

Chromatographic conditions:

1. Stationary phase: Silica gel $60F_{254}$ pre-coated TLC plates glass, 20 × 10 cm (250 μm) – Merck
2. Mobile phase (MP): Toluene–acetone–methanol–25% ammonia (6 : 4 : 3 : 1 v/v)
3. Standard/Sample application:
   Band length: 8 mm Volume applied: 10 μl Spacing: 10 mm
4. Chamber saturation: 20 min (MP)
5. RH (%): 55 ± 5
6. Temperature °C: 25 ± 2
7. Separation technique: Ascending
8. Quantity of mobile phase: 28 ml
9. Migration distance: 70 mm
10. Migration time: 18 min

Densitometric evaluation:

Wavelength: UV–210 nm Scanning mode: Reflectance/Absorbance

HRF: Ramipril—28; Hydrochlorothiazide—43

Linearity: 500–2000 ng/band for both the compounds

Recovery (%): —

References: —

Comments: The method was optimized and analytical work carried out at **Anchrom's HPTLC Application Laboratory**, Mumbai, India.

HPTLC : High Performance Thin Layer Chromatography
HPTLC Densitogram

No. 64

Hydrochlorothiazide

Ramipril

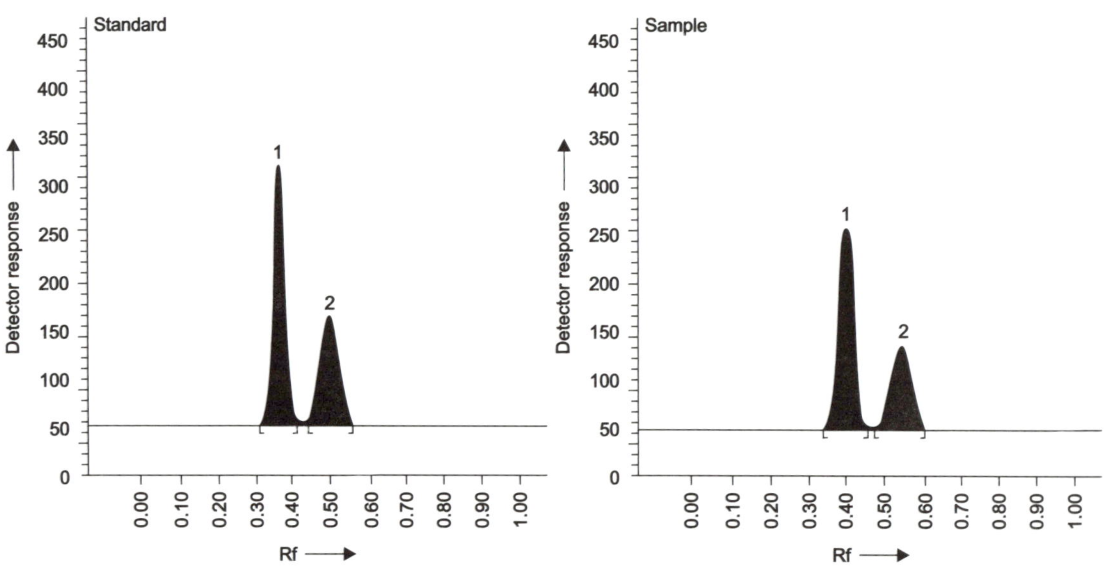

Typical densitogram of the sample and standard containing hydrochlorothiazide and ramipril. For detailed experimental and chromatographic conditions, refer to Protocol No. 64. Peaks identification: 1. Hydrochlorothiazide; 2. Ramipril.

PROTOCOL FOR HPTLC ANALYSIS OF PHARMACEUTICAL FORMULATION

Protocol No. 64

Formulation: Hydrochlorothiazide, Ramipril

Classification: Cardiovascular System **Dosage form:** Tablets

Standard preparation: Weigh accurately 20 mg of ramipril and 25 mg of hydrochlorothiazide, dissolve in methanol to produce 10 ml. Further dilute 0.5 ml of each solution to 10 ml with methanol and proceed with chromatographic analysis.

Sample preparation: Powdered sample equivalent to 12.5 mg of hydrochlorothiazide suspended in methanol, sonicated for 15 min, diluted to 10 ml, filtered and 1 ml of filtrate diluted to 10 ml with methanol and use the solution for analysis.

Chromatographic equipments:

Sample applicator: Camag Linomat–V

Development chamber: Camag twin-trough glass chamber, 10 × 10 cm

Densitometric scanner: Camag TLC Scanner–III

Chromatographic conditions:

1. Stationary phase: Silica gel $60F_{254}$ pre-coated HPTLC plates, 10 × 10 cm (200 μm), Merck
2. Mobile phase (MP): Toluene–methanol–25% ammonia (6 : 4 : 0.1 v/v)
3. Standard/Sample application:
   Band length: 8 mm Volume applied: 10 μl Spacing: 10 mm
4. Chamber saturation: 20 min (MP)
5. RH (%): 55 ± 5
6. Temperature °C: 22
7. Separation technique: Ascending
8. Quantity of mobile phase: 10 ml
9. Migration distance: 80 mm
10. Migration time: 15 min

Densitometric evaluation:

Wavelength: UV–210 nm Scanning mode: Reflectance/Absorbance

HRF: Hydrochlorothiazide—37; Ramipril—50

Linearity: —

Recovery (%): 98.75–101.5 for both the drugs

References: —

Comments:

- The method was optimized and analytical work carried out at **Anchrom's HPTLC Application Laboratory**, Mumbai, India.
- The method is suitable for content uniformity of both the drugs.

HPTLC : High Performance Thin Layer Chromatography
HPTLC Densitogram

No. 65

Hydrochlorothiazide

Telmisartan

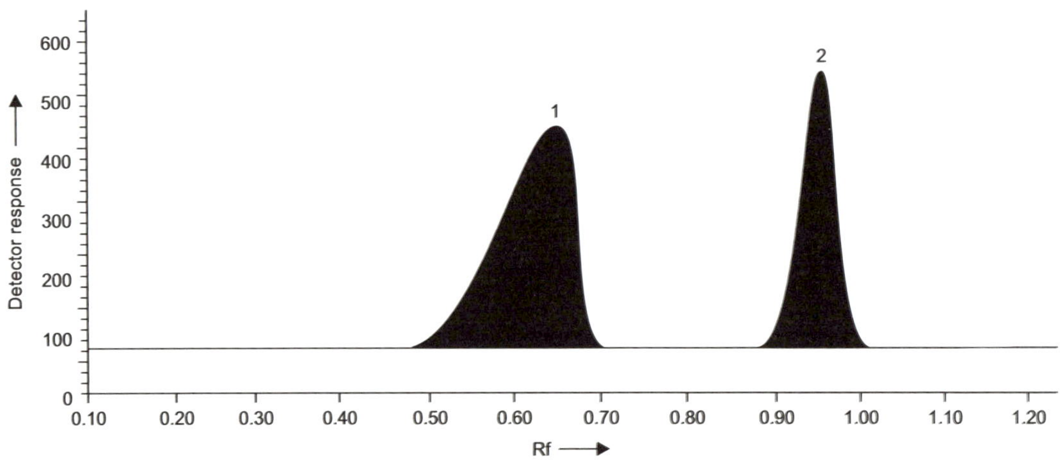

Typical densitogram of the sample containing hydrochlorothiazide and telmisartan. For detailed experimental and chromatographic conditions, refer to Protocol No. 65. Peaks identification: 1. Hydrochlorothiazide; 2. Telmisartan.

PROTOCOL FOR HPTLC ANALYSIS OF PHARMACEUTICAL FORMULATION

Protocol No. 65

Formulation: Hydrochlorothiazide, Telmisartan

Classification: Cardiovascular System **Dosage form:** Tablets

Standard preparation: Dissolve 12.5 mg of hydrochlorothiazide and 40 mg of telmisartan in 20 ml of diluent and use for chromatographic analysis.

Diluent: Mixture of methanol–chloroform (1 : 1 v/v).

Sample preparation: Powdered sample equivalent to 12.5 mg of hydrochlorothiazide or 40 mg of telmisartan suspended in 15 ml of diluent, sonicated for 15 min, diluted to 20 ml with diluent and filtered through Whatman filter paper No. 42 and filtrate used for analysis.

Chromatographic equipments:

Sample applicator: Camag Linomat–V

Development chamber: Camag twin-trough glass chamber, 10 × 10 cm

Densitometric scanner: Camag TLC Scanner–III

Chromatographic conditions:

1. Stationary phase: Silica gel $60F_{254}$ pre-coated TLC plates (250 μm) – Merck, pre-washed with methanol and dried prior to use
2. Mobile phase (MP): Ethyl acetate–chloroform–methanol (10 : 3 : 1 v/v)
3. Standard/Sample application:
   Band length: 10 mm Volume applied: 5 μl Spacing: 14 mm
4. Chamber saturation: 20 min (MP)
5. RH (%): 55 ± 5
6. Temperature °C: 25 ± 2
7. Separation technique: Ascending
8. Quantity of mobile phase: 14 ml
9. Migration distance: 100 mm
10. Migration time: 40 min

Densitometric evaluation:

Wavelength: UV–270 nm Scanning mode: Reflectance/Absorbance

HRF: Hydrochlorothiazide—65; Telmisartan—95

Linearity: Hydrochlorothiazide—500–750 μg/ml; Telmisartan—1600–2400 μg/ml

Recovery (%): 99.49–99.61 for both the compounds

References: R. Maheswari, S.D. Mageswari, K. Surendra, V. Gunasekaran and P. Shanmugasundaram, *Asian J. Chem.*, **19(7)**, 5582–5586, 2007.

Comments: The method validated for accuracy, precision, linearity and system suitability.

HPTLC : High Performance Thin Layer Chromatography
HPTLC Densitogram

No. 66

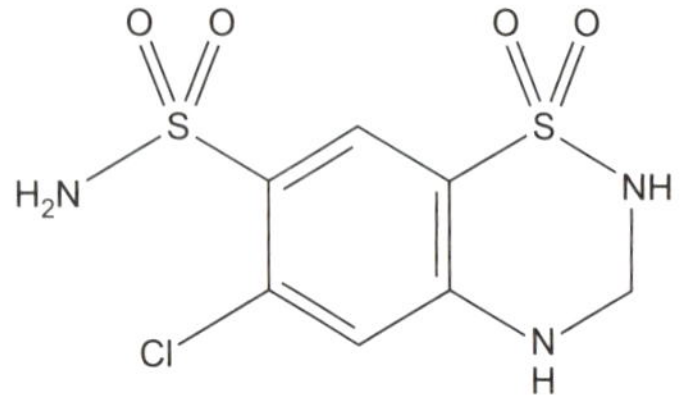

Hydrochlorothiazide

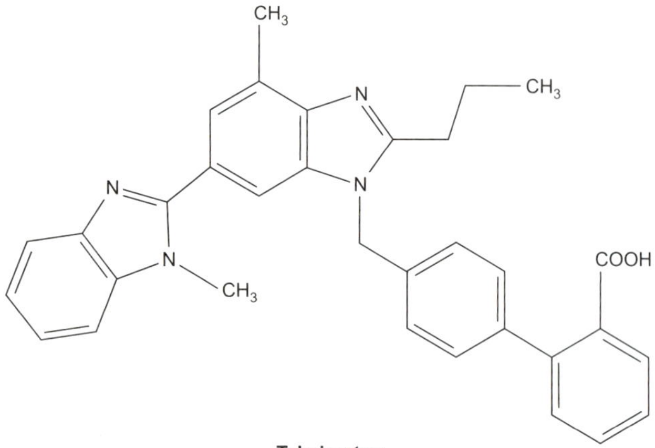

Telmisartan

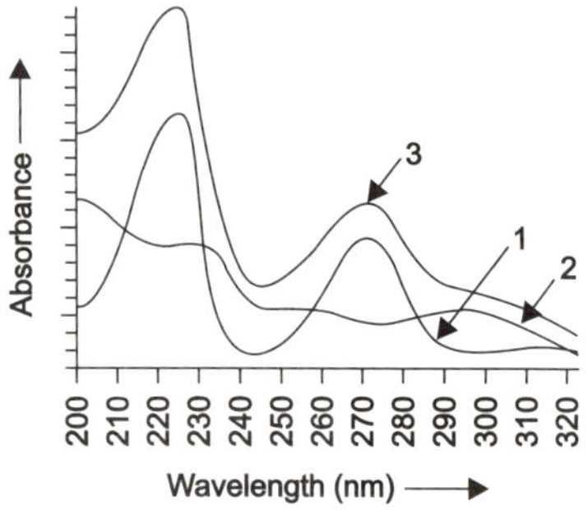

Overlaid UV-spectra of hydrochlorothiazide (1) and telmisartan (2) and mixture of both drugs (3) for selection of suitable wavelength for densitometric scanning

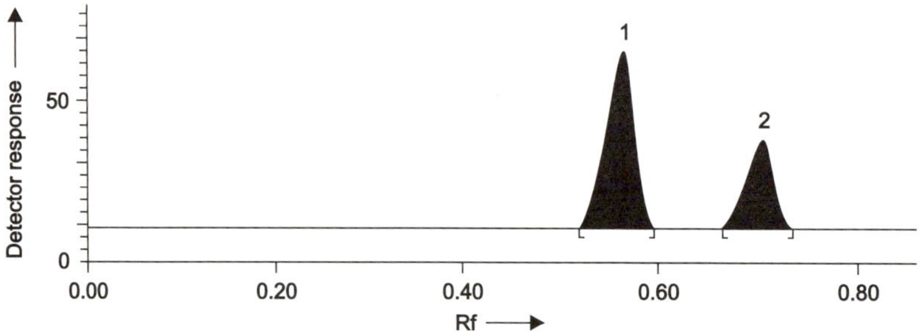

Typical densitogram of the sample containing hydrochlorothiazide and telmisartan. For detailed experimental and chromatographic conditions, refer to Protocol No. 66. Peaks identification: 1. Hydrochlorothiazide; 2. Telmisartan.

PROTOCOL FOR HPTLC ANALYSIS OF PHARMACEUTICAL FORMULATION

Protocol No. 66

Formulation: Hydrochlorothiazide, Telmisartan

Classification: Cardiovascular System **Dosage form:** Tablets

Standard preparation: Prepare 100 μg/ml solution of each compound in chloroform and use for chromatographic application.

Sample preparation: Powdered sample equivalent to 25 mg of telmisartan suspended in chloroform, shake for 15 min, filter through Whatman No. 41 filter paper. Further dilutions suitably made with chloroform for chromatographic analysis.

Chromatographic equipments:

Sample applicator: Camag Linomat–V

Development chamber: Camag twin-trough glass chamber, 10 × 10 cm

Densitometric scanner: Camag TLC Scanner–III

Chromatographic conditions:

1. Stationary phase: Silica gel 60F_{254} pre-coated TLC plates, 10 × 10 cm (250 μm) – Merck, pre-washed with methanol, activatcd at 50°C for 5 min prior to use
2. Mobile phase (MP): Chloroform–methanol–toluene (2 : 5 : 5 v/v)
3. Standard/Sample application:

   Band length: 5 mm Volume applied: 4 μl Spacing: 5 mm
4. Chamber saturation: 30 min (MP)
5. RH (%): 55 ± 5
6. Temperature °C: Ambient
7. Separation technique: Ascending
8. Quantity of mobile phase: 12 ml
9. Migration distance: 72 mm
10. Migration time: 25 min

Densitometric evaluation:

Wavelength: UV–272 nm Scanning mode: Reflectance/Absorbance

HRF: Hydrochlorothiazide—55; Telmisartan—70

Linearity (ng/band): Hydrochlorothiazide—200–700; Telmisartan—250–500

Recovery (%): Hydrochlorothiazide—98.55–100.1; Telmisartan—99.81–101.16

References: N.J. Shah, B.N. Suhagia, R.R. Shah and P.B. Shah, *Ind. J. Pharm, Sci.*, **69(2)**, 202–205, 2005.

Comments: The method validated for accuracy, precision, linearity, LOD, LOQ and specificity.

HPTLC : High Performance Thin Layer Chromatography
HPTLC Densitogram

No. 67

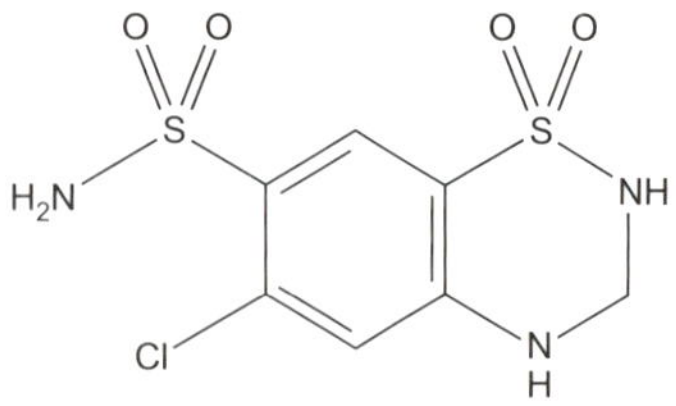

Hydrochlorothiazide

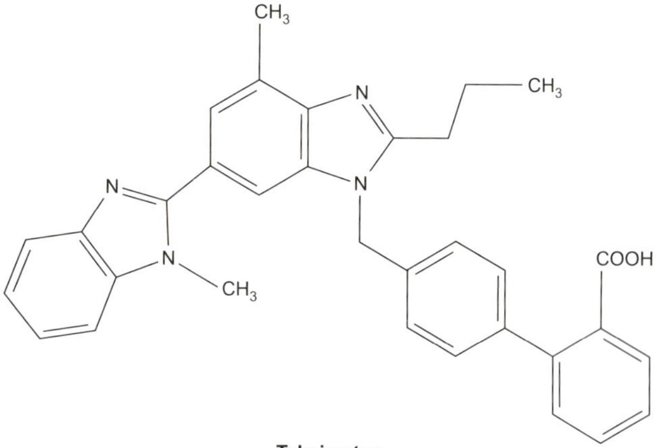

Telmisartan

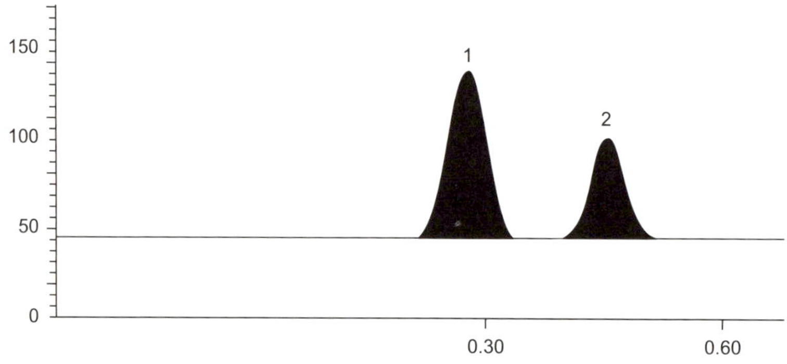

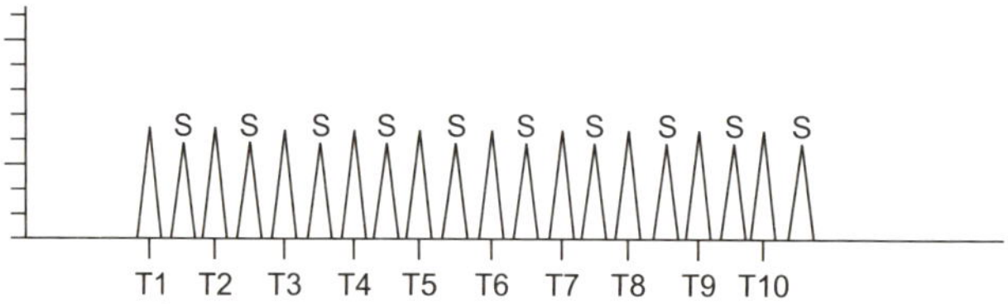

Content uniformity test (T_1–T_{10}–Sample) S–Standards

Typical densitogram of the sample containing hydrochlorothiazide and telmisartan. For detailed experimental and chromatographic conditions, refer to Protocol No. 67. Peaks identification: 1. Telmisartan; 2. Hydrochlorothiazide.

PROTOCOL FOR HPTLC ANALYSIS OF PHARMACEUTICAL FORMULATION

Protocol No. 67

Formulation: Hydrochlorothiazide, Telmisartan

Classification: Cardiovascular System **Dosage form:** Tablets

Standard preparation: Mixed standard solution of both the compounds was prepared in methanol to get 200 μg/ml of telmisartan and 62 μg/ml of hydrochlorothiazide. Apply 2–10 μl of solution for linearity studies.

Sample preparation: Powdered sample equivalent to 40 mg of telmisartan suspended in 20 ml of methanol, sonicate for 10 min, dilute to 5 ml with methanol, filter through Whatman filter paper No. 1, dilute 5 ml of the filtrate to 20 ml with methanol and use for assay.

Chromatographic equipments:

Sample applicator: Camag Linomat–V

Development chamber: Camag twin-trough glass chamber, 20 × 10 cm

Densitometric scanner: Camag TLC Scanner–III

Chromatographic conditions:

1. Stationary phase: Silica gel $60F_{254}$ pre-coated HPTLC plates, 20 × 10 cm (200 μm) – Merck
2. Mobile phase (MP): Ethyl acetate–chloroform–acetone–methanol (3 : 3 : 3 : 0.5 v/v)
3. Standard/Sample application:
   Band length: 6 mm Volume applied: 5 μl Spacing: 10 mm
4. Chamber saturation: 10 min (MP)
5. RH (%): 55 ± 5
6. Temperature °C: 25 ± 5
7. Separation technique: Ascending
8. Quantity of mobile phase: 19 ml
9. Migration distance: 80 mm
10. Migration time: 20 min

Densitometric evaluation:

Wavelength: UV–280 nm Scanning mode: Reflectance/Absorbance

HRF: Telmisartan—27; Hydrochlorothiazide—45

Linearity (μg/band): Hydrochlorothiazide—25–125; Telmisartan—80–400

Recovery (%): Hydrochlorothiazide—99.39–100.71; Telmisartan—98.74–99

References: S.B. Morge and B.H. Mehta, *J. Pharm. Res.*, **7(2)**, 126–128, 2008.

Comments:

- The method validated for accuracy, precision, linearity, LOD, LOQ, specificity and ruggedness.
- The method is suitable for content uniformity test.

HPTLC : High Performance Thin Layer Chromatography
HPTLC Densitogram

No. 68

Hydrochlorothiazide

Olmesartan medoxomil

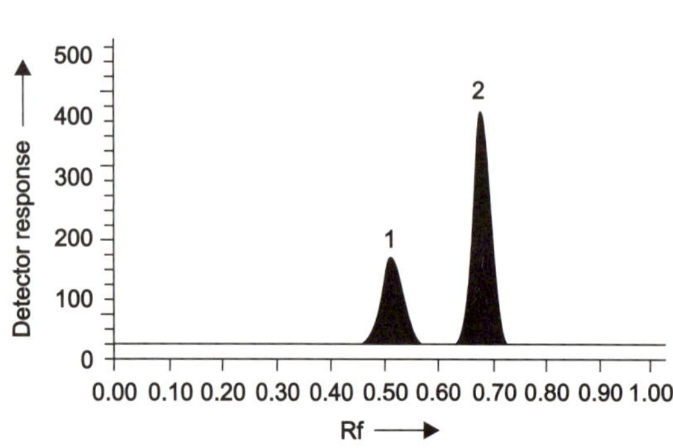

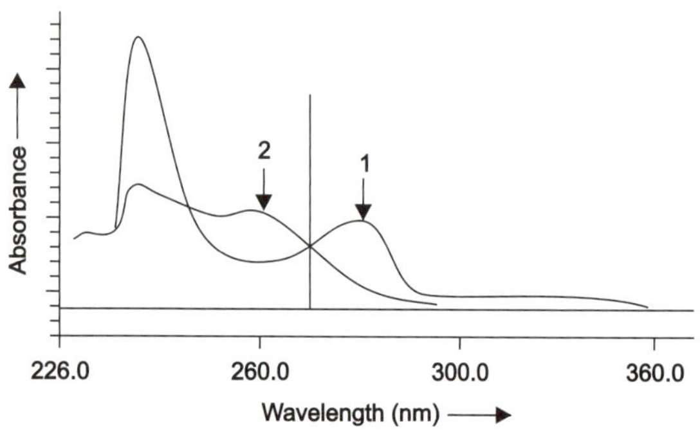

Overlaid UV-spectra of hydrochlorothiazide (1) and olmesartan (2) for selection of suitable wavelength for densitometric scanning

Typical densitogram of the sample containing hydrochlorothiazide and olmesartan medoxomil. For detailed experimental and chromatographic conditions, refer to Protocol No. 68. Peaks identification: 1. Olmesartan medoxomil; 2. Hydrochlorothiazide.

PROTOCOL FOR HPTLC ANALYSIS OF PHARMACEUTICAL FORMULATION

Protocol No. 68

Formulation: Hydrochlorothiazide, Olmesartan medoxomil

Classification: Cardiovascular System **Dosage form:** Tablets

Standard preparation: Prepare 100 μg/ml solution of each compound in methanol. Apply 5–7.5 μl of olmesartan solution and 1–6 ml of hydrochlorothiazide for linearity studies.

Sample preparation: Powdered sample equivalent to 25 mg olmesartan medoxomil suspended in 100 ml of methanol, sonicated for 15 min, diluted to 250 ml, filtered and filtrate suitably diluted to get 100 μg/ml of olmesartan medoxomil and use for chromatographic analysis.

Chromatographic equipments:

Sample applicator: Camag Linomat–V

Development chamber: Camag twin-trough glass chamber, 10 × 10 cm

Densitometric scanner: Camag TLC Scanner–III

Chromatographic conditions:

1. Stationary phase: Silica gel $60F_{254}$ pre-coated HPTLC plates, 10 × 10 cm (200 μm) – Merck, pre-washed with methanol, activated (50°C) for 5 min prior to use
2. Mobile phase (MP): Acetonitrile–chloroform–glacial acetic acid (7 : 2 : 0.5 v/v)
3. Standard/Sample application:
   Band length: 5 mm Volume applied: 6 μl Spacing: 5 mm
4. Chamber saturation: 30 min (MP)
5. RH (%): 55 ± 5
6. Temperature °C: 25 ± 2
7. Separation technique: Ascending
8. Quantity of mobile phase: 9.5 ml
9. Migration distance: 72 mm
10. Migration time: 25 min

Densitometric evaluation:

Wavelength: UV–260 nm or 272.8 nm Scanning mode: Reflectance/Absorbance

HRF: Olmesartan—52; Hydrochlorothiazide—68

Linearity (ng/band): Hydrochlorothiazide—100–600; Olmesartan medoxomil—500–750

Recovery (%): Hydrochlorothiazide—99.86–101.14; Olmesartan medoxomil—99.03–100.04

References: N.J. Shah, B.N. Suhagia, R.R. Shah and N.M. Patel, *Indian J. Pharm. Sci.*, **70(6)**, 834–836, 2007.

Comments: The method validated for accuracy, precision, linearity, LOD, LOQ and specificity.

HPTLC : High Performance Thin Layer Chromatography
HPTLC Densitogram

No. 69

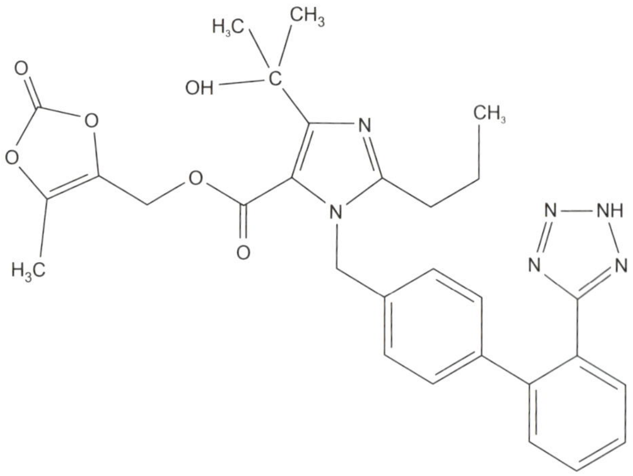

Olmesartan medoxomil

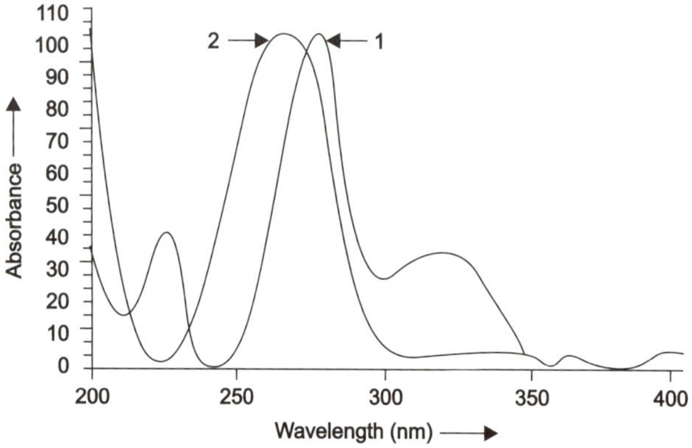

Overlaid UV-spectra of HCZ (1) and OM (2) for selection of suitable wavelength for densitometric scanning

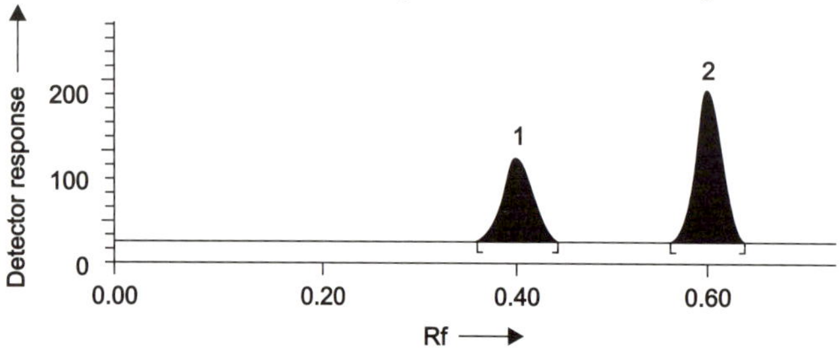

Typical densitogram of the sample containing hydrochlorothiazide and olmesartan medoxomil. For detailed experimental and chromatographic conditions, refer to Protocol No. 69. Peaks identification: 1. Hydrochlorothiazide; 2. Olmesartan medoxomil.

PROTOCOL FOR HPTLC ANALYSIS OF PHARMACEUTICAL FORMULATION

Protocol No. 69

Formulation: Hydrochlorothiazide, Olmesartan medoxomil

Classification: Cardiovascular System **Dosage form:** Tablets

Standard preparation: Prepare 500 μg/ml solution of each compound in methanol. Further dilutions made to get 25 μg/ml solution of each. Apply varying volumes of these solutions for linearity profile.

Sample preparation: Powdered sample equivalent to 12.5 mg of hydrochlorothiazide suspended in 30 ml of methanol, sonicated for 5 min, diluted to 50 ml, filtered and the filtrate suitably diluted with methanol. Apply 10 μl for assay.

Chromatographic equipments:

Sample applicator: Camag Linomat–V

Development chamber: Camag twin-trough glass chamber, 20 × 10 cm

Densitometric scanner: Camag TLC Scanner–III

Chromatographic conditions:

1. Stationary phase: Silica gel $60F_{254}$ pre-coated HPTLC plates, 20 × 10 cm (250 μm) – Merck, pre-washed with methanol, activated at 110°C for 5 min prior to use
2. Mobile phase (MP): (i) Chloroform–methanol–toluene (6 : 4 : 5 v/v); (ii) Chloroform–methanol (8 : 2 v/v)
3. Standard/Sample application:
   Band length: 6 mm Volume applied: 10 μl Spacing: 12.1 mm
4. Chamber saturation: 15 min (MP)
5. RH (%): 55 ± 5
6. Temperature °C: 22 ± 2
7. Separation technique: Ascending
8. Quantity of mobile phase: 15 ml
9. Migration distance: 90 mm
10. Migration time: 20 min

Densitometric evaluation:

Wavelength: UV–258 nm; 270 nm

Scanning mode: Reflectance/Absorbance

HRF: Hydrochlorothiazide—40, 30; Olmesartan medoxomil—58, 40

Linearity (ng/band): Hydrochlorothiazide—50–300; Olmesartan medoxomil—200–600

Recovery (%): 99.92–100.82 for both the drugs

References: Sayali S. Kadukar, Santosh V. Gandhi, Poonam N. Ranjana and Sandeep S. Ranher, *J. Planar. Chromatography*, **22(6)**, 425–428, 2009; Prabhu Dessai D.S. et al., Abstract No. F-287, 63rd IPC, 2011.

Comments: The method validated for accuracy, precision, linearity, LOD, LOQ, specificity and robustness.

HPTLC : High Performance Thin Layer Chromatography
HPTLC Densitogram

No. 70

Hydrochlorothiazide

Olmesartan medoxomil

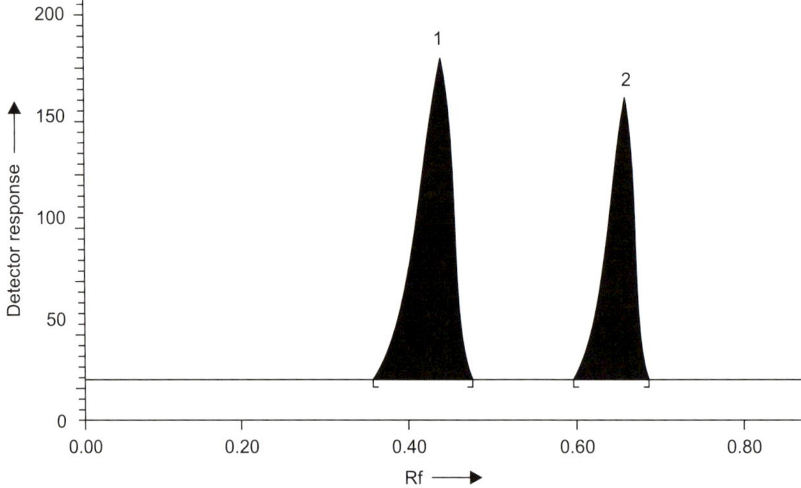

Typical densitogram of the sample containing hydrochlorothiazide and olmesartan medoxomil. For detailed experimental and chromatographic conditions, refer to Protocol No. 70. Peaks identification: 1. Olmesartan medoxomil; 2. Hydrochlorothiazide.

PROTOCOL FOR HPTLC ANALYSIS OF PHARMACEUTICAL FORMULATION

Protocol No. 70

Formulation: Hydrochlorothiazide, Olmesartan medoxomil

Classification: Cardiovascular System **Dosage form:** Tablets

Standard preparation: Prepare separately 1 mg/ml solution of each compound in methanol. Further serial dilutions made with methanol for linearity profile.

Sample preparation: An adequate quantity of the powdered sample suspended in methanol to get 1 mg/ml, filter and dilute the filtrate suitably for analysis.

Chromatographic equipments:

Sample applicator: Camag Linomat–V

Development chamber: Camag twin-trough glass chamber, 20 × 10 cm

Densitometric scanner: Camag TLC Scanner–III

Chromatographic conditions:

1. Stationary phase: Silica gel 60F_{254} pre-coated HPTLC plates, 20 × 10 cm (200 μm) – Merck, pre-washed with methanol, dried at 120°C for 20 min prior to use
2. Mobile phase (MP): (i) Acetonitrile–ethyl acetate–glacial acetic acid (7 : 3 : 0.4); (ii) Ethyl acetate–chloroform–methanol (4 : 4 : 2 v/v)
3. Standard/Sample application:
   Band length: 10 mm Volume applied: 5 μl Spacing: 11.4 mm
4. Chamber saturation: 20 min (MP)
5. RH (%): 55 ± 5
6. Temperature °C: 23 ± 2
7. Separation technique: Ascending
8. Quantity of mobile phase: 20 ml
9. Migration distance: 70 mm
10. Migration time: 20 min

Densitometric evaluation:

Wavelength: UV–254 nm, 274 nm Scanning mode: Reflectance/Absorbance

HRF: Olmesartan medoxomil—44, 39; Hydrochlorothiazide—64, 63

Linearity (ng/band): Hydrochlorothiazide—125–375; Olmesartan medoxomil—200–600

Recovery (%): 99.77–100.09 for both the drugs

References: P.D. Bari and A.R. Rote, *Chromatographia*, **69(11–12)**, 1469–1472, 2009; A.K. Sen, D.B. Sen, U. Sahoo and A.K. Seth, Abstract No. 277, 63rd IPC, 2011.

Comments: The analytical data reported by the authors by HPLC and HPTLC methods was comparable.

HPTLC : High Performance Thin Layer Chromatography
HPTLC Densitogram

No. 71

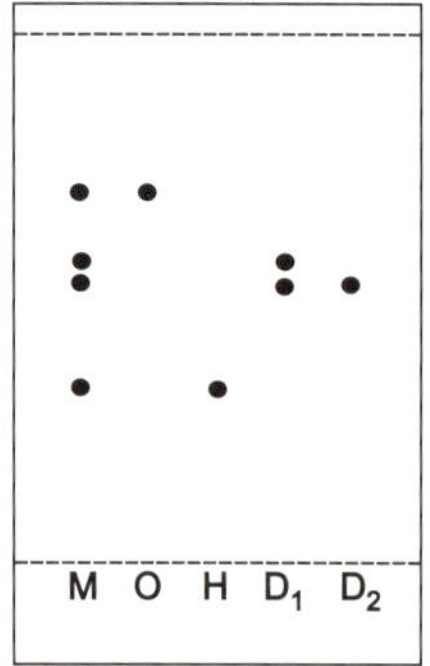

Thin layer chromatogram of both the drugs and degradation products.
M = Mixture of both the drugs and degradation products
O = Olmesartan,
H = Hydrochlorothiazide
D_1 = Acidic degradation
D_2 = Alkaline degradation

(A)

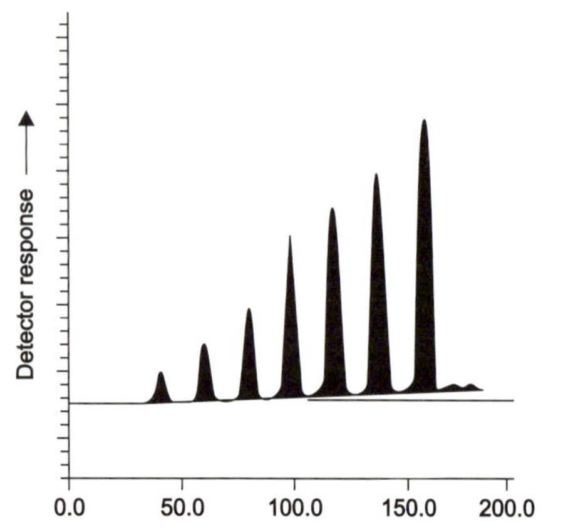

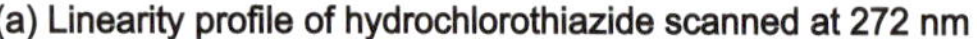
(a) Linearity profile of hydrochlorothiazide scanned at 272 nm

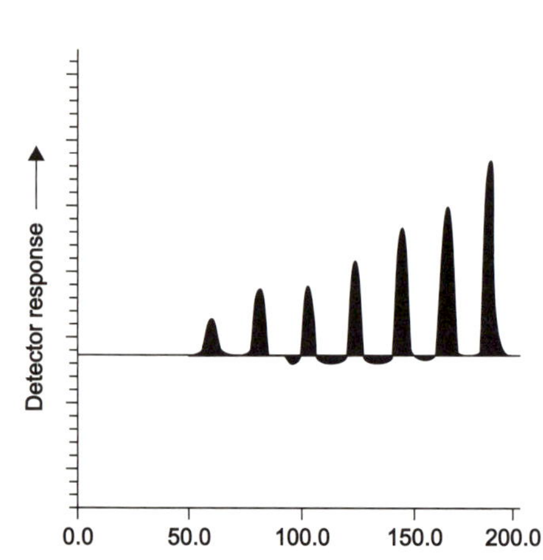

(b) Linearity profile of olmesartan medoxomil scanned at 260 nm

Typical densitogram of the standards containing hydrochlorothiazide (A) and olmesartan medoxomil (B). For detailed experimental and chromatographic conditions, refer to Protocol No. 71. Peaks identification: 1. Hydrochlorothiazide; 2. Olmesartan medoxomil.

PROTOCOL FOR HPTLC ANALYSIS OF PHARMACEUTICAL FORMULATION

Protocol No. 71

Formulation: Hydrochlorothiazide, Olmesartan medoxomil

Classification: Cardiovascular System **Dosage form:** Tablets

Standard preparation: Prepare standard solution of each drug in methanol to get 1 mg/ml of olmesartan medoxomil (OLM) and 0.625 mg/ml of hydrochlorothiazide (HTZ). Further serial dilutions made with methanol for linearity profile.

Sample preparation: Coating of the tablets was removed with cotton moistened with ethanol, dried, powdered and weighed sample equivalent to 100 mg of olmesartan medoxomil (OLM) and suspended in 80 ml of methanol, sonicate for 30 min, dilute to 100 ml with methanol. Filter and dilute suitable with methanol for assay.

Chromatographic equipments:

Sample applicator: Hamilton 25 μl syringe

Development chamber: Flat-bottom glass chamber, 20 × 20 × 10 cm

Densitometric scanner: Shimadzu CS-930 densitometer

Chromatographic conditions:

1. Stationary phase: NanoSilica gel 60F_{254} pre-coated HPTLC plates, 20 × 20 cm (200 μm) – M & N
2. Mobile phase (MP): Chloroform–methanol–formic acid (8 : 1.5 : 0.5 v/v)
3. Standard/Sample application:
   Band length: 10 mm Volume applied: 10 μl Spacing: 20 mm
4. Chamber saturation: 60 min (MP)
5. RH (%): —
6. Temperature °C: 22 ± 1
7. Separation technique: Ascending
8. Quantity of mobile phase: 20 ml
9. Migration distance: 170 mm
10. Migration time: —

Densitometric evaluation:

Wavelength: UV–260 nm (OLM); 272 nm (HTZ)

Scanning mode: Reflectance/Absorbance

HRF: See Figure A

Linearity: 500–10,000 ng/band for both the compounds

Recovery (%): 99.88–100.16 for both the drugs

References: Bahia Moussa, Marwa Mohamed and Nadia Youssef, *J. Planar Chromatog.*, **24(1)**, 35–39, 2011.

Comments:

- The method validated for accuracy, precision, linearity, LOD, LOQ, specificity, robustness and ruggedness.
- The results comparable with reported RP-HPLC method (*J. Chromatogr.*, **66**, 213–218, 2007).
- The method is stability indicating (acid, base, oxidative, thermal, photolytic). The degradation products were separated from main compounds.

HPTLC : High Performance Thin Layer Chromatography
HPTLC Densitogram

No. 72

Irbesartan

Hydrochlorothiazide

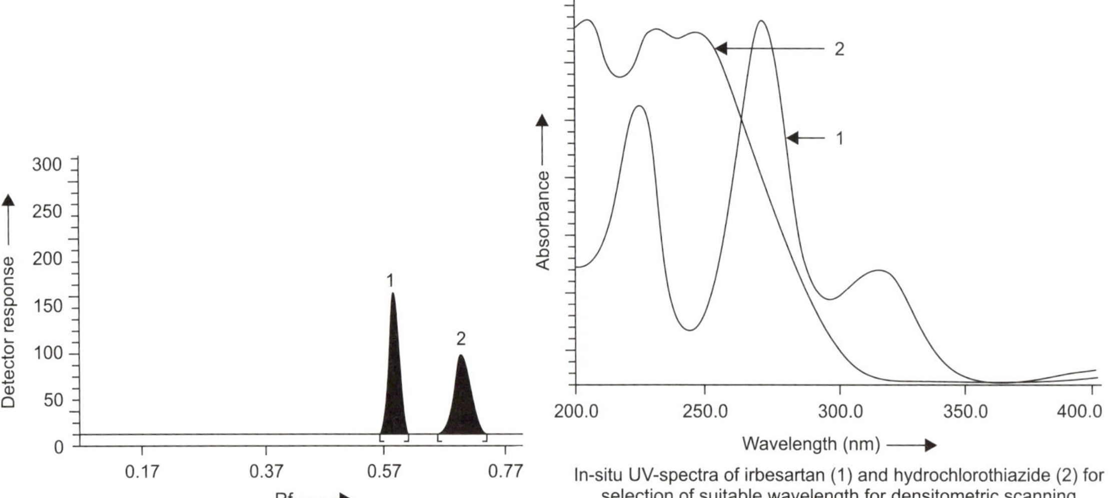

In-situ UV-spectra of irbesartan (1) and hydrochlorothiazide (2) for selection of suitable wavelength for densitometric scanning

Typical densitogram of the standard containing hydrochlorothiazide and irbesartan. For detailed experimental and chromatographic conditions, refer to Protocol No. 72. Peaks identification: 1. Irbesartan; 2. Hydrochlorothiazide.

PROTOCOL FOR HPTLC ANALYSIS OF PHARMACEUTICAL FORMULATION

Protocol No. 72

Formulation: Hydrochlorothiazide, Irbesartan

Classification: Cardiovascular System **Dosage form:** Tablets

Standard preparation: Prepare 100 μg/ml solution of each drug in methanol. Apply varying volumes for linearity profile.

Sample preparation: Powdered sample equivalent to 25 mg of irbesartan suspended in methanol, sonicated for 15 min, filtered through Whatman No. 41 filter paper and diluted with methanol to get 100 μg/ml of irbesartan and 8.33 μg/ml of hydrochlorothiazide and used for assay.

Chromatographic equipments:

Sample applicator: Camag Linomat–V

Development chamber: Camag twin-trough glass chamber, 10 × 10 cm

Densitometric scanner: Camag TLC Scanner–III

Chromatographic conditions:

1. Stationary phase: Silica gel $60F_{254}$ pre-coated HPTLC plates, 10 × 10 cm (200 μm) – Merck, pre-washed with methanol, activated at 50°C for 5 min before use
2. Mobile phase (MP): (i) Acetonitrile–chloroform–glacial acetic acid (7 : 3 : 0.1 v/v); (ii) Chloroform–methanol (8 : 2 v/v)
3. Standard/Sample application:
   Band length: 6 mm Volume applied: 4 μl Spacing: 4 mm
4. Chamber saturation: 30 min (MP)
5. RH (%): 55 ± 5
6. Temperature °C: 22 ± 2
7. Separation technique: Ascending
8. Quantity of mobile phase: 10 ml
9. Migration distance: 72 mm
10. Migration time: 30 min

Densitometric evaluation:

Wavelength: UV–260 nm Scanning mode: Reflectance/Absorbance

HRF: Irbesartan—60, 45; Hydrochlorothiazide—70, 30

Linearity (ng/band): Hydrochlorothiazide—100–350; Irbesartan—100–700 ng

Recovery (%): Hydrochlorothiazide—99.14–102.53; Irbesartan—99.59–101.82

References: N.J. Shah, B.N. Suhagia, R.R. Shah and N.M. Patel, *Indian J. Pharm. Sci.*, **69(2)**, 240–243, 2007; P.C. Sardessai et al., Abstract No. F–295, 63rd IPC, 2011.

Comments: The method validated for accuracy, precision, linearity, LOD and LOQ as per ICH guidelines.

HPTLC : High Performance Thin Layer Chromatography
HPTLC Densitogram

No. 73

Irbesartan

Hydrochlorothiazide

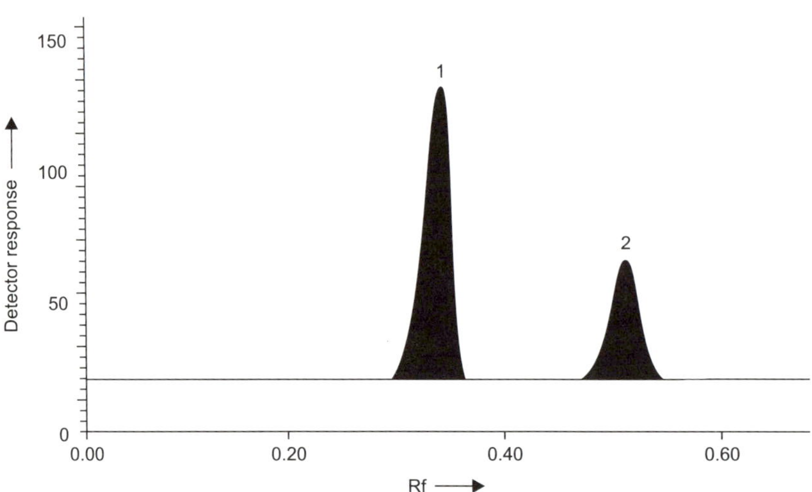

Typical densitogram of the sample containing hydrochlorothiazide and irbesartan. For detailed experimental and chromatographic conditions, refer to Protocol No. 73. Peaks identification: 1. Irbesartan; 2. Hydrochlorothiazide.

PROTOCOL FOR HPTLC ANALYSIS OF PHARMACEUTICAL FORMULATION

Protocol No. 73

Formulation: Hydrochlorothiazide, Irbesartan

Classification: Cardiovascular System **Dosage form:** Tablets

Standard preparation: Standard solution of both the compounds prepared separately in methanol to get 250 μg/ml of hydrochlorothiazide and 300.4 μg/ml of irbesartan. Further dilute 2–12 ml of above solutions to 20 ml with methanol and apply 5 μl of each solution for linearity.

Sample preparation: Powdered sample equivalent to 12.5 mg of hydrochlorothiazide suspended in 25 ml of methanol, sonicated for 10 min, diluted to 50 ml with methanol, filtered through Whatman filter paper No. 1. 5 ml of the filtrate further diluted to 20 ml with methanol and apply 5 μl for assay.

Chromatographic equipments:

Sample applicator: Camag Linomat–IV

Development chamber: Camag twin-trough glass chamber, 10 × 10 cm

Densitometric scanner: Camag TLC Scanner–III

Chromatographic conditions:

1. Stationary phase: Silica gel $60F_{254}$ pre-coated HPTLC plates, 10 × 10 cm (200 μm) – Merck
2. Mobile phase (MP): Acetonitrile–chloroform–ethyl acetate–methanol (3 : 3 : 3 : 0.5 v/v)
3. Standard/Sample application:
   Band length: 6 mm Volume applied: 5 μl Spacing: 10 mm
4. Chamber saturation: 10 min (MP)
5. RH (%): 55 ± 5.6
6. Temperature °C: 25 ± 2°C
7. Separation technique: Ascending
8. Quantity of mobile phase: 9.5 ml
9. Migration distance: 80 mm
10. Migration time: 22 min

Densitometric evaluation:

Wavelength: UV–250 nm Scanning mode: Reflectance/Absorbance

HRF: Irbesartan—35; Hydrochlorothiazide—50

Linearity (ng/ml): Hydrochlorothiazide—25–150; Irbesartan—300.4–1802.4

Recovery (%): 98.5–99.2 for both the compounds

References: B.H. Mehta and S.B. Morgan, *Indian Drugs*, **47(2)**, 71–74, 2010.

Comments: The method validated for accuracy, precision, linearity, LOD, LOQ and specificity.

HPTLC : High Performance Thin Layer Chromatography
HPTLC Densitogram

No. 74

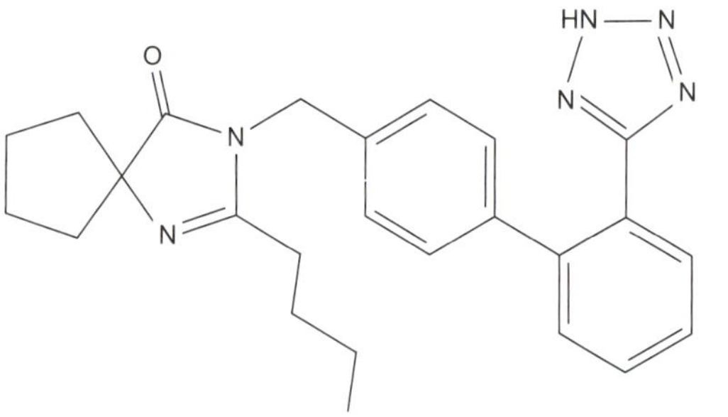

Irbesartan

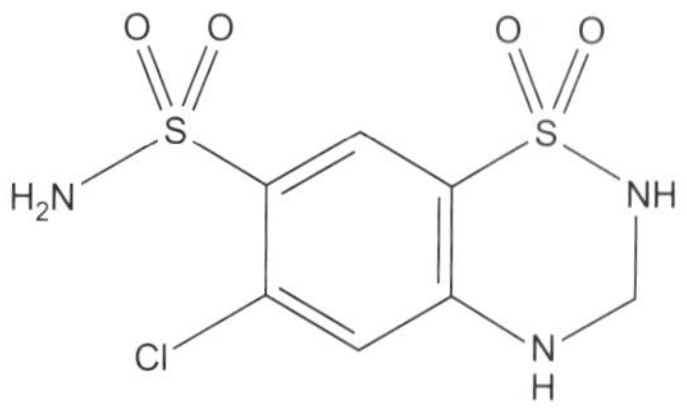

Hydrochlorothiazide

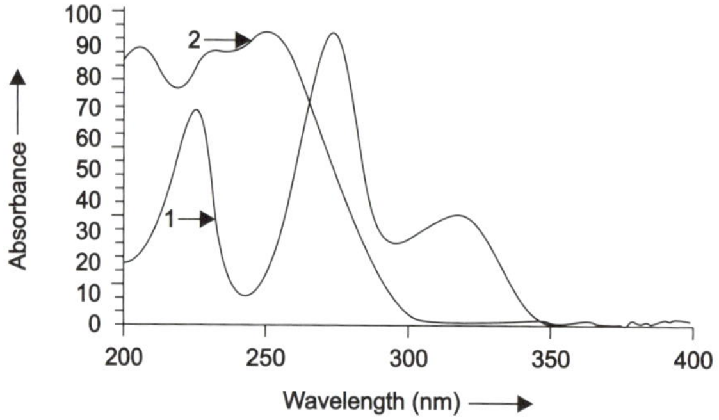

Overlaid UV-spectra of hydrochlorothiazide (I) and irbesartan (2) for selection of suitable wavelength for densitometric scanning

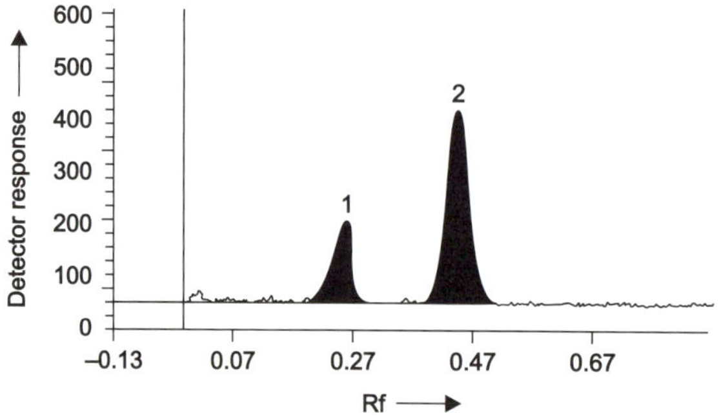

Typical densitogram of the sample containing hydrochlorothiazide and irbesartan. For detailed experimental and chromatographic conditions, refer to Protocol No. 74. Peaks identification: 1. Irbesartan; 2. Hydrochlorothiazide.

PROTOCOL FOR HPTLC ANALYSIS OF PHARMACEUTICAL FORMULATION

Protocol No. 74

Formulation: Hydrochlorothiazide, Irbesartan

Classification: Cardiovascular System **Dosage form:** Tablets

Standard preparation: Prepare 1 mg/ml solution of each compound in methanol. Further dilution of each solution made with methanol to get 100 μg/ml. Apply varying volumes (2–10 μl) for linearity studies.

Sample preparation: Powdered sample equivalent to 10 mg of hydrochlorothiazide suspended in methanol, sonicated for 10 min, diluted to 25 ml with methanol. Filter and dilute further to get 100 μg/ml in respect of hydrochlorothiazide. Apply 2 μl of final solution for assay.

Chromatographic equipments:

Sample applicator: Camag Linomat–IV

Development chamber: Camag twin-trough glass chamber, 10 × 10 cm

Densitometric scanner: Camag TLC Scanner–III

Chromatographic conditions:

1. Stationary phase: Silica gel 60F_{254} pre-coated TLC plates, 10 × 10 cm (250 μm) – Merck
2. Mobile phase (MP): (i) Acetonitrile–chloroform (5 : 6 v/v); (ii) Toluene–ethyl acetate–acetic acid–methanol (7 : 3 : 0.2 : 0.5 v/v)
3. Standard/Sample application:
   Band length: 4 mm Volume applied: 2–10 μl Spacing: 10 mm
4. Chamber saturation: 15 min (MP)
5. RH (%): 55 ± 5
6. Temperature °C: 22 ± 2
7. Separation technique: Ascending
8. Quantity of mobile phase: 11 ml
9. Migration distance: 90 mm
10. Migration time: 20 min

Densitometric evaluation:

Wavelength: UV–270 nm Scanning mode: Reflectance/Absorbance

HRF: Irbesartan—25, 45; Hydrochlorothiazide—46, 15

Linearity (ng/band): Hydrochlorothiazide—200–600; Irbesartan—200–1000

Recovery (%): 98.0–102.0 for both the compounds

References: (i) Amol S. Khodke, Laxman V. Potale, M.C. Damle and K.G. Bothara, Pharmaceutical Methods, an addendum to *J. Young Pharmacist*, **1(1)**, 39–43, 2010; (ii) M.U. Trvambake et al., Abstract No. F343, 62nd IPC, 2010.

Comments:

- The method validated for accuracy, precision, linearity, LOD, LOQ, specificity, robustness and ruggedness.
- The method is stability indicating (acid, base, oxidative, thermal, photolytic). The degradation products were separated from main compounds.
- Reversal of retention factor in two mobile phases reported.

HPTLC : High Performance Thin Layer Chromatography
HPTLC Densitogram

No. 75

Hydrochlorothiazide

Valsartan

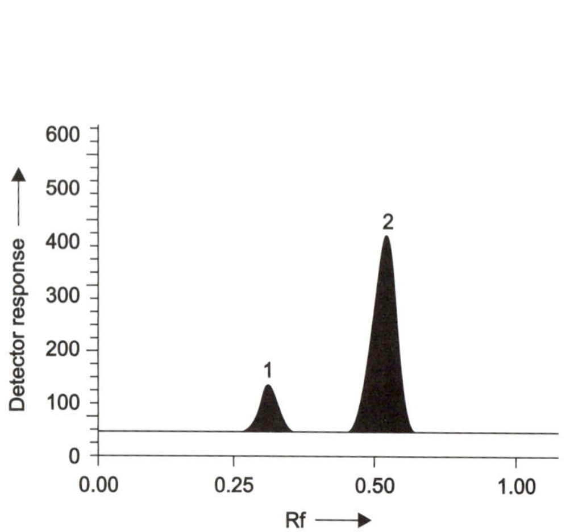

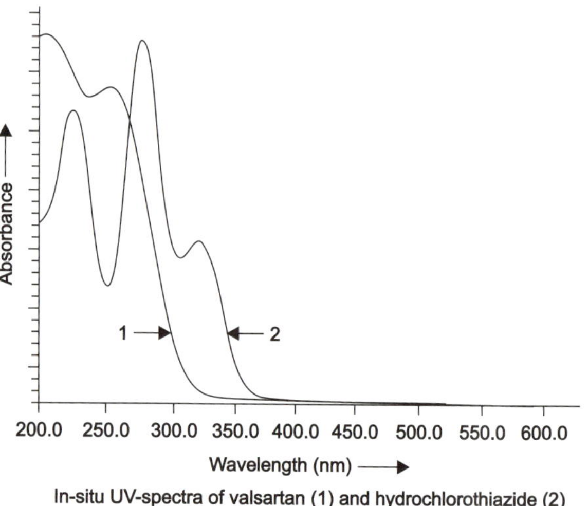

In-situ UV-spectra of valsartan (1) and hydrochlorothiazide (2) for selection of suitable wavelength for densitometric scanning

Typical densitogram of the standard containing hydrochlorothiazide and valsartan. For detailed experimental and chromatographic conditions, refer to Protocol No. 75. Peaks identification: 1. Hydrochlorothiazide; 2. Valsartan.

PROTOCOL FOR HPTLC ANALYSIS OF PHARMACEUTICAL FORMULATION

Protocol No. 75

Formulation: Hydrochlorothiazide, Valsartan

Classification: Cardiovascular System **Dosage form:** Tablets

Standard preparation: Prepare 8 mg/ml solution of valsartan and 1.25 mg/ml solution of hydrochlorothiazide, both in ethanol or methanol. Further dilute to get 800 ng/µl (valsartan) and 125 ng/µl (hydrochlorothiazide) and use for application.

Sample preparation: Powdered sample equivalent to 80 mg of valsartan or 12.5 mg of hydrochlorothiazide suspended in 10 ml of methanol, sonicate, filter and dilute further to get 800 ng/µl (valsartan) and 125 ng/µl (hydrochlorothiazide).

Chromatographic equipments:

Sample applicator: Camag Linomat–IV

Development chamber: Camag twin-trough glass chamber, 20 × 20 cm

Densitometric scanner: Camag TLC Scanner–III

Chromatographic conditions:

1. Stationary phase: Silica gel $60F_{254}$ pre-coated HPTLC plates, 10 × 20 cm (200 µm) – Merck, pre-washed with methanol and stored in desiccator before use
2. Mobile phase (MP): Chloroform–ethyl acetate–acetic acid (5 : 5 : 0.2 v/v)
3. Standard/Sample application:
   Band length: 6 mm Volume applied: 5 µl Spacing: 11.6 mm
4. Chamber saturation: 30 min (MP)
5. RH (%): 55 ± 5
6. Temperature °C: 25 ± 5
7. Separation technique: Ascending
8. Quantity of mobile phase: 20 ml
9. Migration distance: 70 mm
10. Migration time: 35 min

Densitometric evaluation:

Wavelength: UV–248 nm Scanning mode: Reflectance/Absorbance

HRF: Hydrochlorothiazide—27; Valsartan—56

Linearity (ng/band): Valsartan—800–5600; Hydrochlorothiazide—125–875ng

Recovery (%): Valsartan—100.36–100.79; Hydrochlorothiazide—100.41–101.46

References: B.R. Kadam and S.B. Bari, *Acta Chromatographica*, **18**, 260–269, 2007.

Comments: The method validated for accuracy, precision, linearity, LOD, LOQ and specificity as per ICH guidelines.

HPTLC : High Performance Thin Layer Chromatography
HPTLC Densitogram

No. 76

Hydrochlorothiazide

Valsartan

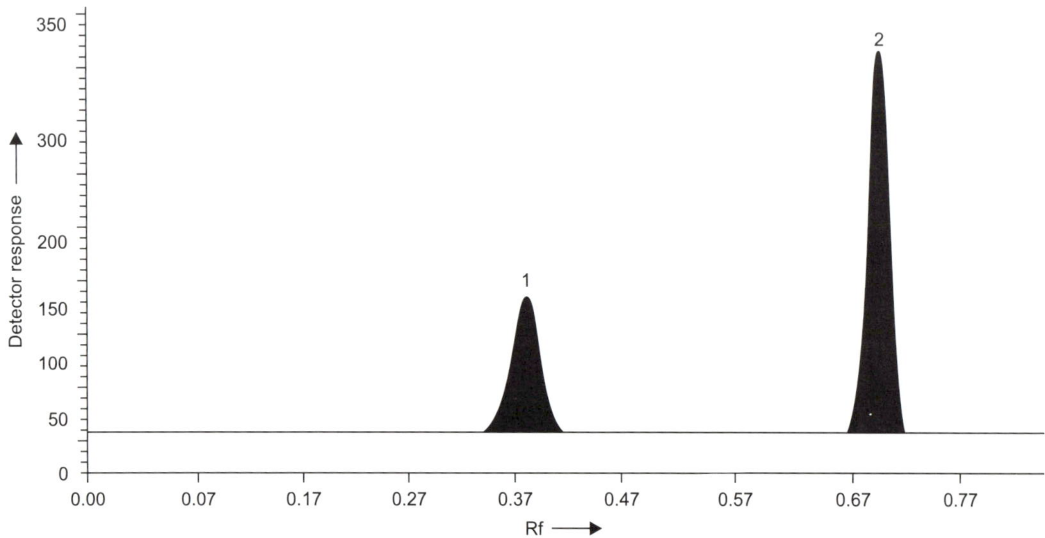

Typical densitogram of the standard containing hydrochlorothiazide and valsartan. For detailed experimental and chromatographic conditions, refer to Protocol No. 76. Peaks identification: 1. Valsartan; 2. Hydrochlorothiazide.

PROTOCOL FOR HPTLC ANALYSIS OF PHARMACEUTICAL FORMULATION

Protocol No. 76

Formulation: Hydrochlorothiazide, Valsartan

Classification: Cardiovascular System **Dosage form:** Tablets

Standard preparation: Prepare separately 100 μg/ml solution of each compound in methanol. Apply 3–8 μl of standard solution of valsartan and 1–6 μl of hydrochlorothiazide for linearity profile.

Sample preparation: Powdered sample equivalent to 25 mg of valsartan suspeneded in methanol, sonicated for 15 min, diluted, filtered and filtrate suitably diluted with methanol to get 100 μg/ml of each. Apply 5 μl for assay.

Chromatographic equipments:

Sample applicator: Camag Linomat–V

Development chamber: Camag twin-trough glass chamber, 10 × 10 cm

Densitometric scanner: Camag TLC Scanner–III

Chromatographic conditions:

1. Stationary phase: Silica gel 60F_{254} pre-coated TLC plates, 10 × 10 cm (200 μm) – Merck, pre-washed with methanol, activated at 50°C for 5 min prior to use
2. Mobile phase (MP): Toluene–chloroform–methanol–glacial acetic acid (1 : 6 : 2 : 0.1 v/v)
3. Standard/Sample application:
   Band length: 5 mm Volume applied: 5 μl Spacing: 10 mm
4. Chamber saturation: 30 min (MP)
5. RH (%): 55 ± 5
6. Temperature °C: 22 ± 2
7. Separation technique: Ascending
8. Quantity of mobile phase: 9 ml
9. Migration distance: 72 mm
10. Migration time: 22 min

Densitometric evaluation:

Wavelength: UV–260 nm Scanning mode: Reflectance/Absorbance

HRF: Valsartan—39; Hydrochlorothiazide—69

Linearity (ng/band): Hydrochlorothiazide—100–600; Valsartan—300–800

Recovery (%): 99.81–100.78 for both the compounds

References: N.J. Shaha, B.N. Suhagia, R.R. Shah and N.M. Patel, *Indian J. Pharm. Sci.*, **71(1)**, 72–74, 2009.

Comments: The method validated for accuracy, precision, linearity, LOD, LOQ and specificity.

HPTLC : High Performance Thin Layer Chromatography
HPTLC Densitogram

No. 77

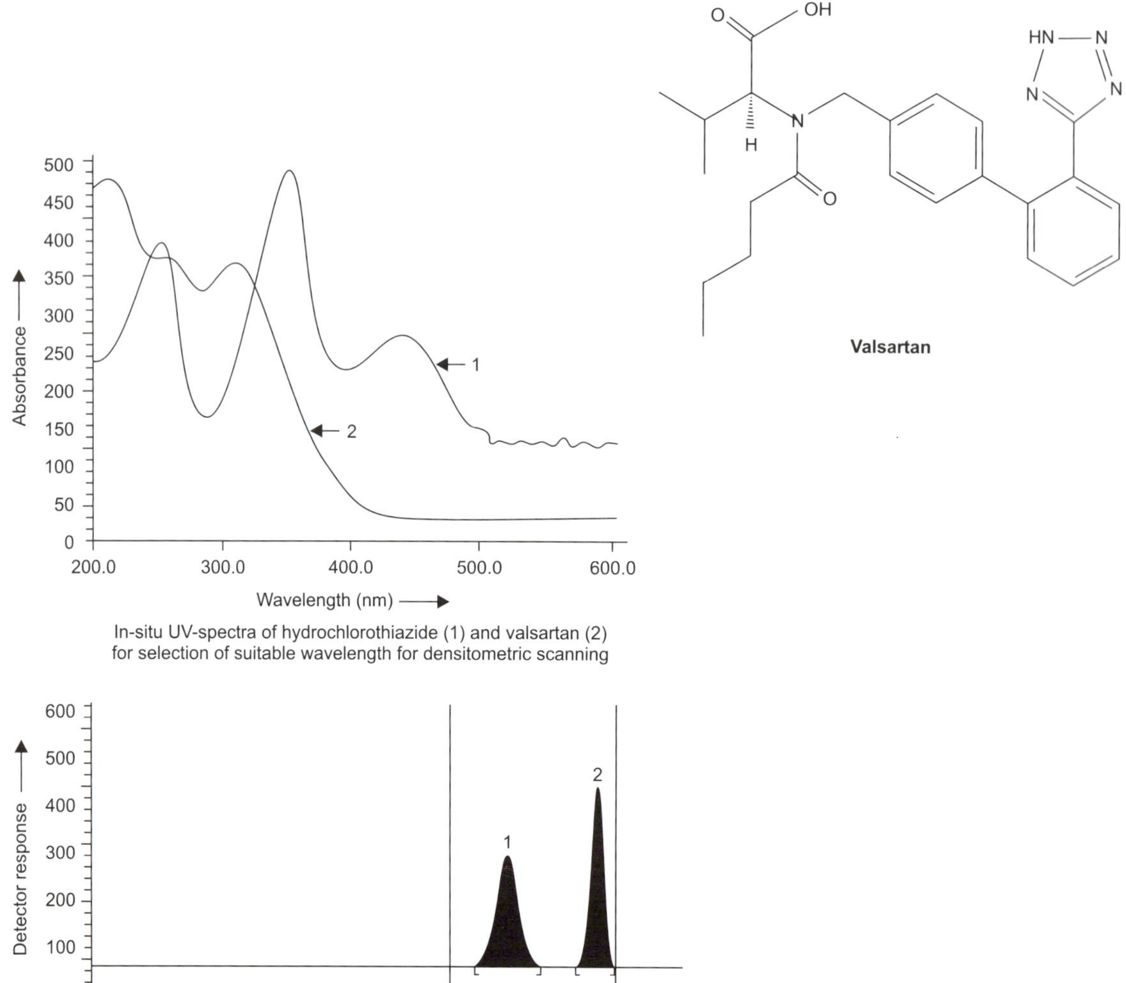

In-situ UV-spectra of hydrochlorothiazide (1) and valsartan (2) for selection of suitable wavelength for densitometric scanning

Typical densitogram of the sample containing hydrochlorothiazide and valsartan. For detailed experimental and chromatographic conditions, refer to Protocol No. 77. Peaks identification: 1. Hydrochlorothiazide; 2. Valsartan.

PROTOCOL FOR HPTLC ANALYSIS OF PHARMACEUTICAL FORMULATION

Protocol No. 77

Formulation: Hydrochlorothiazide (H), Valsartan (V)

Classification: Cardiovascular System **Dosage form:** Tablets

Standard preparation: Standard solution of each compound prepared in methanol to get 4 mg/ml of valsartan and 0.125 mg/ml of hydrochlorothiazide and used for analysis.

Sample preparation: An appropriate quantity of the powdered sample shaken with 10 ml of methanol for 15 min, centrifuged and supernatant used for application. The final solution contained 4 mg/ml of valsartan and 0.125 mg/ml of of hydrochlorothiazide.

Chromatographic equipments:

Sample applicator: Camag Linomat–IV

Development chamber: Sigma Aldrich glass chamber, 18 × 9 × 18 cm

Densitometric scanner: Camag TLC Scanner–III

Chromatographic conditions:

1. Stationary phase: Silica gel 60F_{254} pre-coated HPTLC plates, 10 × 10 cm (200 μm) – Merck
2. Mobile phase (MP): Ethyl acetate–tetrahydrofuran–acetic acid (8 : 2 : 0.5 v/v)
3. Standard/Sample application:
   Band length: 10 mm   Volume applied: 5 μl   Spacing: 10 mm
4. Chamber saturation: 30 min (MP)
5. RH (%): 55 ± 5
6. Temperature °C: 22 ± 2
7. Separation technique: Ascending
8. Quantity of mobile phase: 20 ml
9. Migration distance: 95 mm
10. Migration time: —

Densitometric evaluation:

Wavelength: UV–252 nm (V), 274 nm (H)

Scanning mode: Reflectance/Absorbance

HRF: Hydrochlorothiazide—74; Valsartan—88

Linearity (ng/band): Hydrochlorothiazide—75–1250; Valsartan—385–6150

Recovery (%): Hydrochlorothiazide—96.7–100.8; Valsartan—92.1–95.1

References: Mariusz Stolarczyk, Maslanka Anna and Jan Krzek, *J. Liq. Chromatogr. and Rel. Technol.*, **31**, 1892–1902, 2008.

Comments: The method validated for accuracy, precision, linearity, LOD and LOQ.

HPTLC : High Performance Thin Layer Chromatography
HPTLC Densitogram

No. 78

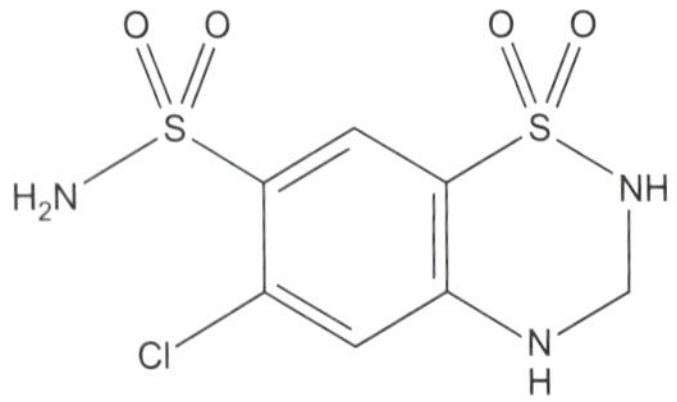

Hydrochlorothiazide

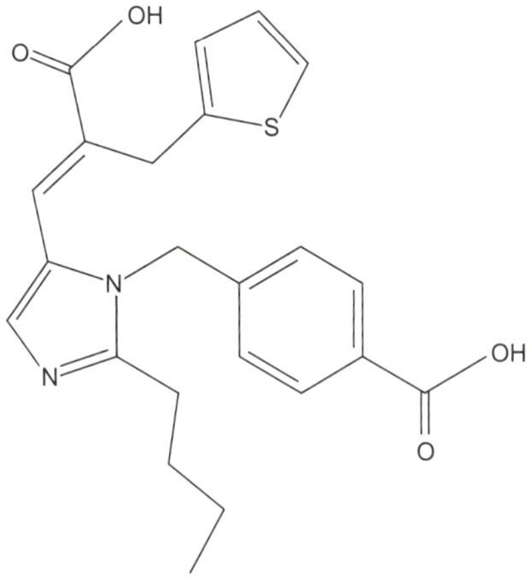

Eprosartan

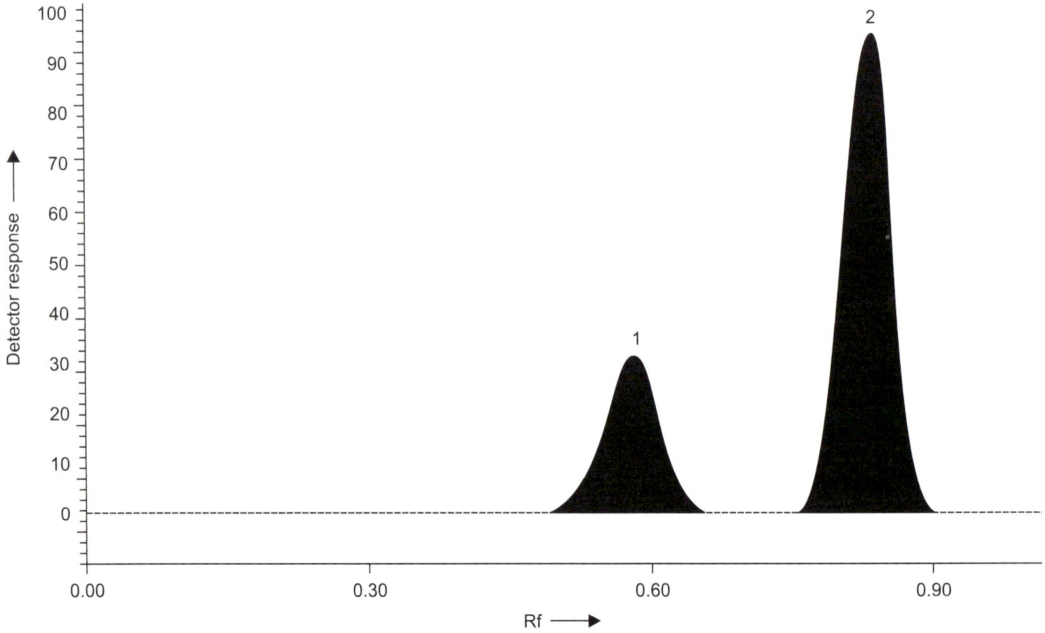

Typical densitogram of the sample containing hydrochlorothiazide and eprosartan. For detailed experimental and chromatographic conditions, refer to Protocol No. 78. Peaks identification: 1. Eprosartan; 2. Hydrochlorothiazide.

PROTOCOL FOR HPTLC ANALYSIS OF PHARMACEUTICAL FORMULATION

Protocol No. 78

Formulation: Hydrochlorothiazide, Eprosartan

Classification: Cardiovascular System **Dosage form:** Tablets

Standard preparation: Prepare stock solution of hydrochlorothiazide (0.5 mg/ml) and eprosartan (12 mg/ml), both in methanol. Apply different volumes of each solution for linearity studies.

Sample preparation: Powdered sample equivalent to 600 mg of eprosartan and 25 mg of hydrochlorothiazide suspeneded in 40 ml of methanol, sonicated for 15 min, diluted to 50 ml with methanol, filtered through 0.45 μm nylon membrane filter and used for assay.

Chromatographic equipments:

Sample applicator: Desaga AS 30 Win

Development chamber: Flat-bottomed glass chamber, 10 × 10 cm

Densitometric scanner: Desaga–60 Densitometer

Chromatographic conditions:

1. Stationary phase: Silica gel $60F_{254}$ pre-coated HPTLC plates, 5 × 5 cm (200 μm) – Merck, pre-washed with methanol, dreid and stored in desiccator
2. Mobile phase (MP): Benzene–methanol–formic acid (70 : 30 : 1 v/v)
3. Standard/Sample application:
   Band length: 3 mm Volume applied: 10 μl Spacing: 6 mm
4. Chamber saturation: 30 min (MP)
5. RH (%): 55 ± 5
6. Temperature °C: 22 ± 2
7. Separation technique: Ascending
8. Quantity of mobile phase: 25 ml
9. Migration distance: 45 mm
10. Migration time: 25 min

Densitometric evaluation:

Wavelength: UV–272 nm Scanning mode: Reflectance/Absorbance

HRF: Eprosartan—57; Hydrochlorothiazide—88

Linearity (μg/band): Eprosartan—4.8–43.2; Hydrochlorothiazide—0.15–1.35

Recovery (%): 99.45–100.68 for both the compounds.

References: H.U. Patel, B.N. Suhagia and C.N. Patel, *Acta Chromatographica*, **21(2)**, 319–326, 2009.

Comments: The method validated for accuracy, precision, linearity, LOD and LOQ.

HPTLC : High Performance Thin Layer Chromatography
HPTLC Densitogram

No. 79

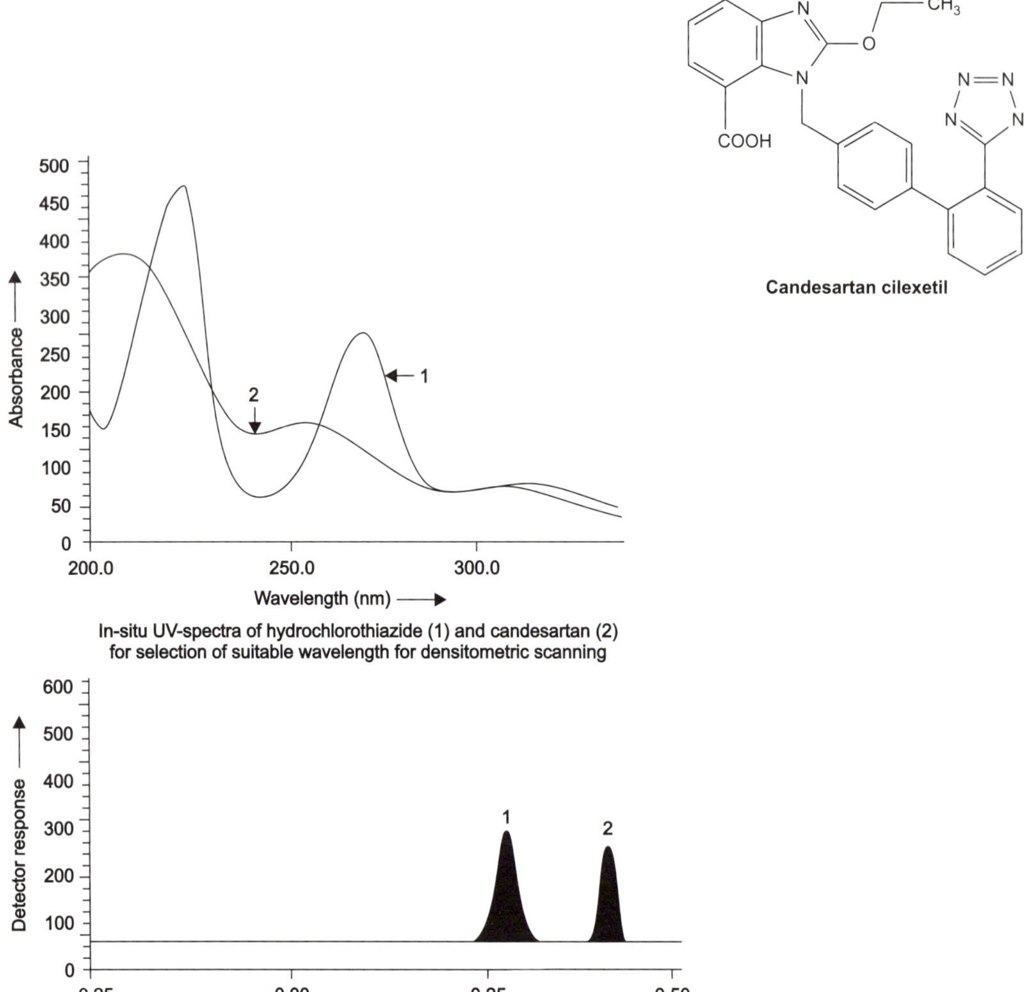

Typical densitogram of the sample containing hydrochlorothiazide and candesartan cilexetil. For detailed experimental and chromatographic conditions, refer to Protocol No. 79. Peaks identification: 1. Candesartan cilexetil; 2. Hydrochlorothiazide.

PROTOCOL FOR HPTLC ANALYSIS OF PHARMACEUTICAL FORMULATION

Protocol No. 79

Formulation: Hydrochlorothiazide, Candesartan cilexetil

Classification: Cardiovascular System **Dosage form:** Tablets

Standard preparation: Dissolve 32.5 mg of candesartan cilexetil and 25.3 mg of hydrochlorothiazide in methanol to produce 50 ml. Further serial dilutions suitably made with methanol for linearity studies. Apply 10 μl of each solution for chromatographic analysis.

Sample preparation: Powdered sample equivalent to 16 mg of candesartan cilexetil and 12.5 mg of hydrochlorothiazide suspended in 15 ml of methanol, sonicated, diluted to 20 ml, filtered and 5 ml of filtrate diluted to 20 ml with methanol for analysis.

Chromatographic equipments:

Sample applicator: Camag Linomat–IV

Development chamber: Camag twin-trough glass chamber, 10 × 10 cm

Densitometric scanner: Camag TLC scanner III

Chromatographic conditions:

1. Stationary phase: Silica gel $60F_{254}$ pre-coated HPTLC plates, 10 × 10 cm (200 μm) – Merck
2. Mobile phase (MP): Ethyl acetate–chloroform–acetone–methanol (3 : 3 : 3 : 0.5 v/v)
3. Standard/Sample application:
   Band length: 6 mm Volume applied: 10 μl Spacing: 6 mm
4. Chamber saturation: 10 min (MP)
5. RH (%): 55 ± 5
6. Temperature °C: 25 ± 2
7. Separation technique: Ascending
8. Quantity of mobile phase: 9 ml
9. Migration distance: 80 mm
10. Migration time: 30 min

Densitometric evaluation:

Wavelength: UV–280 nm Scanning mode: Reflectance/Absorbance

HRF: Candesartan cilexetil—27; Hydrochlorothiazide—45

Linearity (ng/band): Hydrochlorothiazide—50.6–253 μg; Candesartan cilexetil—65–325 μg

Recovery (%): 99.39–100.26 for both the compounds

References: B.H. Mehta and S.B. Morge, *J. Planar Chromatogr.*, **21(3)**, 173–176, 2008.

Comments: The method validated for accuracy, precision, linearity, LOD and LOQ.

HPTLC : High Performance Thin Layer Chromatography
HPTLC Densitogram

No. 80

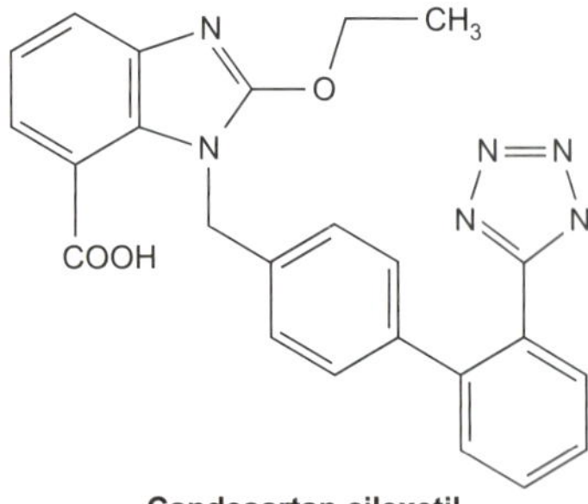

Candesartan cilexetil

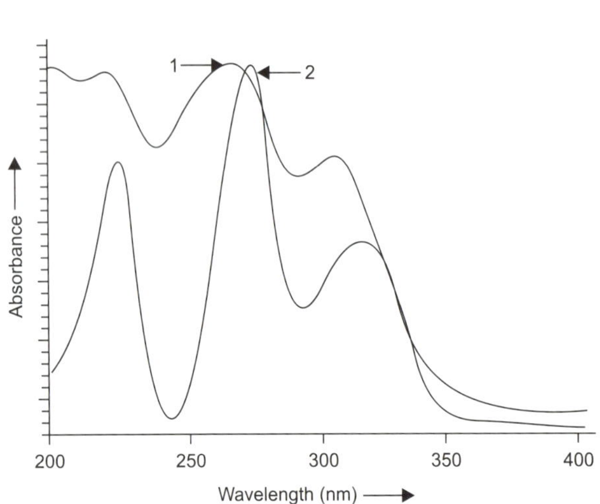

Overlaid UV-spectra of hydrochlorothiazide (2) and candesartan (1) for selection of suitable wavelength for densitometric scanning

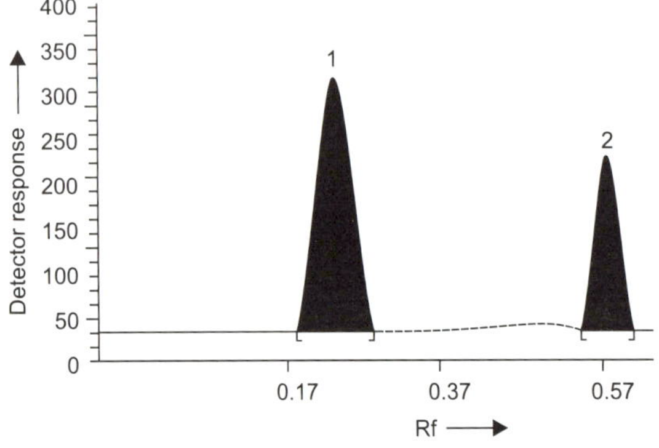

Typical densitogram of the sample containing hydrochlorothiazide and candesartan cilexetil. For detailed experimental and chromatographic conditions, refer to Protocol No. 80. Peaks identification: 1. Candesartan cilexetil; 2. Hydrochlorothiazide.

PROTOCOL FOR HPTLC ANALYSIS OF PHARMACEUTICAL FORMULATION

Protocol No. 80

Formulation: Hydrochlorothiazide, Candesartan cilexetil

Classification: Cardiovascular System **Dosage form:** Tablets

Standard preparation: Prepare 100 µg/ml solution of each compound in methanol; apply different volumes of each solution (1–8 µl) for linearity studies.

Sample preparation: Powdered sample equivalent to 25 mg of candesartan suspended in 100 ml of methanol, sonicated for 15 min, filtered through Whatman No. 41 filter paper. The filtrate suitably diluted with methanol to get 100 µg/ml of candesartan. Apply 4 µl for chromatographic assay.

Chromatographic equipments:

Sample applicator: Camag Linomat–V

Development chamber: Camag twin-trough glass chamber, 10 × 10 cm

Densitometric scanner: Camag TLC scanner III

Chromatographic conditions:

1. Stationary phase: Silica gel $60F_{254}$ pre-coated TLC plates, 10 × 10 cm (250 µm) – Merck, pre-washed with methanol, dried (50°C) for 5 min, prior to use.
2. Mobile phase (MP): Chloroform–methanol–toluene–glacaial acetic acid (6 : 2 : 2 : 0.1 v/v)
3. Standard/Sample application:
   Band length: 5 mm Volume applied: 4 µl Spacing: 6 mm
4. Chamber saturation: 30 min (MP)
5. RH (%): 55 ± 5
6. Temperature °C: 22 ± 2
7. Separation technique: Ascending
8. Quantity of mobile phase: 10 ml
9. Migration distance: 72 mm
10. Migration time: 20 min

Densitometric evaluation:

Wavelength: UV–260 nm Scanning mode: Reflectance/Absorbance

HRF: Candesartan cilexetil—22; Hydrochlorothiazide—60

Linearity (ng/band): Candesartan cilexetil—100–800; Hydrochlorothiazide—100–600

Recovery (%): Candesartan cilexetil—99.24–100.32; Hydrochlorothiazide—99.30–108.80

References: N.J. Shah, B.N. Suhagia, R.R. Shah and N.M. Patel, *Int. J. Chem. Sci.*, **4(2)**, 337–342, 2006.

Comments: The method validated for accuracy, precision, linearity, LOD, LOQ and specificity.

HPTLC : High Performance Thin Layer Chromatography
HPTLC Densitogram

No. 81

Hydrochlorothiazide

Candesartan cilexetil

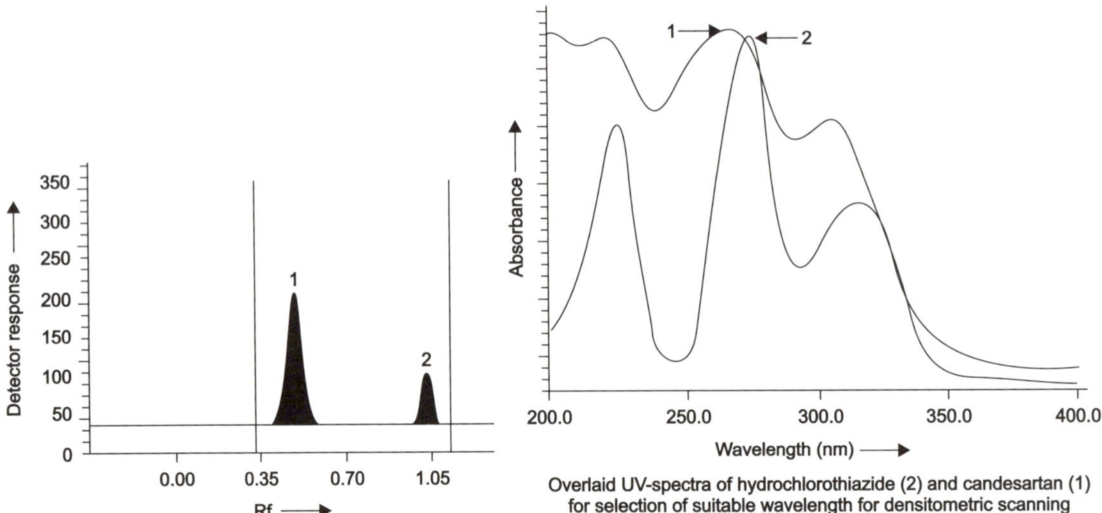

Overlaid UV-spectra of hydrochlorothiazide (2) and candesartan (1) for selection of suitable wavelength for densitometric scanning

Typical densitogram of the sample containing hydrochlorothiazide and candesartan cilexetil. For detailed experimental and chromatographic conditions, refer to Protocol No. 81. Peaks identification: 1. Hydrochlorothiazide; 2. Candesartan cilexetil.

PROTOCOL FOR HPTLC ANALYSIS OF PHARMACEUTICAL FORMULATION

Protocol No. 81

Formulation: Hydrochlorothiazide, Candesartan cilexetil

Classification: Cardiovascular System **Dosage form:** Tablets

Standard preparation: Dissolve 15 mg of hydrochlorothiazide and 10 mg of candesartan in 10 ml of methanol. 1 ml of the solution was further diluted to ml with methanol and used for analysis.

Sample preparation: Powdered sample equivalent to 12.5 mg of hydrochlorothiazide or 8 mg of candesartan suspeneded in 10 ml of methanol, sonicated, filtered and 1 ml of the filtrate diluted to 10 ml with methanol. Spot 1.5 μl of the resulting solution for assay.

Chromatographic equipments:

Sample applicator: Camag Linomat–V

Development chamber: Camag twin-trough glass chamber,

Densitometric scanner: Camag TLC scanner III

Chromatographic conditions:

1. Stationary phase: Silica gel $60F_{254}$ pre-coated TLC plates, 20 × 10 cm (250 μm) – Merck, pre-washed with methanol, activated at 60°C for min, prior to use
2. Mobile phase (MP): Toluene–ethyl acetate–glacial acetic acid (2 : 5 : 0.1 v/v)
3. Standard/Sample application:
   Band length: 6 mm Volume applied: 0.5–2.5 μl Spacing: 5 mm
4. Chamber saturation: 30 min (MP)
5. RH (%): 55 ± 5
6. Temperature °C: 25 ± 2
7. Separation technique: Ascending
8. Quantity of mobile phase: 14 ml
9. Migration distance: 75 mm
10. Migration time: 25 min

Densitometric evaluation:

Wavelength: UV–273 nm Scanning mode: Reflectance/Absorbance

HRF: Hydrochlorothiazide—30; Candesartan cilexetil—68

Linearity (ng/band): Hydrochlorothiazide—75–375; Candesartan cilexetil—50–250

Recovery (%): 98.73–102.85 for both the compounds

References: M. Gandhimathi and T.K. Ravi, *Indian Drugs*, **46(2)**, 151–153, 2009.

Comments: The method validated for accuracy, precision, linearity, LOD, LOQ and robustness.

HPTLC : High Performance Thin Layer Chromatography
HPTLC Densitogram

No. 82

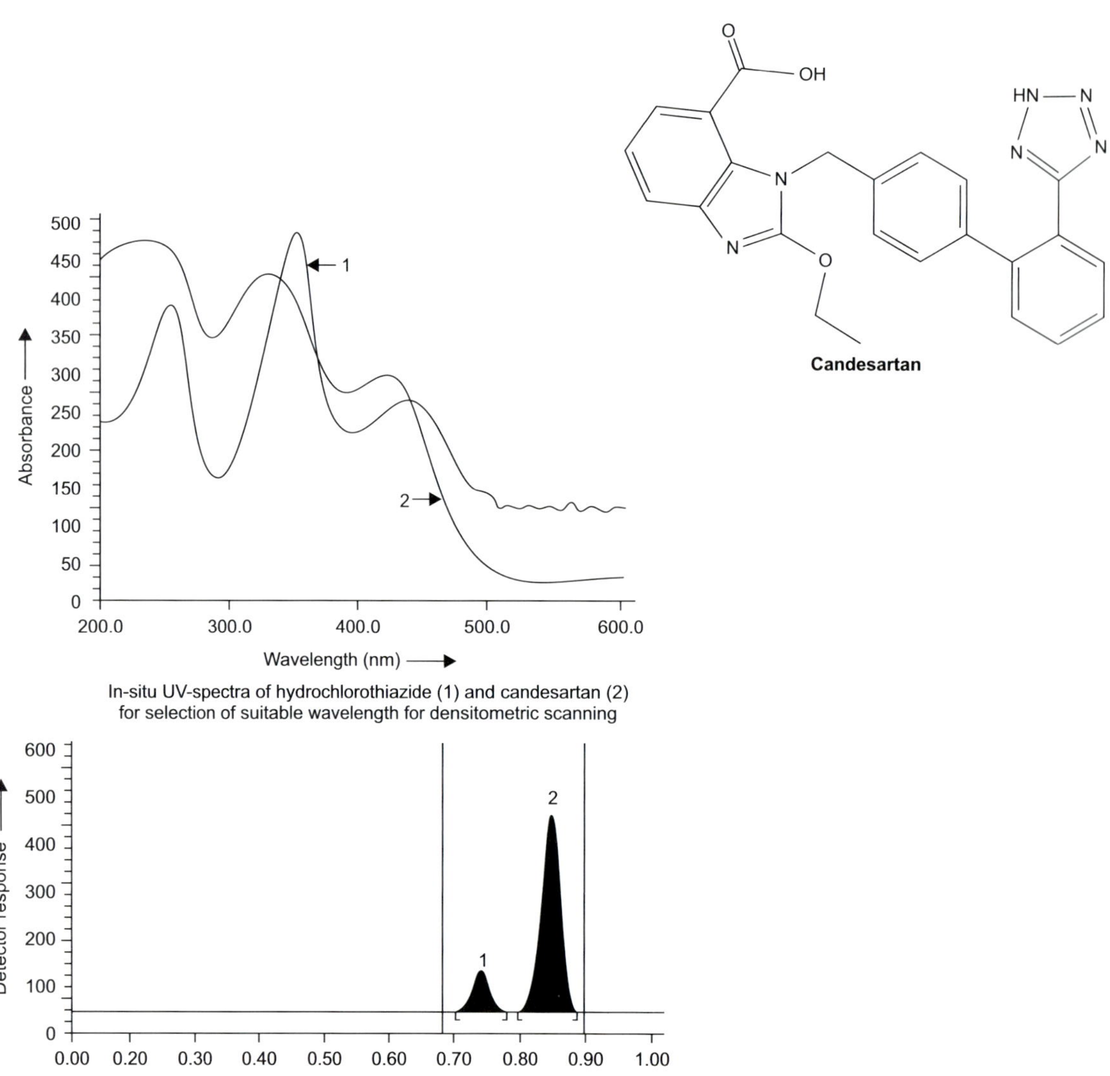

Typical densitogram of the standard containing hydrochlorothiazide and candesartan. For detailed experimental and chromatographic conditions, refer to Protocol No. 82. Peaks identification: 1. Hydrochlorothiazide; 2. Candesartan.

PROTOCOL FOR HPTLC ANALYSIS OF PHARMACEUTICAL FORMULATION

Protocol No. 82

Formulation: Hydrochlorothiazide (H), Candesartan (C)

Classification: Cardiovascular System **Dosage form:** Tablets

Standard preparation: Prepare standard solution of each compound in methanol to get 160 μg/ml of candesartan and 125 mg/ml of hydrochlorothiazide and use for analysis.

Sample preparation: An appropriate quantity of powdered sample shaken with 10 ml of methanol for 15 min, centrifuged and supernatant used for direct determination. The solution contained 160 μg/ml of kandesartan and 125 μg/ml of hydrochlorothiazide

Chromatographic equipments:

Sample applicator: Camag Linomat–IV

Development chamber: Sigma Aldrich glass chamber, 18 × 9 × 18 cm

Densitometric scanner: Camag TLC Scanner–III

Chromatographic conditions:

1. Stationary phase: Silica gel 60F$_{254}$ pre-coated HPTLC plates, 10 × 10 cm (200 μm) – Merck
2. Mobile phase (MP): Ethyl acetate–tetrahydrofuran–acetic acid (8 : 2 : 0.5 v/v)
3. Standard/Sample application:
   Band length: 10 mm Volume applied: 5 μl Spacing: 10 mm
4. Chamber saturation: 30 min (MP)
5. RH (%): 55 ± 5
6. Temperature °C: 22 ± 2
7. Separation technique: Ascending
8. Quantity of mobile phase: 20 ml
9. Migration distance: 95 mm
10. Migration time: 25 min

Densitometric evaluation:

Wavelength: UV–252 nm (C), 274 nm (H)

Scanning mode: Reflectance/Absorbance

HRF: Hydrochlorothiazide—71; Candesartan—84

Linearity (ng/band): Candesartan—226–1810; Hydrochlorothiazide—78–1250

Recovery (%): Candesartan—92.1–95.1; Hydrochlorothiazide—96.4–100.8

References: Mariusz Stólarczyk, Maslanka Anna and Jan Krzek, *J. Liq. Chromatogr. and Rel. Technol.*, **31**, 1892–1902, 2008.

Comments: The method validated for accuracy, precision, linearity, LOD and LOQ.

HPTLC : High Performance Thin Layer Chromatography
HPTLC Densitogram

No. 83

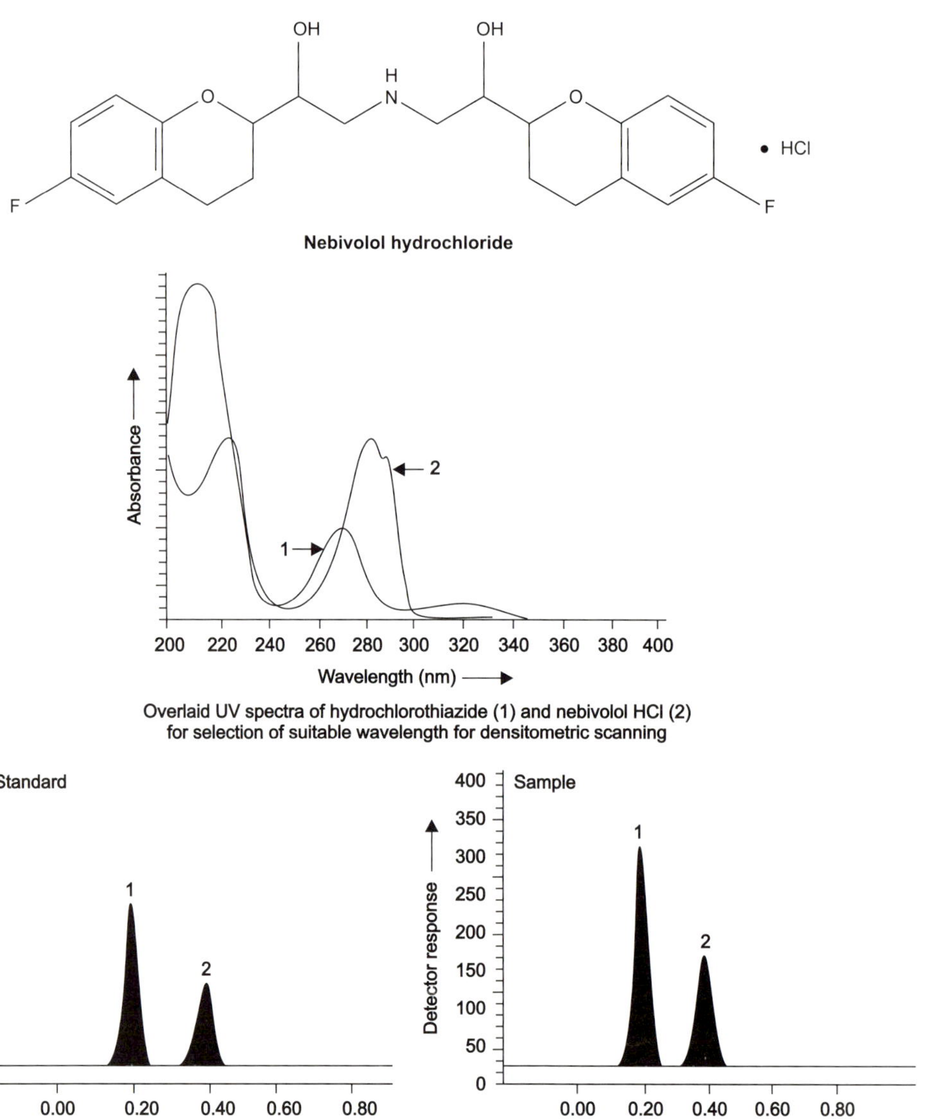

Typical densitogram of the sample and standard containing hydrochlorothiazide and nebivolol hydrochloride. For detailed experimental and chromatographic conditions, refer to Protocol No. 83. Peaks identification: 1. Hydrochlorothiazide; 2. Nebivolol HCl.

PROTOCOL FOR HPTLC ANALYSIS OF PHARMACEUTICAL FORMULATION

Protocol No. 83

Formulation: Hydrochlorothiazide, Nebivolol hydrochloride

Classification: Cardiovascular System **Dosage form:** Tablets

Standard preparation: Prepare 1 mg/ml solution of each compound in methanol. Further dilutions made with methanol to get 500 μg/ml (nebivolol HCl) and 100 μg/ml (hydrochlorothiazide). Apply 10 μl for analysis.

Sample preparation: Powdered sample equivalent to 25 mg of nebivolol HCl suspended in 20 ml of methanol, shake for 5 min, dilute to 25 ml, filter through Whatman No. 41 filter paper and dilute the filtrate suitably for assay.

Chromatographic equipments:

Sample applicator: Camag Linomat–IV

Development chamber: Camag twin-trough glass chamber, 10 × 10 cm

Densitometric scanner: Camag TLC scanner III

Chromatographic conditions:

1. Stationary phase: Silica gel $60F_{254}$ pre-coated TLC plates, 10 × 10 cm (250 μm) – Merck, pre-washed with methanol and dried
2. Mobile phase (MP): Ethyl acetate–methanol–25% ammonia (8.5 : 1 : 0.5 v/v)
3. Standard/Sample application:
   Band length: 7 mm Volume applied: 10 μl Spacing: 8 mm
4. Chamber saturation: 15 min (MP)
5. RH (%): 55 ± 5
6. Temperature °C: 25 ± 2
7. Separation technique: Ascending
8. Quantity of mobile phase: 10 ml
9. Migration distance: 90 mm
10. Migration time: 20 min

Densitometric evaluation:

Wavelength: UV–280 nm Scanning mode: Reflectance/Absorbance

HRF: Hydrochlorothiazide—20; Nebivolol HCl—40

Linearity (μg/ml): Hydrochlorothiazide—100–500; Nebivolol HCl—500–1300

Recovery (%): Hydrochlorothiazide—99.41–99.72; Nebivolol HCl—99.26–101.95

References: L.R. Bhat, K.G. Bothara and M.C. Damle, *Indian Drugs*, **45(12)**, 948–951, 2008.

Comments: The method validated for accuracy, precision, linearity, LOD, LOQ and robustness.

HPTLC : High Performance Thin Layer Chromatography
HPTLC Densitogram

No. 84

Nebivolol hydrochloride

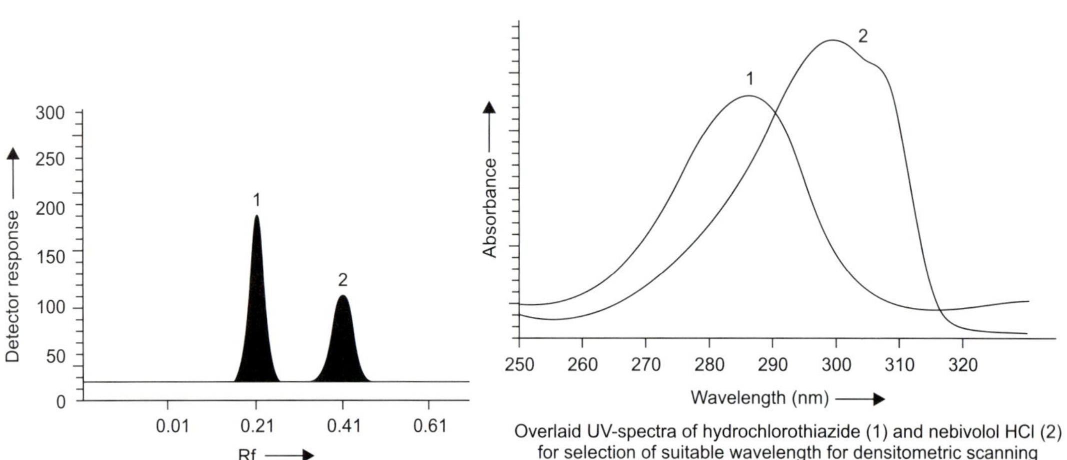

Overlaid UV-spectra of hydrochlorothiazide (1) and nebivolol HCl (2) for selection of suitable wavelength for densitometric scanning

Typical densitogram of the sample containing hydrochlorothiazide and nebivolol hydrochloride. For detailed experimental and chromatographic conditions, refer to Protocol No. 84. Peaks identification: 1. Hydrochlorothiazide; 2. Nebivolol HCl.

PROTOCOL FOR HPTLC ANALYSIS OF PHARMACEUTICAL FORMULATION

Protocol No. 84

Formulation: Hydrochlorothiazide, Nebivolol hydrochloride

Classification: Cardiovascular System **Dosage form:** Tablets

Standard preparation: Prepare 1 mg/ml solution of each compound in methanol. Further dilutions made to get serial dilutions of 100–500 μg/ml (nebivolol) and 250–1250 μg/ml (hydrochlorothiazide) for application on the plate.

Sample preparation: Powdered sample equivalent to 125 mg of hydrochlorothiazide suspended in methanol, sonicated, diluted, filtered and the filtrate suitably diluted for spotting and chromatographic evaluation.

Chromatographic equipments:

Sample applicator: Camag Linomat–IV

Development chamber: Camag twin-trough glass chamber, 20 × 10 cm

Densitometric scanner: Camag TLC scanner III

Chromatographic conditions:

1. Stationary phase: Silica gel $60F_{254}$ pre-coated, pre-washed with methanol dried and activated
2. Mobile phase (MP): Ethyl acetate–methanol–25% ammonia (8.5 : 1 : 0.5 v/v)
3. Standard/Sample application:
   Band length: 8 mm Volume applied: 2 μl Spacing: 10 mm
4. Chamber saturation: 10 min (MP)
5. RH (%): 60 ± 5
6. Temperature °C: 26 ± 2
7. Separation technique: Ascending
8. Quantity of mobile phase: 20 ml
9. Migration distance: 80 mm
10. Migration time: 20 min

Densitometric evaluation:

Wavelength: UV–285 nm Scanning mode: Reflectance/Absorbance

HRF: Hydrochlorothiazide—21; Nebivolol HCl—41

Linearity (ng/band): Hydrochlorothiazide—100–500; Nebivolol HCl—50–250

Recovery (%): 98.43–100.92 for both the drugs

References: B. Dhandapani, N. Thirumoorthyl and D. Jose Prakash, *E. Journal of Chem.*, **7(2)**, 341–348, 2010.

Comments:

- The method validated for accuracy, precision, linearity, LOD and LOQ.
- The authors simultaneously carried out analysis by UV and HPLC methods with comparable results.

HPTLC : High Performance Thin Layer Chromatography
HPTLC Densitogram

No. 85

Degradation profile of both the drugs under different stress conditions				
	Standard drug (amount of degradation, %)		Marketed formulation (amount of degradation, %)	
Stress condition	Hydro-chlorothiazide	Nebivolol hydro-chlorothiazide	Hydro-chlorothiazide	Nebivolol hydrochlorothiazide
Acidic hydrolysis (5 M/10 M, reflux, 60°C, 1 h)	17.61	52.58	23.51	(5 N) 37.95
Basic hydrolysis (5 M/10 M, reflux, 60°C, 1 h)	5.67	13.64	8.59	(5 N) 43.27
Neutral hydrolysis (reflux, 60°C, 1 h)	1.09	0.59	0.2	1.69
Oxidation (30% H_2O_2, reflux, 60°C, 1 h)	62.67	1.02	58.49	0.87
Heat 80°C (4 h)		15.90	0.31	3.29 2.67
Photolysis				
UV fluorescent lamp (320 nm to 400 nm)	3.53	0.78	1.5	0.50
Cool white fluorescent lamp	0.36	0.21	0.05	0.23

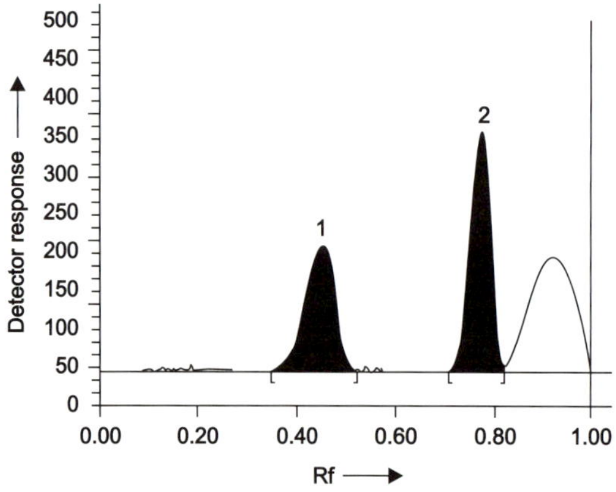

Typical densitogram of the sample containing hydrochlorothiazide and nebivolol HCl. For detailed experimental and chromatographic conditions, refer to Protocol No. 85. Peaks identification: 1. Nebivolol HCl; 2. Hydrochlorothiazide.

PROTOCOL FOR HPTLC ANALYSIS OF PHARMACEUTICAL FORMULATION

Protocol No. 85

Formulation: Hydrochlorothiazide, Nebivolol hydrochloride

Classification: Cardiovascular System **Dosage form:** Tablets

Standard preparation: Prepare 1 mg/ml solution of each compound in methanol. Further dilutions made to get 50 μg/ml hydrochlorothiazide and 200 μg/ml of nebivolol hydrochloride. Apply varying volume of each solution for linearity profile.

Sample preparation: Powdered sample equivalent to 10 mg of hydrochlorothiazide suspended in methanol, sonicated, diluted to 10 ml with methanol. Filtered and diluted suitably to get 200 μg/ml of nebivolol hydrochloride and 50 μg/ml of hyrochlorothiazide. Apply 10 μl for chromatographic analysis.

Chromatographic equipments:

Sample applicator: Camag Linomat–V

Development chamber: Camag twin–trough glass chamber, 10 × 10 cm

Densitometric scanner: Camag TLC Scanner–III

Chromatographic conditions:

1. Stationary phase: Silica gel 60F_{254} pre-coated TLC plates, 10 × 10 cm (250 μm) – Merck
2. Mobile phase (MP): Ethyl acetate–methanol–glacial acetic acid (6.5 : 1 : 0.5 v/v)
3. Standard/Sample application:
   Band length: 5 mm Volume applied: 10 μl Spacing: 10 mm
4. Chamber saturation: 15 min (MP)
5. RH (%): 55 ± 5.6
6. Temperature °C: 25 ± 2
7. Separation technique: Ascending
8. Quantity of mobile phase: 16 ml
9. Migration distance: 90 mm
10. Migration time: 20 min

Densitometric evaluation:

Wavelength: UV–250 nm Scanning mode: Reflectance/Absorbance

HRF: Nebivolol—46; Hydrochlorothiazide—78

Linearity (ng/band): Hydrochlorothiazide—250–2000; Nebivolol HCl—1200–2800

Recovery (%): 99.67—100.43 for both the compounds

References: M.C. Damle, K.S. Topagi and K.G. Bothara, *Acta. Chromatographica*, **22(3)**, 433–443, 2010.

Comments:

- The method validated for accuracy, precision, linearity, LOD, LOQ, specificity, robustness and ruggedness.
- The method is stability indicating (acid, base, oxidative, thermal, photolytic). The degradation products were separated from main compounds.

HPTLC : High Performance Thin Layer Chromatography
HPTLC Densitogram

No. 86

Nebivolol hydrochloride

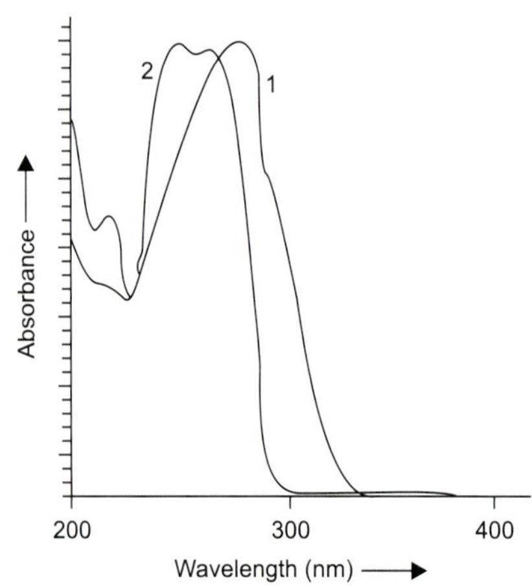

Overlaid UV-spectra of hydrochlorothiazide (2) and nebivolol HCl (1) for selection of suitable wavelength for densitometric scanning

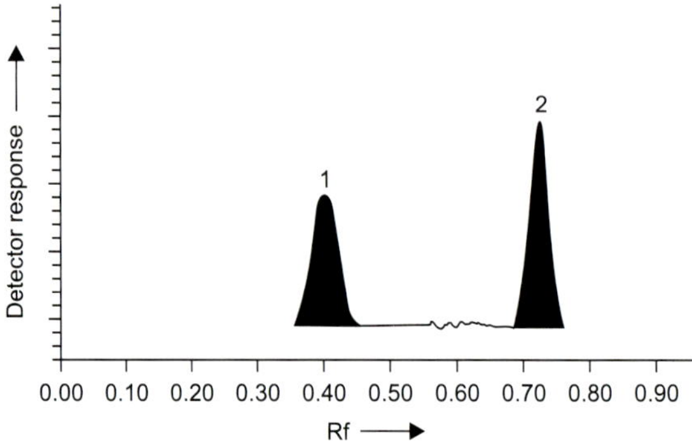

Typical densitogram of the standard containing hydrochlorothiazide and nebivolol hydrochloride. For detailed experimental and chromatographic conditions, refer to Protocol No. 86. Peaks identification: 1. Hydrochlorothiazide; 2. Nebivolol HCl.

PROTOCOL FOR HPTLC ANALYSIS OF PHARMACEUTICAL FORMULATION

Protocol No. 86

Formulation: Hydrochlorothiazide, Nebivolol hydrochloride

Classification: Cardiovascular System **Dosage form:** Tablets

Standard preparation: Prepare standard solution of both the compounds in methanol to get 1000 μg/ml of nebivolol hydrochloride and 400 μg/ml of hydrochlorothiazide. Apply 1–5 μl of each solution for linearity profile.

Sample preparation: Powdered sample equivalent to 100 mg of nebivolol or 40 mg of hydrochlorothiazide suspended in 40 ml of methanol, sonicated for 10 min, diluted to 100 ml with methanol, filtered and apply 3 μl of resulting solution for assay.

Chromatographic equipments:

Sample applicator: Camag Linomat–V

Development chamber: Camag twin–trough glass chamber, 10 × 10 cm

Densitometric scanner: Camag TLC scanner III

Chromatographic conditions:

1. Stationary phase: Silica gel $60F_{254}$ pre-coated HPTLC plates, 10 × 10 cm (200 μm), pre-washed with methanol, dried at 110°C for 5 min, prior to use
2. Mobile phase (MP): 1,4-dioxane–toluene–triethylamine (5 : 3 : 0.1 v/v)
3. Standard/Sample application:
   Band length: 6 mm Volume applied: 1–5 μl Spacing: 11.6 mm
4. Chamber saturation: 30 min (MP)
5. RH (%): 55 ± 5
6. Temperature °C: 25 ± 2
7. Separation technique: Ascending
8. Quantity of mobile phase: 16 ml
9. Migration distance: 80 mm
10. Migration time: 15 min

Densitometric evaluation:

Wavelength: UV–281 nm Scanning mode: Reflectance/Absorbance

HRF: Hydrochlorothiazide—40; Nebivolol HCl—73

Linearity (ng/band): Hydrochlorothiazide—400–2000; Nebivolol HCl—1000–5000;

Recovery (%): Hydrochlorothiazide—99.90–101.10; Nebivolol HCl—99.80–100.10

References: S.T. Kumbhar, G.K. Chougule, V.S. Tegeli, G.B. Gajeli, Y.S. Thorat, U.S. Shivsharan, *Int. J. Pharm. Sci and Drug Res.*, **3(1)**, 62–66, 2011.

Comments: The method validated for accuracy, precision, linearity, LOD, LOQ, specificity, robustness and ruggedness.

HPTLC : High Performance Thin Layer Chromatography
HPTLC Densitogram

No. 87

Nebivolol hydrochloride

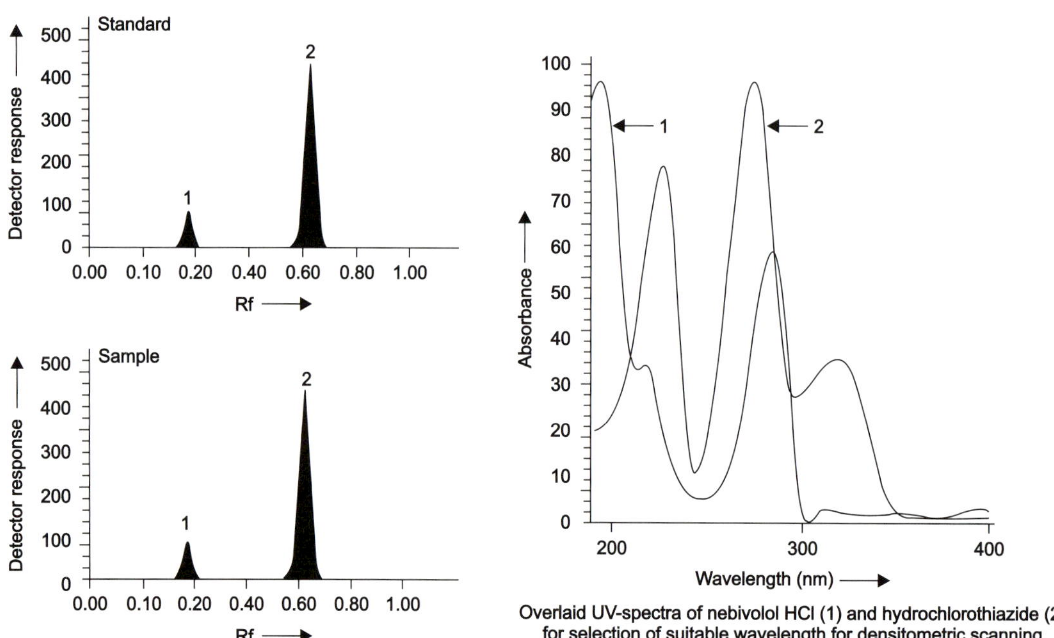

Overlaid UV-spectra of nebivolol HCl (1) and hydrochlorothiazide (2) for selection of suitable wavelength for densitometric scanning

Typical densitogram of the standard and the sample containing nebivolol hydrochloride and hydrochlorothiazide. For detailed experimental and chromatographic conditions, refer to Protocol No. 87. Peaks identification: 1. Nebivolol HCl; 2. Hydrochlorothiazide.

PROTOCOL FOR HPTLC ANALYSIS OF PHARMACEUTICAL FORMULATION

Protocol No. 87

Formulation: **Hydrochlorothiazide, Nebivolol hydrochloride**

Classification: Cardiovascular System **Dosage form:** Tablets

Standard preparation: Prepare separately 1 mg/ml solution of each compound in methanol. Further serial dilutions made with methanol for linearity studies. Apply 10 μl of each solution for chromatographic analysis.

Sample preparation: Powdered sample equivalent to 5 mg of nebivolol hydrochloride suspended in 15 ml of methanol, sonicated for 10 min, diluted to 20 ml with methanol, filtered and 1 ml of filtrate diluted to 10 ml with methanol. Apply 10 μl for chromatographic analysis.

Chromatographic equipments:

Sample applicator: Camag Linomat–IV

Development chamber: Camag automatic development chamber, saturated with camag saturatic pad

Densitometric scanner: Camag TLC scanner III

Chromatographic conditions:

1. Stationary phase: Silica gel $60F_{254}$ pre-coated TLC plates glass, 20 × 10 cm (250 μm) – Merck
2. Mobile phase (MP): Ethyl acetate–methanol–glacial acetic acid (6.5 : 1 : 0.5 v/v)
3. Standard/Sample application:
   Band length: 8 mm Volume applied: 10 μl Spacing: 10 mm
4. Chamber saturation: 20 min (MP)
5. RH (%): 55 ± 5
6. Temperature °C: 25 ± 2
7. Separation technique: Ascending
8. Quantity of mobile phase: 20 ml
9. Migration distance: 70 mm
10. Migration time: 10 min

Densitometric evaluation:

Wavelength: UV–285 nm Scanning mode: Reflectance/Absorbance

HRF: Nebivolol HCl—17; Hydrochlorothiazide—63

Linearity (ng/band): Nebivolol HCl—100–500; Hydrochlorothiazide—200–1600

Recovery (%): —

References: —

Comments: The method was optimized and analytical work carried out at **Anchrom's HPTLC Application Laboratory**, Mumbai, India.

HPTLC : High Performance Thin Layer Chromatography
HPTLC Densitogram

No. 88

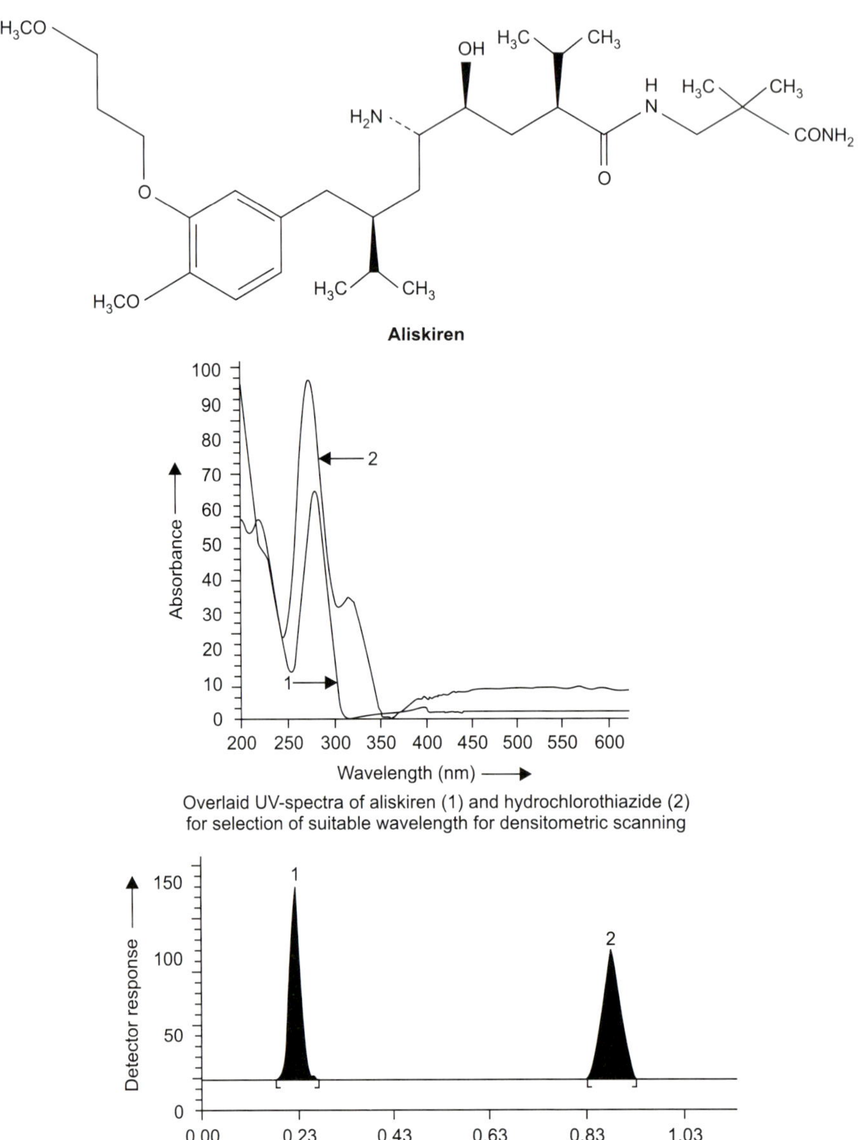

Overlaid UV-spectra of aliskiren (1) and hydrochlorothiazide (2) for selection of suitable wavelength for densitometric scanning

Typical densitogram of the standard containing hydrochlorothiazide and aliskiren. For detailed experimental and chromatographic conditions, refer to Protocol No. 88. Peaks identification: 1. Aliskiren; 2. Hydrochlorothiazide.

PROTOCOL FOR HPTLC ANALYSIS OF PHARMACEUTICAL FORMULATION

Protocol No. 88

Formulation: Hydrochlorothiazide, Aliskiren hemifumarate

Classification: Cardiovascular System **Dosage form:** Tablets

Standard preparation: Prepare 100 μg/ml solution of each compound in methanol. Apply varying volumes of each solution for linearity profile. Carry out chromatographic separation under specified conditions.

Sample preparation: Powdered sample equivalent to 12.5 mg of aliskiren suspended in 40 ml of methanol, sonicated for 10 min, diluted to 50 ml. Filtered and the filtrate suitably diluted and used for chromatographic separation and analysis.

Chromatographic equipments:

Sample applicator: Camag Linomat–V

Development chamber: Camag twin-trough glass chamber, 20 × 10 cm

Densitometric scanner: Camag TLC scanner III

Chromatographic conditions:

1. Stationary phase: Silica gel $60F_{254}$ pre-coated TLC plates, 20 × 10 cm (250 μm) – Merck
2. Mobile phase (MP): Ethyl acetate–methanol–glacial acetic acid (9 : 1 : 0.5 v/v)
3. Standard/Sample application:
   Band length: 10 mm Volume applied: 10 μl Spacing: 15.4 mm
4. Chamber saturation: 30 min (MP)
5. RH (%): 55 ± 5
6. Temperature °C: Ambient
7. Separation technique: Ascending
8. Quantity of mobile phase: 20 ml
9. Migration distance: 80 mm
10. Migration time: 20 min

Densitometric evaluation:

Wavelength: UV–281 nm Scanning mode: Reflectance/Absorbance

HRF: Aliskiren—22; Hydrochlorothiazide—85

Linearity (ng/band): Hydrochlorothiazide—300–800; Aliskiren—2000–12000

Recovery (%): Hydrochlorothiazide—99.97–100.21; Aliskiren—99.79–100.42

References: S.S. Bhise, A. Shah, V.P. Choudhari and B.S. Kuchekar, Abstract No. F–282, 63rd IPC, 2011, *Courtesy:* Prof. V.P. Choudhari.

Comments: The method validated for accuracy, precision, linearity, LOD, LOQ, specificity and robustness as per ICH guidelines.

HPTLC : High Performance Thin Layer Chromatography
HPTLC Densitogram

No. 90

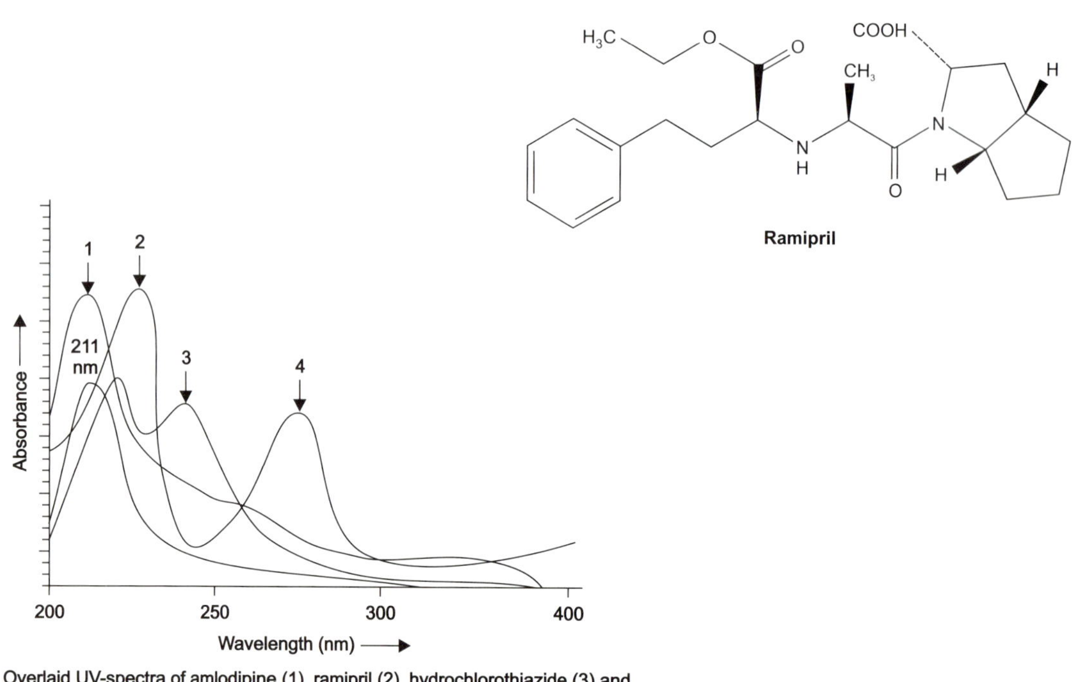

Overlaid UV-spectra of amlodipine (1), ramipril (2), hydrochlorothiazide (3) and losartan (4) for selection of suitable wavelength for densitometric scanning

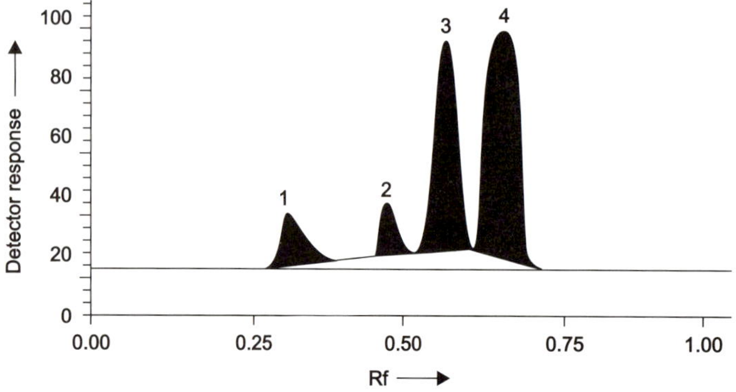

Typical densitogram of the standard containing hydrochlorothiazide, losartan K^+ and ramipril. For detailed experimental and chromatographic conditions, refer to Protocol No. 90. Peaks identification: 1. Amlodipine besylate (IS); 2. Ramipril; 3. Hydrochlorothiazide; 4. Losartan potassium.

PROTOCOL FOR HPTLC ANALYSIS OF PHARMACEUTICAL FORMULATION

Protocol No. 90

Formulation: Hydrochlorothiazide, Losartan potassium, Ramipril

Classification: Cardiovascular System **Dosage form:** Tablets

Standard preparation: Prepare 10 mg/ml solution of each compound in methanol. Solution of amlodipine besylate (10 mg/ml) also prepared in methanol. Further suitably dilute with methanol for linearity studies. Apply 10 µl of each solution.

Sample preparation: Powdered sample equivalent to average weight of one tablet taken in 8 ml of methanol, add 0.5 ml of (IS) solution, dilute to 10 ml with methanol, filter and apply 10 µl for assay.

Chromatographic equipments:

Sample applicator: Camag Linomat–V

Development chamber: Camag twin-trough glass chamber, 20 × 10 cm

Densitometric scanner: Camag TLC scanner III

Chromatographic conditions:

1. Stationary phase: Silica gel $60F_{254}$ pre-coated HPTLC plates, 20 × 20 cm (200 µm) – Merck, pre-washed with methanol, activated at 110°C for 60 min prior to use
2. Mobile phase (MP): Toluene–acetonitrile–formic acid (5 : 5 : 0.3 v/v)
3. Standard/Sample application:
   Band length: 8 mm Volume applied: 10 µl Spacing: 7 mm
4. Chamber saturation: 15 min (MP)
5. RH (%): 55 ± 5
6. Temperature °C: 25 ± 2
7. Separation technique: Ascending
8. Quantity of mobile phase: 20 ml
9. Migration distance: 80 mm
10. Migration time: 35 min

Densitometric evaluation:

Wavelength: UV–215 nm Scanning mode: Reflectance/Absorbance

HRF: Amlodipine besylate (IS)—32; Ramipril—48; Hydrochlorothiazide—58; Losartan K^+—68

Linearity (ng/ml): Hydrochlorothiazide—750–1625; Ramipril—200–325; Losartan K^+—3000–6500

Recovery (%): 99.20–99.85 for all the three compounds

References: M.M. Baing, V.V. Vaidya, G. Singh, H.Mhaske and O. Dhotre, *Indian Drugs*, **43(4)**, 333–337, 2006.

Comments: The method validated for accuracy, precision, linearity, LOD and LOQ.

HPTLC : High Performance Thin Layer Chromatography
HPTLC Densitogram

No. 91

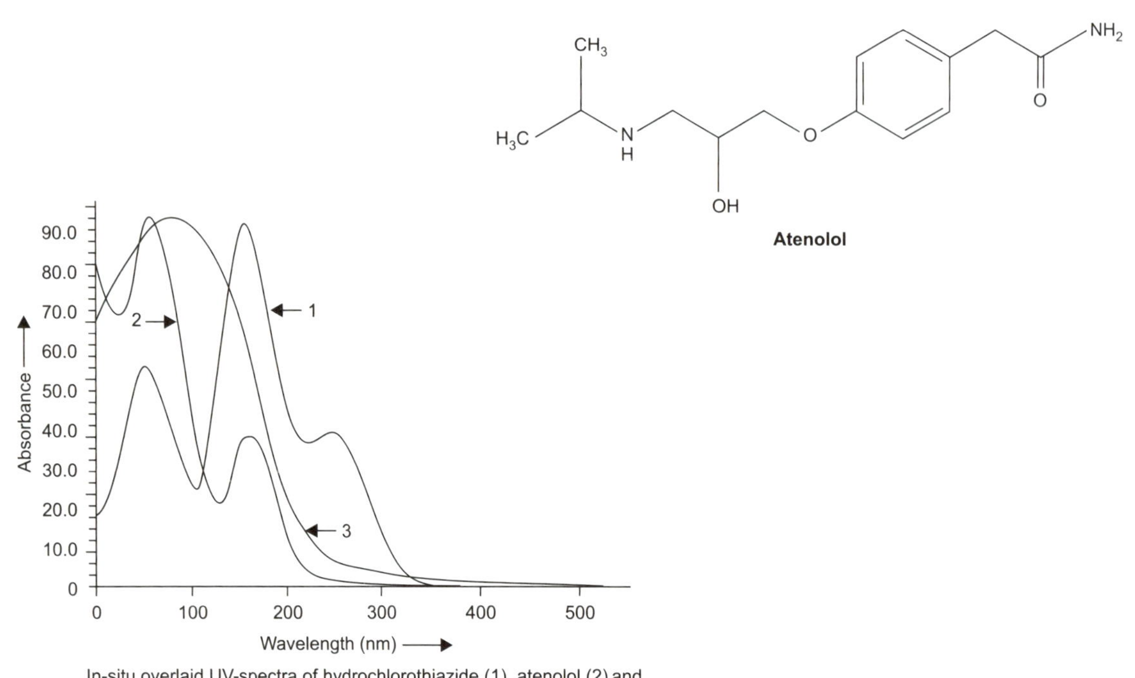

In-situ overlaid UV-spectra of hydrochlorothiazide (1), atenolol (2) and losartan K$^+$(3) for selection of suitable wavelength for densitometric scanning

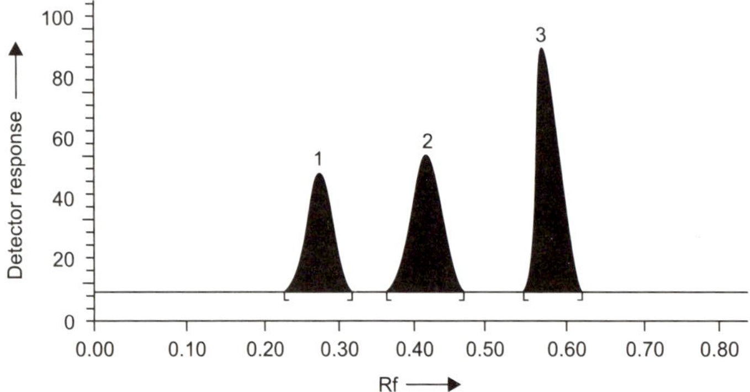

Typical densitogram of the standard containing hydrochlorothiazide, atenolol and losartan K$^+$. For detailed experimental and chromatographic conditions, refer to Protocol No. 91. Peaks identification: 1. Hydrochlorothiazide; 2. Atenolol; 3. Losartan K$^+$.

PROTOCOL FOR HPTLC ANALYSIS OF PHARMACEUTICAL FORMULATION

Protocol No. 91

Formulation: Hydrochlorothiazide, Losartan potassium, Atenolol

Classification: Cardiovascular System **Dosage form:** Tablets

Standard preparation: Prepare solution of all the compounds in methanol to get 1 mg/ml of atenolol and losartan potassium and 0.25 mg/ml of hydrochlorothiazide and use for chromatographic application.

Sample preparation: Powdered sample equivalent to 50 mg of atenolol, 50 mg of losartan potassium and 12.5 mg of hydrochlorothiazide suspended in methanol, sonicated for 35–40 min, diluted to 50 ml, filtered through 0.45 μm membrane filter. Apply 2 μl of solution for chromatographic analysis.

Chromatographic equipments:

Sample applicator: Camag Linomat–V

Development chamber: Camag twin-trough glass chamber, 20 × 10 cm

Densitometric scanner: Camag TLC Scanner–III

Chromatographic conditions:

1. Stationary phase: Silica gel 60F_{254} pre-coated HPTLC plates, 20 × 10 cm (200 μm) – Merck, pre-washed with methanol, dried (50°C) for 5 min prior to use
2. Mobile phase (MP): Toluene–methnol–triethylamine (6.5 : 4 : 0.5 v/v)
3. Standard/Sample application:
   Band length: 6 mm Volume applied: 2 μl Spacing: 13 mm
4. Chamber saturation: 30 min (MP)
5. RH (%): 55 ± 2
6. Temperature °C: 25 ± 2
7. Separation technique: Ascending
8. Quantity of mobile phase: 22 ml
9. Migration distance: 70 mm
10. Migration time: 25 min

Densitometric evaluation:

Wavelength: UV–274 nm Scanning mode: Reflectance/Absorbance

HRF: Hydrochlorothiazide—29; Atenolol—43; Losartan K^+—60

Linearity (ng/band): Atenolol and Losartan K^+—1000–5000; Hydrochlorothiazide—250–1250

Recovery (%): Hydrochlorothiazide—99.18–100.33; Atenolol—99.81–100.30; Losartan K^+—99.33–100.2

References: S.R. Sathe and S.B. Bari, *Acta Chromatographica*, **19**, 270–278, 2007.

Comments: The method validated for accuracy, precision, linearity, LOD, LOQ and specificity.

HPTLC : High Performance Thin Layer Chromatography
HPTLC Densitogram

No. 92

Amlodipine besylate

Losartan potassium

Overlaid UV-spectra of hydrochlorothiazide (1), amlodipine (2) and losartan K$^+$(3) for selection of suitable wavelength for densitometric scanning

Typical densitogram of the standard containing hydrochlorothiazide, amlodipine besylate and losartan K$^+$. For detailed experimental and chromatographic conditions, refer to Protocol No. 92. Peaks identification: 1. Losartan K$^+$; 2. Amlodipine besylate; 3. Hydrochlorothiazide.

PROTOCOL FOR HPTLC ANALYSIS OF PHARMACEUTICAL FORMULATION

Protocol No. 92

Formulation: Hydrochlorothiazide, Amlodipine besylate, Losartan potassium

Classification: Cardiovascular System **Dosage form:** Tablets

Standard preparation: Prepare solution of each compound separately in methanol to get 400 μg/ml (amlodipine besylate), 1 mg/ml (hydrochlorothiazide) and 4 mg/ml (losartan potassium). Further each solution was diluted appropriately with methanol for application to study linearity profile.

Sample preparation: Powdered sample equivalent to 5 mg of amlodipine suspended in 15 ml of methanol, sonicated for 10 min, diluted to 25 ml with methanol, filtered and appropriately diluted for chromatographic application.

Chromatographic equipments:

Sample applicator: Camag Linomat–V
Development chamber: Camag twin-trough glass chamber, 10 × 20 cm
Densitometric scanner: Camag TLC Scanner–III

Chromatographic conditions:

1. Stationary phase: Silica gel $60F_{254}$ pre-coated HPTLC plates, 10 × 20 cm (200 μm) – Merck
2. Mobile phase (MP): Chloroform–ethyl acetate–methanol–25% ammonia (4 : 4 : 2 : 0.2 v/v)
3. Standard/Sample application:
   Band length: 10 mm Volume applied: 10 μl Spacing: 10 mm
4. Chamber saturation: 20 min (MP)
5. RH (%): 55 ± 5
6. Temperature °C: 22 ± 2
7. Separation technique: Ascending
8. Quantity of mobile phase: 20 ml
9. Migration distance: 80 mm
10. Migration time: 35 min

Densitometric evaluation:

Wavelength: UV–232 nm Scanning mode: Reflectance/Absorbance
HRF: Losartan K^+—15; Amlodipine besylate—32; Hydrochlorothiazide—52
Linearity: Hydrochlorothiazide—400–2400; Amlodipine besylate—100–800; Losartan K^+—1000–8000
Recovery (%): Hydrochlorothiazide—99.97–100.53; Amlodipine besylate—99.29–99.73; Losartan K^+—99.88–100.62

References: S.B. Wankhede, K.C. Raka, S.B. Wadkar and S.S. Chitlange, *J. Pharm. Res.*, **9(2)**, 60–62, 2010.

Comments:

- The method validated for accuracy, precision, linearity, LOD, LOQ and robustness.
- The method is stability indicated (acid, alkali, photolytic, oxidative and thermal).

HPTLC : High Performance Thin Layer Chromatography
HPTLC Densitogram

No. 93

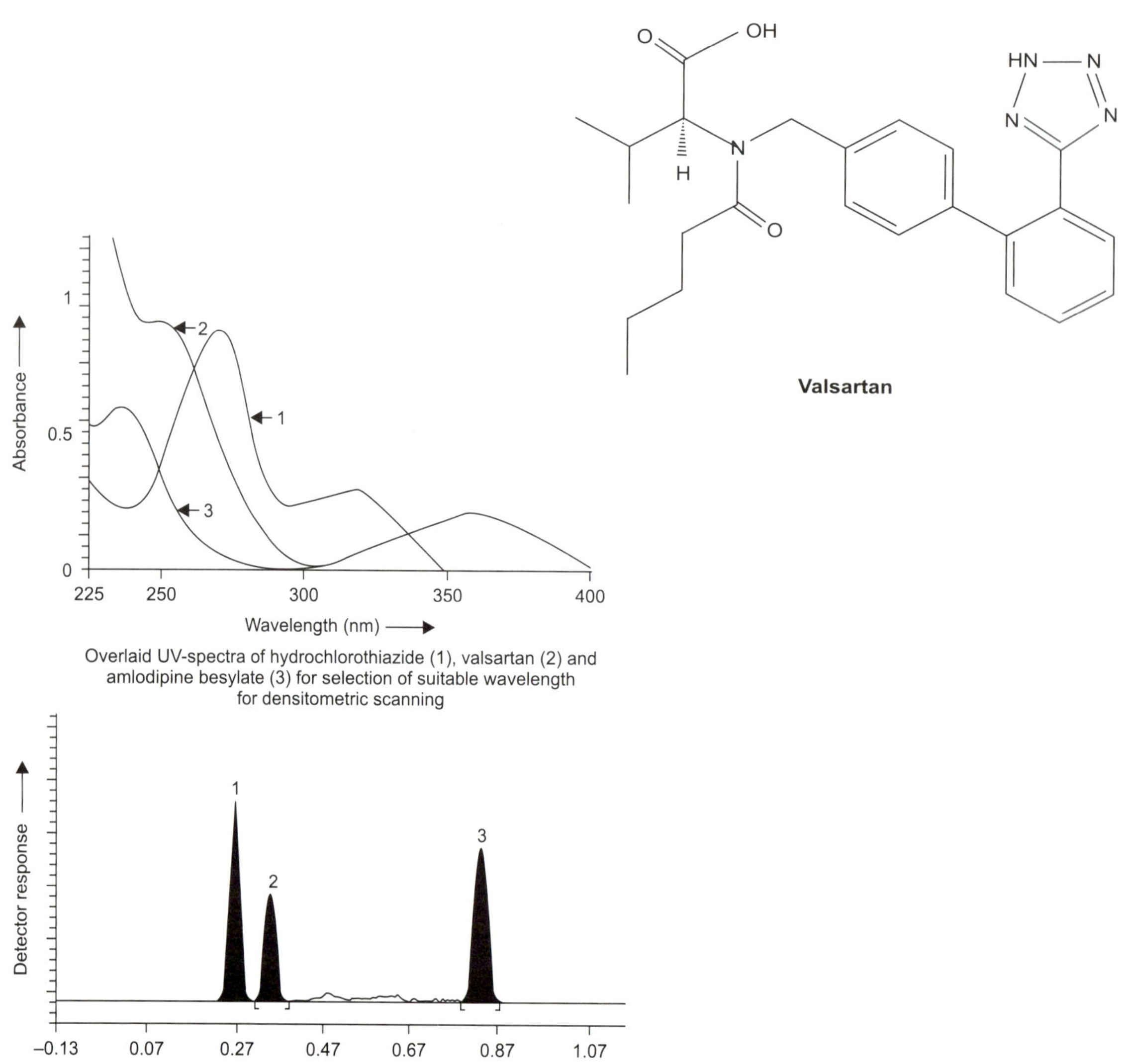

Overlaid UV-spectra of hydrochlorothiazide (1), valsartan (2) and amlodipine besylate (3) for selection of suitable wavelength for densitometric scanning

Typical densitogram of the standard containing hydrochlorothiazide, amlodipine besylate and valsartan. For detailed experimental and chromatographic conditions, refer to Protocol No. 93. Peaks identification: 1. Amlodipine besylate; 2. Valsartan; 3. Hydrochlorothiazide.

PROTOCOL FOR HPTLC ANALYSIS OF PHARMACEUTICAL FORMULATION

Protocol No. 93

Formulation: Hydrochlorothiazide, Amlodipine besylate, Valsartan

Classification: Cardiovascular System **Dosage form:** Tablets

Standard preparation: Prepare 1 mg/ml solution of each compound separately in methanol. Dilute 0.25 ml of amlodipine solution to 10 ml with methanol to get 25 μg/ml; whereas dilute 0.5 ml each of hydrochlorothiazide and valsartan to get 50 μg/ml solution. Apply different volumes of each solution for linearity studies.

Sample preparation: Powdered sample equivalent to 25 mg of amlodipine besylate suspended in 50 ml of methanol, sonicated for 15 min, dilute to 100 ml with methanol, fitler and dilute 5 ml of the filtrate to 20 ml for analysis.

Chromatographic equipments:

Sample applicator: Camag Linomat–V

Development chamber: Camag twin-trough glass chamber, 20 × 10 cm

Densitometric scanner: Camag TLC Scanner–III

Chromatographic conditions:

1. Stationary phase: Silica gel $60F_{254}$ pre-coated HPTLC plates, 20 × 10 cm (200 μm) – Merck
2. Mobile phase (MP): Ethyl acetate–methanol–10% ammonia (8.5 : 2.0 : 1.0 v/v)
3. Standard/Sample application:
   Band length: 8 mm Volume applied: 10 μl Spacing: 10 mm
4. Chamber saturation: 30 min (MP)
5. RH (%): 55 ± 5
6. Temperature °C: 25 ± 2
7. Separation technique: Ascending
8. Quantity of mobile phase: 20 ml
9. Migration distance: 80 mm
10. Migration time: 15 min

Densitometric evaluation:

Wavelength: UV–254 nm (hydrochlorothiazide and valsartan); 366 nm (amlodipine besylate)

Scanning mode: Reflectance/Absorbance

HRF: Amlodipine besylate—26; Valsartan—34; Hydrochlorothiazide—84

Linearity (ng/band): Hydrochlorothiazide and Valsartan—100–700; Amlodipine besylate—50–400

Recovery (%): 98.91–100.1 for all the three drugs

References: V.R. Galande, K.G. Baheti and M.H. Dehghan, *Indian Drugs*, **48(4)**, 49–56, 2011.

Comments: The method validated for accuracy, precision, linearity, LOD, LOQ, specificity, robustness and ruggedness.

HPTLC : High Performance Thin Layer Chromatography
HPTLC Densitogram

No. 94

Frusemide

Spironolactone

Triamterene

Overlaid UV-spectra of hydrochlorothiazide (1), triamterene (2), frusemide (3) and spironolactone (4) for selection of suitable wavelength for densitometric scanning

Typical densitogram of the standard containing hydrochlorothiazide, frusemide, triamterene and spironolactone. For detailed experimental and chromatographic conditions, refer to Protocol No. 94. Peaks identification: 1. Triamterene; 2. Hydrochlorothiazide; 3. Frusemide; 4. Spironolactone.

PROTOCOL FOR HPTLC ANALYSIS OF PHARMACEUTICAL FORMULATION

Protocol No. 94

Formulation: **Hydrochlorothiazide, Frusemide, Spironolactone, Triamterene**

Classification: Cardiovascular System **Dosage form:** Tablets

Standard preparation: Standard solution of each compound prepared in methanol to get HCZ—30–520 μg/ml; FUR—30–530 μg/ml; Spr—20–280 μg/ml; Tria—10–350 μg/ml. 5 μl of each solution was applied as bands for analysis.

Sample preparation: Powdered sample equivalent to 1.25 mg of hydrochlorothiazide (HCZ) suspended in 10 ml of methanol, shaken for 10 min, centrifuged (3000 rpm) and supernatant used for further studies and assay.

Chromatographic equipments:

Sample applicator: Camag Linomat–V sample applicator

Development chamber: Sigma-Aldrich glass chamber, 18 × 9 × 18 cm

Densitometric scanner: Camag TLC Scanner–III

Chromatographic conditions:

1. Stationary phase: Silica gel 60F_{254} pre-coated TLC plates, 10 × 10 cm (250 μm) – Merck
2. Mobile phase (MP): n-hexane–ethyl acetate–methanol–water–acetic acid (4 : 8 : 3 : 0.4 : 0.2 v/v)
3. Standard/Sample application:
   Band length: 10 mm Volume applied: 5 μl Spacing: 10 mm
4. Chamber saturation: 30 min (MP)
5. RH (%): 55 ± 5
6. Temperature °C: 22 ± 2
7. Separation technique: Ascending
8. Quantity of mobile phase: 30 ml
9. Migration distance: 95 mm
10. Migration time: 30 min

Densitometric evaluation:

Wavelength: UV–264 nm Scanning mode: Reflectance/Absorbance

HRF: Triamterene—22; Hydrochlorothiazide—46; Frusemide—58; Spironolactone—71

Linearity: 60–250 ng/band for all the four drugs

Recovery (%): 97.10–10.2.0 for all the four drugs

References: Anna Maśianka, Jankrzek and Mariusz Stolarezyk, *J. Planar Chromatogr.*, **22(6)**, 405–410, 2009.

Comments: The method validated for accuracy, precision, linearity, LOD, LOQ, specificity and robustness.

HPTLC : High Performance Thin Layer Chromatography
HPTLC Densitogram

No. 95

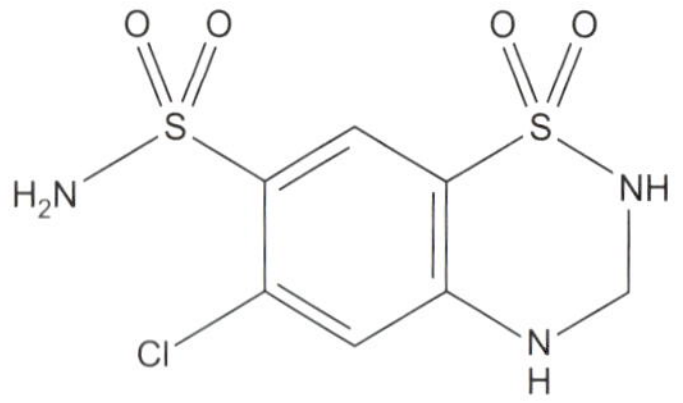

Hydrochlorothiazide

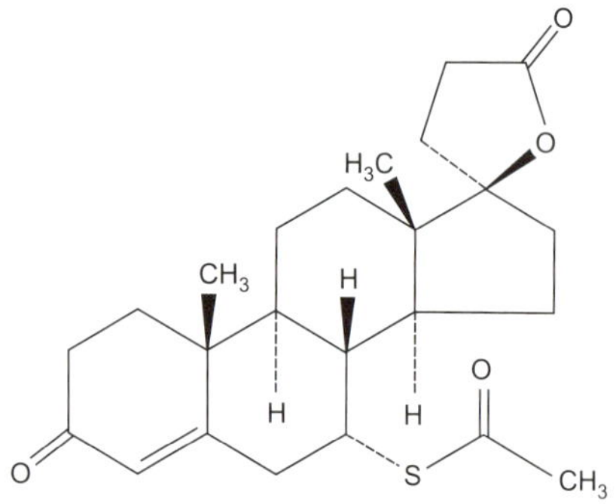

Spironolactone

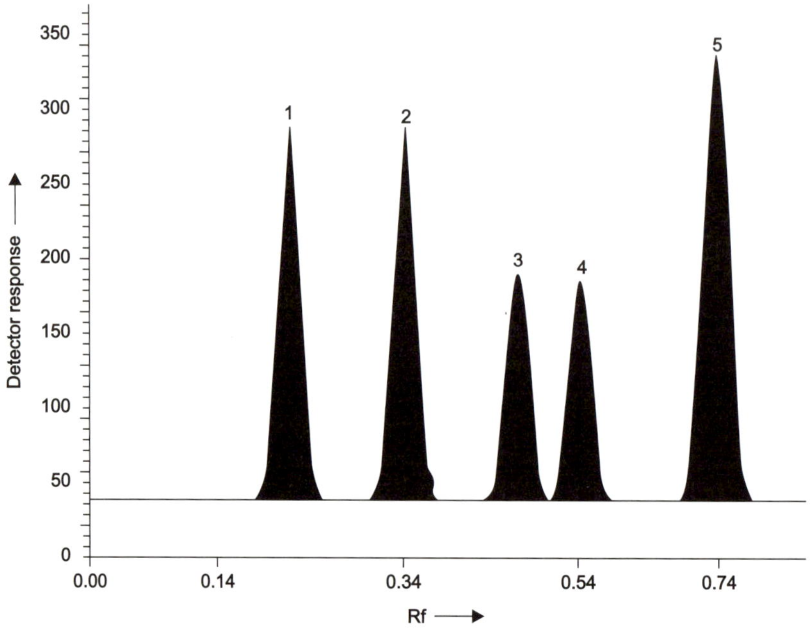

Typical densitogram of the standard containing hydrochlorothiazide and spironolactone. For detailed experimental and chromatographic conditions, refer to Protocol No. 95. Peaks identification: 1. Chlorothiazide; 2. Hydrochlorothiazide; 3. Spironolactone degrade; 4. DSA (degradation product of HCZ); 5. Spironolactone.

PROTOCOL FOR HPTLC ANALYSIS OF PHARMACEUTICAL FORMULATION

Protocol No. 95

Formulation: Hydrochlorothiazide, Spironolactone, their impurities and degradation products

Classification: Cardiovascular System **Dosage form:** Tablets

Standard preparation: Prepare 1 mg/ml solution of all the five compounds in methanol. Further dilutions are made with methanol to get 100 μg/ml. Apply 4–18 μl of HCZ solution and 3–15 μl of SPR solution for linearity profile.

Sample preparation: Powdered sample equivalent to 100 mg of HCZ or SPR suspended in 75 ml of methanol, sonicated for 45 min, diluted to 100 ml with methanol. Filtered and the filtrate diluted with methanol to get 100 μg/ml of each compound. Apply 10 μl for chromatographic analysis.

Chromatographic equipments:

Sample applicator: Camag Linomat–V
Development chamber: Camag twin-trough glass chamber, 20 × 10 cm
Densitometric scanner: Camag TLC Scanner–III

Chromatographic conditions:

1. Stationary phase: Silica gel 60F_{254} pre-coated TLC plates, 20 × 10 cm (250 μm) – Merck, pre-washed with methanol, dried at 100°C for 5 min, prior to use
2. Mobile phase (MP): Ethyl acetate–chloroform–formic acid–triethylamine (7 : 3 : 0.1 : 0.1 v/v)
3. Standard/Sample application:
   Band length: 6 mm Volume applied: 10 μl Spacing: 8.9 mm
4. Chamber saturation: 60 min (MP)
5. RH (%): 55 ± 5
6. Temperature °C: 22 ± 2
7. Separation technique: Ascending
8. Quantity of mobile phase: 20 ml
9. Migration distance: 80 mm
10. Migration time: 20 min

Densitometric evaluation:

Wavelength: UV–235 nm Scanning mode: Reflectance/Absorbance
HRF: See densitogram of the standard mixture
Linearity (ng/band): Hydrochlorothiazide—400–1800; Spironolactone—300–1500
Recovery (%): 99.86–99.88 for both the compounds

References: Maha A. Hegazy, Fadia H. Matwaly and Nada S. Abdelwahab, *J. Chromatogr. Sci.*, **49**, 129–135, 2011.

Comments:

- The method validated for accuracy, precision, linearity, LOD, LOQ, specificity, robustness and ruggedness.
- Analytical results by HPLC and HPTLC methods were comparable.

HPTLC : High Performance Thin Layer Chromatography
HPTLC Densitogram

No. 96

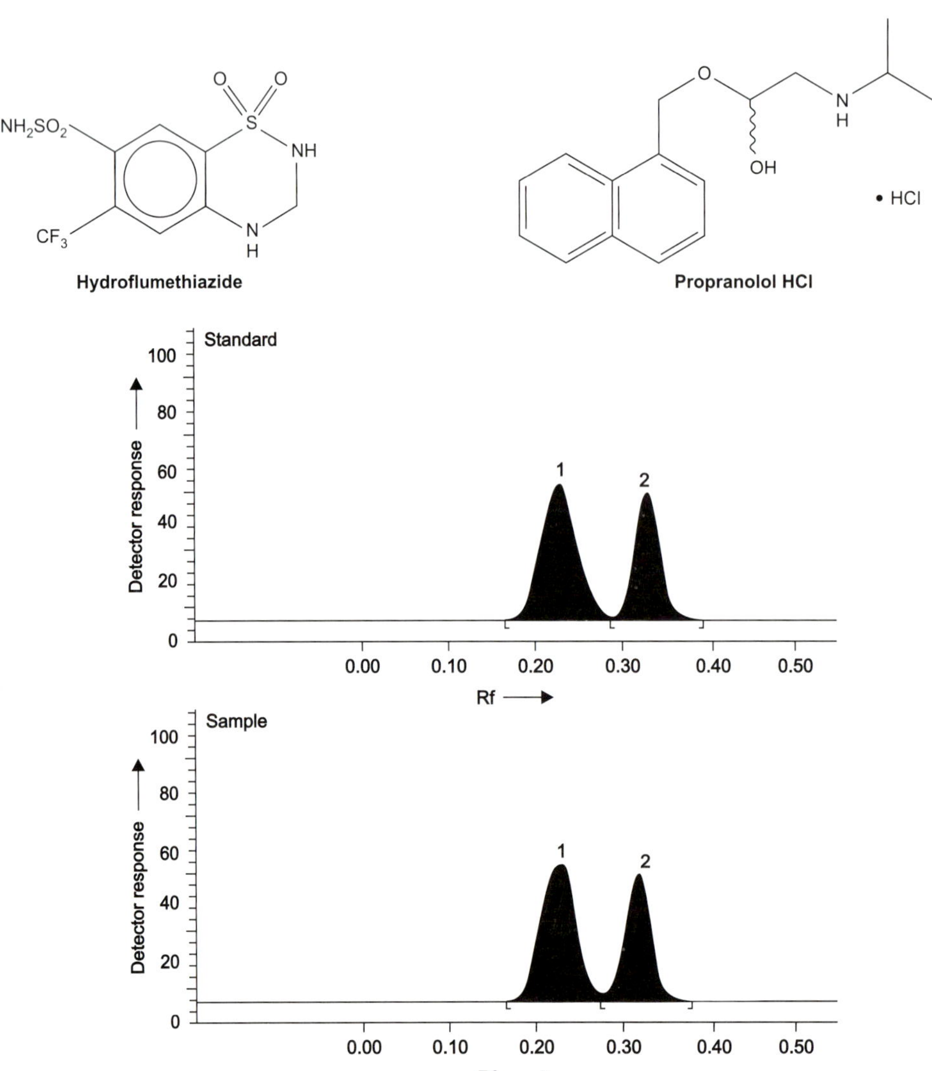

Typical densitogram of the sample and standard containing hydroflumethiazide and propranolol HCl. For detailed experimental and chromatographic conditions, refer to Protocol No. 96. Peaks identification: 1. Hydroflumethiazide; 2. Propranolol HCl.

PROTOCOL FOR HPTLC ANALYSIS OF PHARMACEUTICAL FORMULATION

Protocol No. 96

Formulation: **Hydroflumethiazide, Propranolol hydrochloride**

Classification: Cardiovascular System **Dosage form:** Tablets

Standard preparation: Prepare 1 mg/ml solution of hydroflumethiazide and 1.6 mg/ml solution of propranolol HCl, both in methanol. Further dilute 0.5 ml of stock solution to 10 ml with methanol and use for analysis.

Sample preparation: Powdered sample equivalent to 25 mg of hydroflumethiazide suspended in 30–40 ml of methanol, sonicate for 5 min, dilute to 50 ml with methanol. Filter and dilute 1 ml to 10 ml with methanol for assay.

Chromatographic equipments:

Sample applicator: Camag Linomat–IV

Development chamber: Camag twin–trough glass chamber, 10 × 10 cm

Densitometric scanner: Camag TLC Scanner–II

Chromatographic conditions:

1. Stationary phase: Silica gel $60F_{254}$ pre-coated HPTLC plates, 7 × 10 cm (200 μm) – Merck
2. Mobile phase (MP): Chloroform–methanol–25% ammonia (9 : 1 : 0.05 v/v)
3. Standard/Sample application:
   Band length: 7 mm Volume applied: 4 μl Spacing: 5 mm
4. Chamber saturation: 20 min (MP)
5. RH (%): 55 ± 5
6. Temperature °C: 22 ± 2
7. Separation technique: Ascending
8. Quantity of mobile phase: 10 ml
9. Migration distance: 55 mm
10. Migration time: 16 min

Densitometric evaluation:

Wavelength: UV–275 nm Scanning mode: Reflectance/Absorbance

HRF: Hydroflumethiazide—23; Propranolol hydrochloride—33

Linearity (μg/ml): Hydroflumethiazide—25–200; Propranolol HCl—40–400

Recovery (%): 97.20–99.64 for both the compounds

References: —

Comments: The method was optimized and analytical work carried out at **Anchrom's HPTLC Application Laboratory**, Mumbai, India.

HPTLC : High Performance Thin Layer Chromatography
HPTLC Densitogram

No. 97

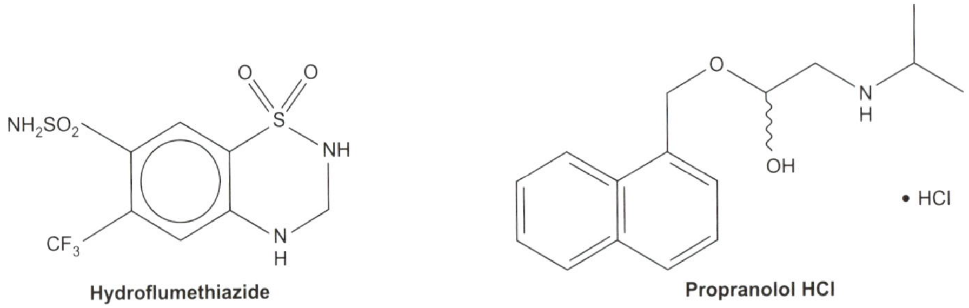

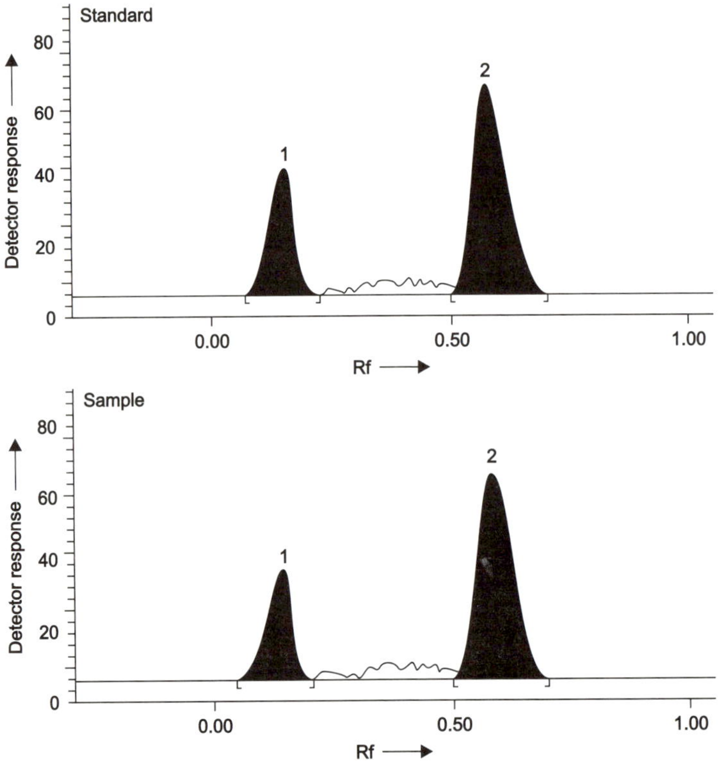

Hydroflumethiazide

Propranolol HCl

Standard

Sample

Typical densitogram of the standard and sample containing hydroflumethiazide and propranolol HCl. For detailed experimental and chromatographic conditions, refer to Protocol No. 97. Peaks identification: 1. Propranolol HCl; 2. Hydroflumethiazide.

PROTOCOL FOR HPTLC ANALYSIS OF PHARMACEUTICAL FORMULATION

Protocol No. 97

Formulation: Hydroflumethiazide, Propranolol hydrochloride

Classification: Cardiovascular System **Dosage form:** Tablets

Standard preparation: Prepare 1 mg/ml solution of hydroflumethiazide and 1.6 mg/ml solution of propranolol HCl, both in methanol. Further dilute 0.5 ml of stock solution to 10 ml with methanol and use for analysis.

Sample preparation: Powdered sample equivalent to 25 mg of hydroflumethiazide suspended in 30–40 ml of methanol, sonicate, dilute to 50 ml with methanol. Filter and dilute 1 ml of the filtrate to 10 ml with methanol for assay.

Chromatographic equipments:

Sample applicator: Camag Linomat–IV

Development chamber: Camag twin–trough glass chamber, 10 × 10 cm

Densitometric scanner: Camag TLC Scanner–II

Chromatographic conditions:

1. Stationary phase: Silica gel 60 RP–18F_{254s} pre-coated HPTLC plates, 7 × 10 cm (200 μm) – Merck
2. Mobile phase (MP): 0.5 M sodium chloride–methanol–glacial acetic acid (12 : 8 : 0.1 v/v)
3. Standard/Sample application:
   Band length: 8 mm Volume applied: 4 μl Spacing: 10 mm
4. Chamber saturation: 30 min (MP)
5. RH (%): 55 ± 5
6. Temperature °C: 22 ± 2
7. Separation technique: Ascending
8. Quantity of mobile phase: 20 ml
9. Migration distance: 50 mm
10. Migration time: 40 min

Densitometric evaluation:

Wavelength: UV–254 or 275 nm Scanning mode: Reflectance/Absorbance

HRF: Propranolol HCl—20; Hydroflumethiazide—65

Linearity (μg/ml): Hydroflumethiazide—25–200; Propranolol HCl—40–400

Recovery (%): 99.0–101.50 for both the compounds

References: —

Comments:

- The method was optimized and analytical work carried out at **Anchrom's HPTLC Application Laboratory**, Mumbai, India.
- Reversed phase chromatography resulted in reversal of retention factor with compared to NP–HPTLC.
- RP-HPTLC carried out on silicon oil impregnated plates (5% silicon oil in pet. ether) gave equally good separation.

HPTLC : High Performance Thin Layer Chromatography
HPTLC Densitogram

No. 98

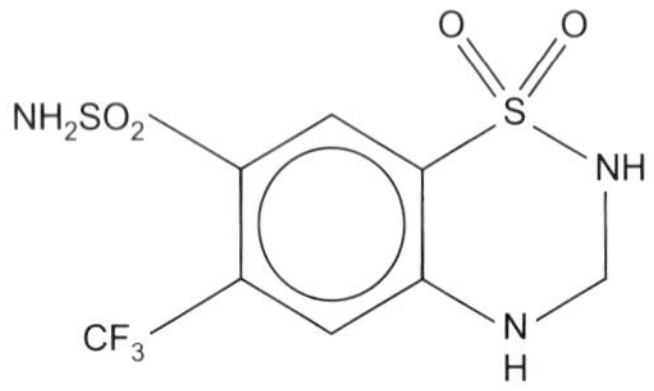

Hydroflumethiazide

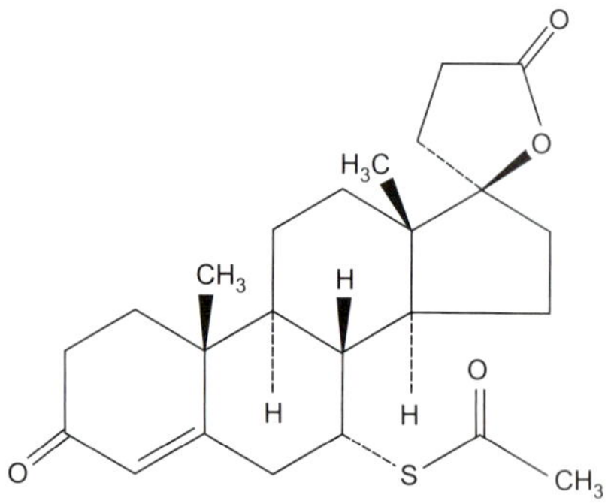

Spironolactone

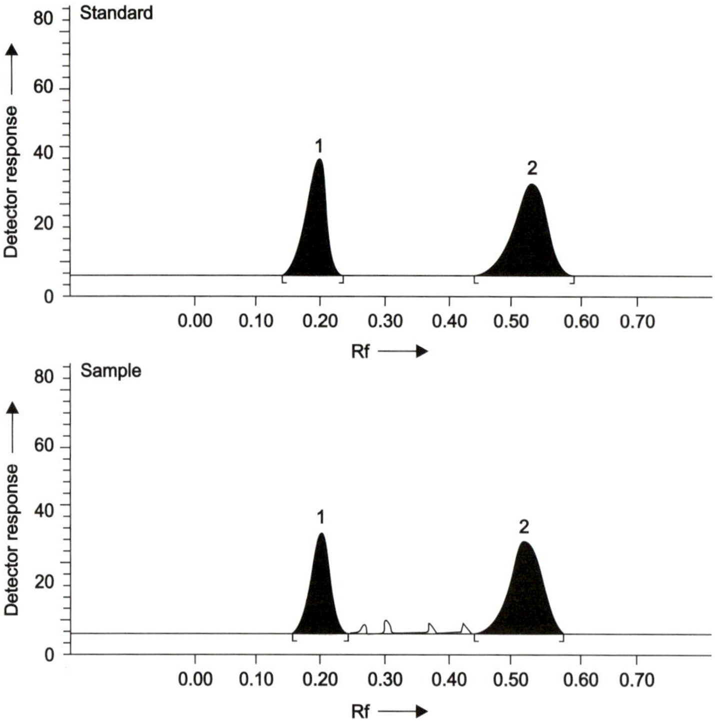

Typical densitogram of the standard and sample containing hydroflumethiazide and spironolactone. For detailed experimental and chromatographic conditions, refer to Protocol No. 98. Peaks identification: 1. Hydroflumethiazide; 2. Spironolactone.

PROTOCOL FOR HPTLC ANALYSIS OF PHARMACEUTICAL FORMULATION

Protocol No. 98

Formulation: **Hydroflumethiazide, Spironolactone**

Classification: Cardiovascular System **Dosage form:** Tablets

Standard preparation: Dissolve 10 mg each of spironolactone and hydroflumethiazide in 10 ml of methanol. Further 0.5 ml of the resulting solution is diluted to 10 ml with methanol for application.

Sample preparation: Powdered sample equivalent to 25 mg of spironolactone suspended in 20 ml of methanol, sonicated for 5 min, diluted to 25 ml with methanol, filtered and 0.5 ml of filtrate diluted to 10 ml with methanol and used for analysis

Chromatographic equipments:

Sample applicator: Camag Linomat–IV

Development chamber: Camag twin–trough glass chamber, 10 × 10 cm

Densitometric scanner: Camag TLC Scanner–II

Chromatographic conditions:

1. Stationary phase: Silica gel $60F_{254}$ pre-coated HPTLC plates, 7 × 10 cm (200 μm) – Merck
2. Mobile phase (MP): n-hexane–ethyl acetate–glacial acetic acid (5 : 5 : 0.05 v/v)
3. Standard/Sample application:
   Band length: 7 mm Volume applied: 5 μl Spacing: 10 mm
4. Chamber saturation: 20 min (MP)
5. RH (%): 55 ± 2
6. Temperature °C: 22 ± 2
7. Separation technique: Ascending
8. Quantity of mobile phase: 10 ml
9. Migration distance: 50 mm
10. Migration time: 15 min

Densitometric evaluation:

Wavelength: UV–260 nm Scanning mode: Reflectance/Absorbance

HRF: Hydroflumethiazide—20; Spironolactone—54

Linearity: 50–500 ng/band for both the drugs

Recovery (%): 98.20–99.60 for both the drugs

References: —

Comments: The method was optimized and analytical work carried out at **Anchrom's HPTLC Application Laboratory**, Mumbai, India.

HPTLC : High Performance Thin Layer Chromatography
HPTLC Densitogram

No. 99

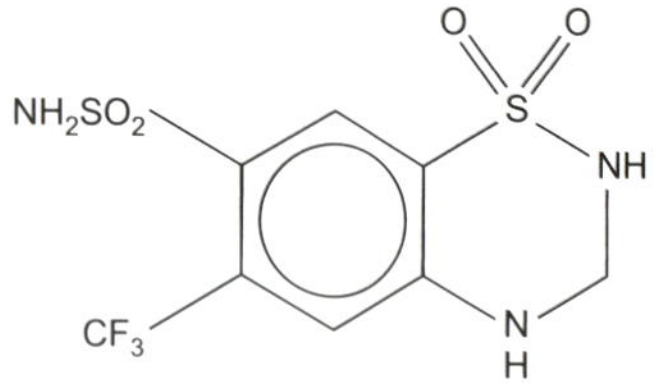

Hydroflumethiazide

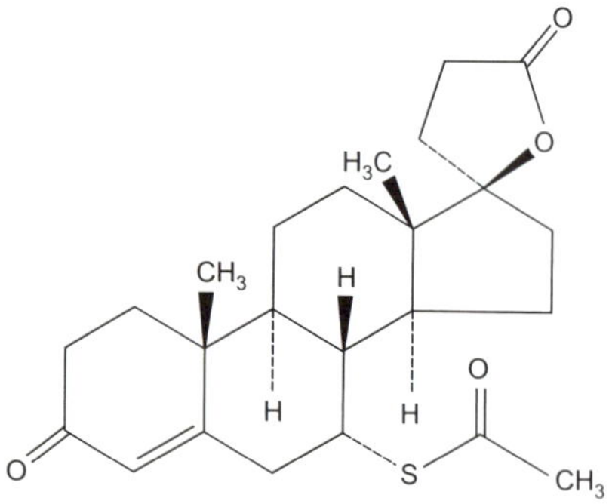

Spironolactone

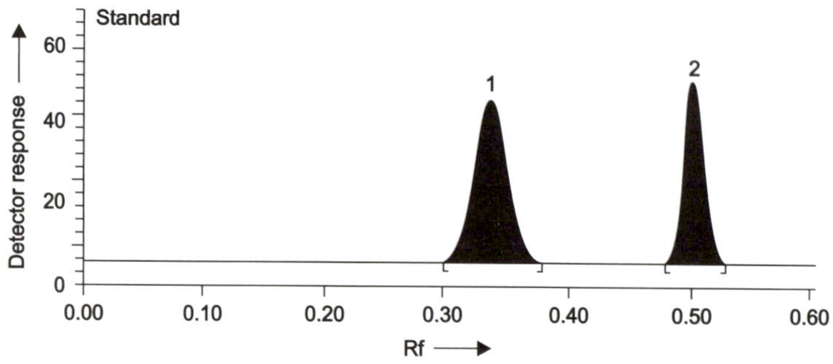

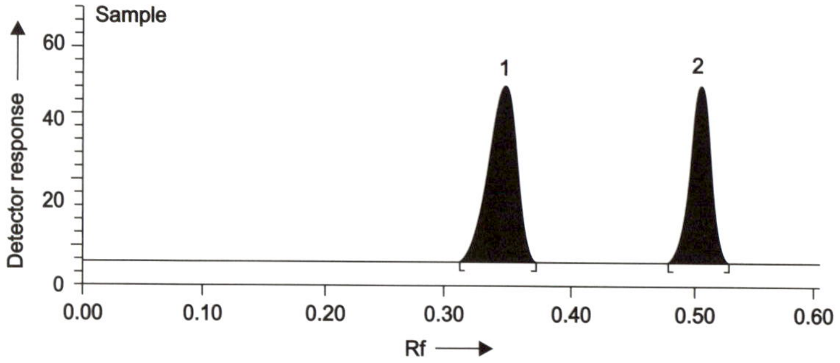

Typical densitogram of the standard and sample containing hydroflumethiazide and spironolactone. For detailed experimental and chromatographic conditions, refer to Protocol No. 99. Peaks identification: 1. Spironolactone; 2. Hydroflumethiazide.

PROTOCOL FOR HPTLC ANALYSIS OF PHARMACEUTICAL FORMULATION

Protocol No. 99

Formulation: Hydroflumethiazide, Spironolactone

Classification: Cardiovascular System **Dosage form:** Tablets

Standard preparation: Dissolve 10 mg each of spironolactone and hydroflumethiazide in 10 ml of methanol. Dilute 0.5 ml of the resulting solution to 10 ml with methanol and use for chromatographic application.

Sample preparation: Powdered sample equivalent to 25 mg of spironolactone suspended in 20 ml of methanol, sonicated for 5 min, dilute to 25 ml, filter and dilute. 0.5 ml of filtrate diluted to 10 ml with methanol to use for chromatographic analysis.

Chromatographic equipments:

Sample applicator: Camag Linomat–IV

Development chamber: Camag twin–trough glass chamber, 10 × 10 cm

Densitometric scanner: Camag TLC Scanner–II

Chromatographic conditions:

1. Stationary phase: Silica gel 60 RP–18 F_{254s} pre-coated HPTLC plates, 10 × 10 cm (200 μm) – Merck
2. Mobile phase (MP): 0.5 M sodium chloride–methanol–acetonitrile–glacial acetic acid (5 : 2 : 3 : 0.1 v/v)
3. Standard/Sample application:
   Band length: 7 mm Volume applied: 5 μl Spacing: 10 mm
4. Chamber saturation: 40 min (MP)
5. RH (%): 55 ± 5
6. Temperature °C: 22 ± 2
7. Separation technique: Ascending
8. Quantity of mobile phase: 10 ml
9. Migration distance: 50 mm
10. Migration time: 25 min

Densitometric evaluation:

Wavelength: UV–260 nm Scanning mode: Reflectance/Absorbance

HRF: Spironolactone—35; Hydroflumethiazide—52;

Linearity: 50–500 ng for both the drugs

Recovery (%): 100.75–101.50 for both the compounds

References: —

Comments:

- The method was optimized and analytical work carried out at **Anchrom's HPTLC Application Laboratory**, Mumbai, India.
- Reversed phase chromatographic method resulted in reversal of retention order when compared to NP chromatographic separation.
- The laboratory made RP-HPTLC plates (impregnated with 5% silicon oil in pet. ether) gave equally good results.

HPTLC : High Performance Thin Layer Chromatography
HPTLC Densitogram

No. 100

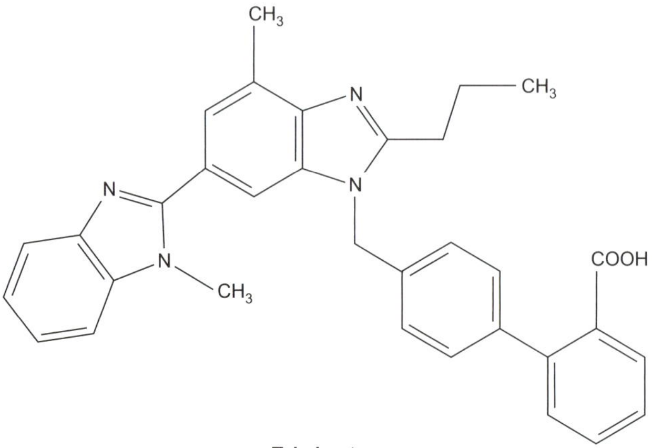
CH3
N
CH3
N
N
N
CH3
COOH

Telmisartan

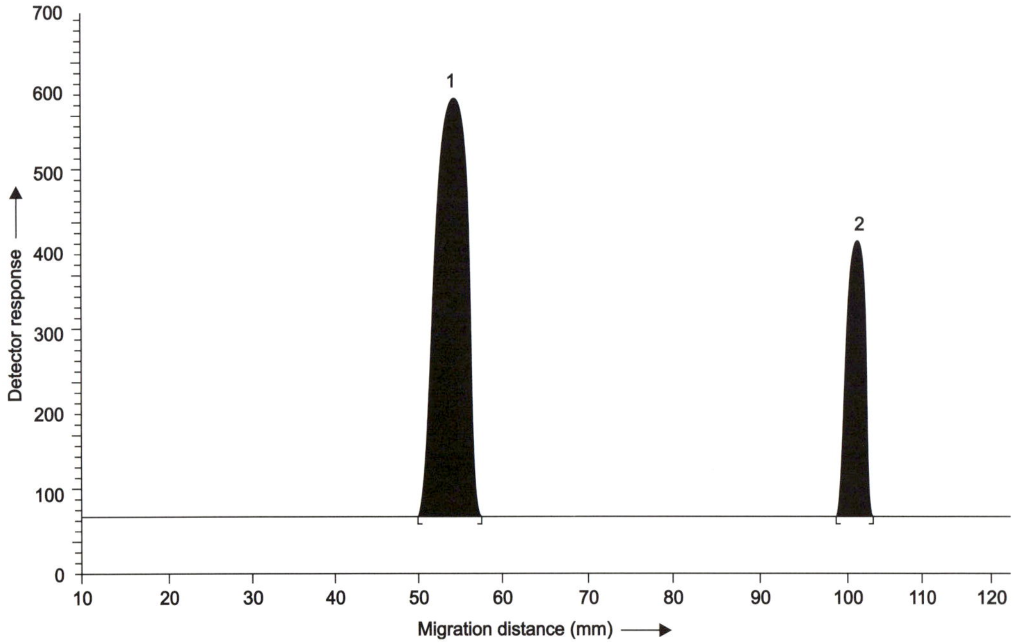
700
600
500
400
300
200
100
0
Detector response
1
2
10
20
30
40
50
60
70
80
90
100
110
120
Migration distance (mm)

Typical densitogram of the sample containing telmisartan and ramipril. For detailed experimental and chromatographic conditions, refer to Protocol No. 100. Peaks identification: 1. Telmisartan; 2. Ramipril.

PROTOCOL FOR HPTLC ANALYSIS OF PHARMACEUTICAL FORMULATION

Protocol No. 100

Formulation: Telmisartan, Ramipril

Classification: Cardiovascular System **Dosage form:** Tablets

Standard preparation: Prepare 1 mg/ml solution of each compound in methanol. Further serial dilutions made with methanol. Apply 10 μl of each solution for linearity profile.

Sample preparation: Powdered sample equivalent to 5 mg of ramipril suspended in methanol, sonicated, diluted, filtered and filtrate suitably diluted with methanol and used for chromatographic application.

Chromatographic equipments:

Sample applicator: Camag Linomat–IV

Development chamber: Camag twin–trough glass chamber, 10 × 10 cm

Densitometric scanner: Camag TLC Scanner–III

Chromatographic conditions:

1. Stationary phase: Silica gel 60F_{254} pre-coated HPTLC plates, 10 × 10 cm (200 μm) – Merck, pre-washed with methanol, dried at 60°C for 5 min prior to use
2. Mobile phase (MP): Ethyl acetate–chloroform–methanol (10 : 3 : 1 v/v)
3. Standard/Sample application:
   Band length: 10 mm Volume applied: 10 μl Spacing: 5 mm
4. Chamber saturation: 30 min (MP)
5. RH (%): 55 ± 5
6. Temperature °C: Ambient
7. Separation technique: Ascending
8. Quantity of mobile phase: 14 ml
9. Migration distance: —
10. Migration time: —

Densitometric evaluation:

Wavelength: UV–272 nm Scanning mode: Reflectance/Absorbance

HRF: See densitogram

Linearity: 50–500 ng for both the drugs

Recovery (%): 100.75–101.50 for both the compounds

References: M.V. Asha Jyoti, et. al., Abstract No. PP099, *Ind. J. Pharm. Sci.*, **71(2)**, 199, 2009.

Comments: The method validated for accuracy, precision, linearity and specificity.

HPTLC : High Performance Thin Layer Chromatography
HPTLC Densitogram

No. 101

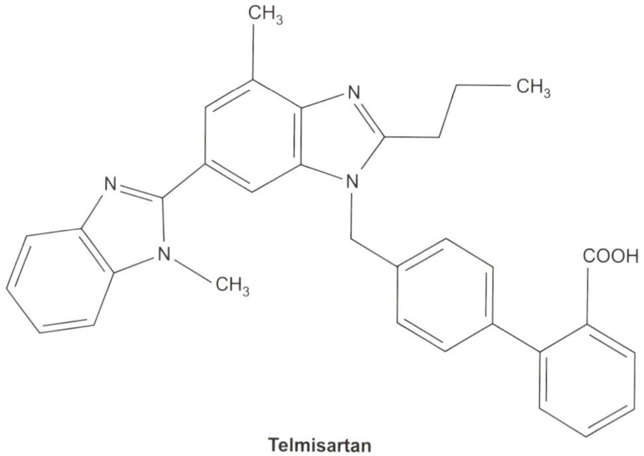

Telmisartan

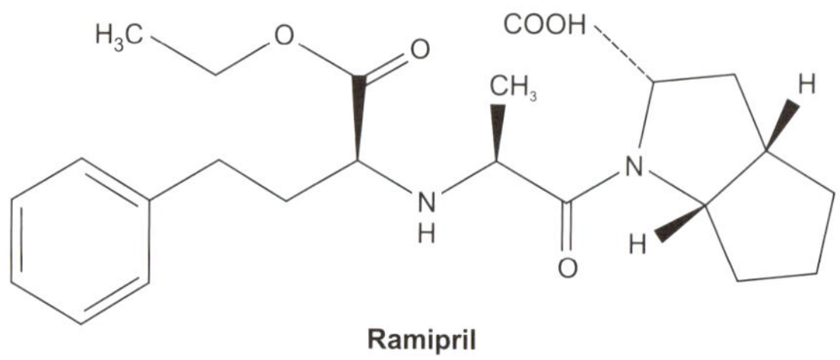

Ramipril

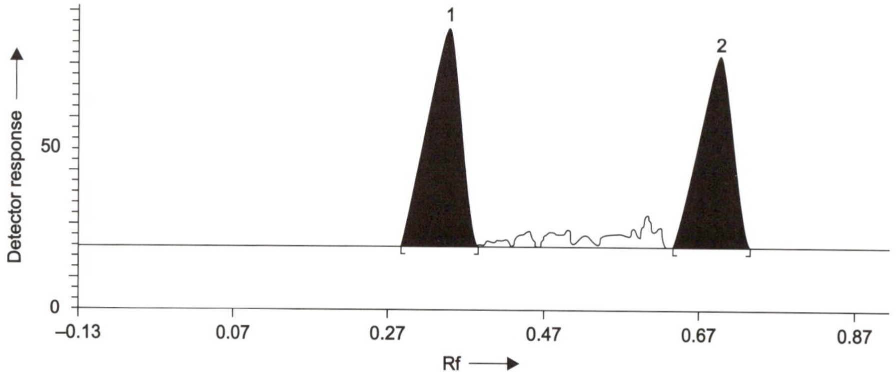

Typical densitogram of the standard containing telmisartan and ramipril. For detailed experimental and chromatographic conditions, refer to Protocol No. 101. Peaks identification: 1. Ramipril; 2. Telmisartan.

PROTOCOL FOR HPTLC ANALYSIS OF PHARMACEUTICAL FORMULATION

Protocol No. 101

Formulation: Telmisartan, Ramipril

Classification: Cardiovascular System **Dosage form:** Capsultes

Standard preparation: Prepare 500 μg/ml solution of each compound in methanol. Apply varying volumes of each solution for linearity profile.

Sample preparation: The sample equivalent to 5 mg of ramipril suspended in water, sonicated for 15 min, diluted to 250 ml with water and filtered through 0.45 μm nylon filter. Dilute 2 ml of filtrate to 10 ml with methanol and use for chromatographic separation and analysis.

Chromatographic equipments:

Sample applicator: Camag Linomat–V

Development chamber: Camag twin–trough glass chamber, 10 × 10 cm

Densitometric scanner: Camag TLC Scanner–III

Chromatographic conditions:

1. Stationary phase: Silica gel $60F_{254}$ pre-coated TLC plates, 10 × 10 cm (250 μm) – Merck, pre-washed with methanol, activated at 60°C for 5 min prior to use
2. Mobile phase (MP): Acetone–benzene–ethyl acetate–glacial acetic acid (5 : 3 : 2 : 0.03 v/v)
3. Standard/Sample application:
   Band length: 6 mm Volume applied: 15 μl Spacing: 10 mm
4. Chamber saturation: 15 min (MP)
5. RH (%): 60 ± 5
6. Temperature °C: 30 ± 1
7. Separation technique: Ascending
8. Quantity of mobile phase: 10 ml
9. Migration distance: —
10. Migration time: —

Densitometric evaluation:

Wavelength: UV–210 nm Scanning mode: Reflectance/Absorbance

HRF: Ramipril—35; Telmisartan—69

Linearity (ng/band): Telmisartan—100–1800; Ramipril—300–1800

Recovery (%): 99.07–100.96 for both the compounds

References: V.A. Patel, P.G. Patel, B.G. Chaudhary, N.B. Rajgor and S.G. Rath, *Int. J. Pharmaceutical and Biological Sciences*, **1(1)**, 18–24, 2010.

Comments: The method validated for accuracy, precision, linearity, LOD, LOQ, specificity, robustness and ruggedness.

HPTLC : High Performance Thin Layer Chromatography
HPTLC Densitogram

No. 102

Telmisartan

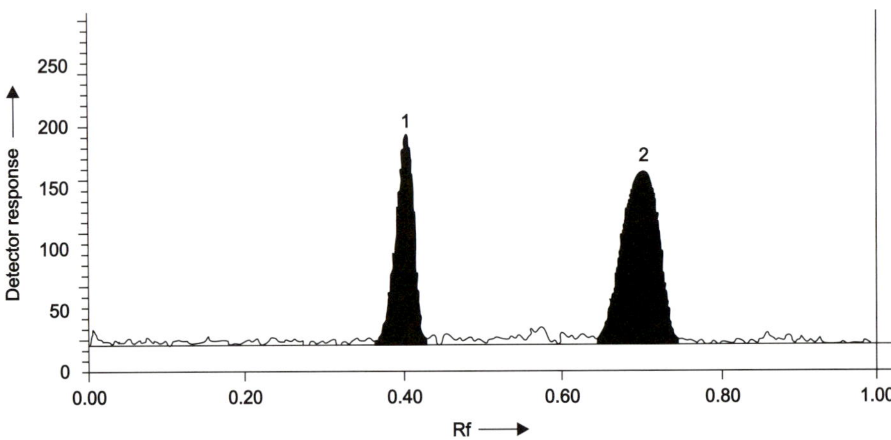

Typical densitogram of the standard containing ramipril and telmisartan. For detailed experimental and chromatographic conditions, refer to Protocol No. 102. Peaks identification: 1. Ramipril; 2. Telmisartan.

PROTOCOL FOR HPTLC ANALYSIS OF PHARMACEUTICAL FORMULATION

Protocol No. 102

Formulation: Telmisartan, Ramipril

Classification: Cardiovascular System **Dosage form:** Tablets

Standard preparation: Prepare 1 mg/ml solution of each compound in methanol. Further dilutions made to get 100 μg/ml of each solution. Dilute 2 ml of telmisartan solution and 0.8 ml of ramipril solution to 10 ml with methanol and apply 5–25 μl for linearity profile.

Sample preparation: Accurately weighed quantity of the powdered sample extracted with methanol by sonication, filtered and suitably diluted to get final concentration of each compound within linearity range. Apply 10 μl for chromatographic analysis.

Chromatographic equipments:

Sample applicator: Camag Linomat–V

Development chamber: Camag twin–trough glass chamber, 10 × 10 cm

Densitometric scanner: Camag TLC Scanner–III

Chromatographic conditions:

1. Stationary phase: Silica gel $60F_{254}$ pre-coated HPTLC plates, 10 × 10 cm (200 μm) – Merck
2. Mobile phase (MP): Chloroform–methanol (6 : 1 v/v)
3. Standard/Sample application:
   Band length: 4 mm Volume applied: 5–25 μl Spacing: 10 mm
4. Chamber saturation: —
5. RH (%): 55 ± 5
6. Temperature °C: 22 ± 2
7. Separation technique: Ascending
8. Quantity of mobile phase: 14 ml
9. Migration distance: —
10. Migration time: —

Densitometric evaluation:

Wavelength: UV–210 nm Scanning mode: Reflectance/Absorbance

HRF: Ramipril—38; Telmisartan—68

Linearity (ng/band): Ramipril—400–2000; Telmisartan—1000–5000

Recovery (%): 98–102 for both the drugs

References: Laxman V. Potale, M.C. Damle, Amol S. Khodke and K.G. Bothara, *Int. J. Pharmaceutical Sci. Review and Research*, **2(2)**, 35–39, 2010.

Comments:

- The method validated for accuracy, precision, linearity, LOD, LOQ, specificity, robustness and ruggedness.
- The method is stability indicating (acid, base, oxidative, thermal, photolytic). The degradation products were separated from main compounds.

HPTLC : High Performance Thin Layer Chromatography
HPTLC Densitogram

No. 103

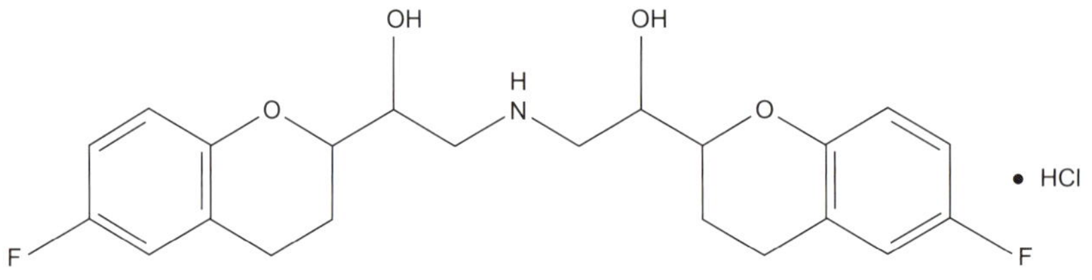

Nebivolol hydrochloride

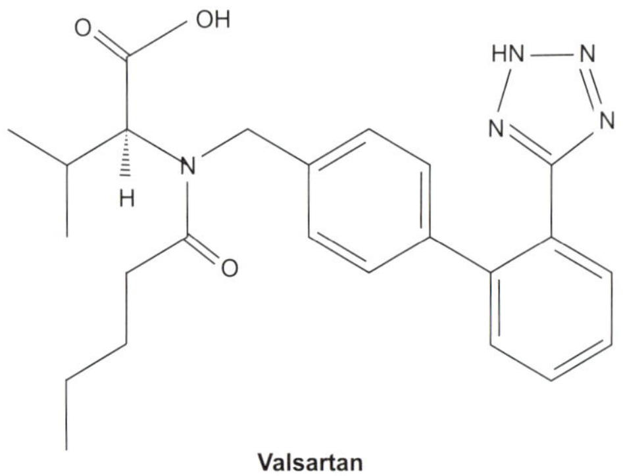

Valsartan

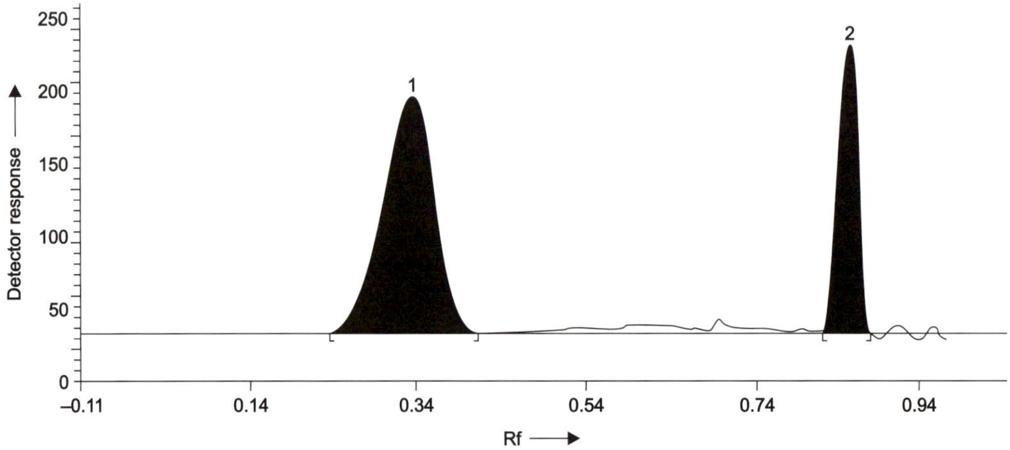

Typical densitogram of the sample containing nebivolol hydrochloride and valsartan. For detailed experimental and chromatographic conditions, refer to Protocol No. 103. Peaks identification: 1. Nebivolol HCl; 2. Valsartan.

PROTOCOL FOR HPTLC ANALYSIS OF PHARMACEUTICAL FORMULATION

Protocol No. 103

Formulation: Nebivolol hydrochloride, Valsartan

Classification: Cardiovascular System **Dosage form:** Tablets

Standard preparation: Prepare 1 mg/ml solution of each compound in methanol with sonication. Further dilutions were ade to get 200 μg/ml (nebivolol HCl) and 100 μg/ml (valsartan).

Sample preparation: Powdered sample equivalent to 4 mg of nebivolol and 64 mg of valsartan suspended in methanol, sonicated for 5 min and diluted to 10 ml with methanol, filtered and further diluted to get 200 μg/ml (nebivolol) and 100 μg/ml (valsartan) and used for analysis.

Chromatographic equipments:

Sample applicator: Camag Linomat–IV

Development chamber: Camag twin–trough glass chamber, 10 × 10 cm

Densitometric scanner: Camag TLC Scanner–III

Chromatographic conditions:

1. Stationary phase: Silica gel $60F_{254}$ pre-coated HPTLC plates, 10 × 10 cm (200 μm) – Merck
2. Mobile phase (MP): Ethyl acetate–methanol–acetic acid (6 : 1 : 0.5 v/v) pre-washed with methanol, dried (60°C) for 5 min prior to use
3. Standard/Sample application:
   Band length: 6 mm Volume applied: 10 μl Spacing: 12 mm
4. Chamber saturation: 15 min (MP)
5. RH (%): 55 ± 5
6. Temperature °C: 22 ± 2
7. Separation technique: Ascending
8. Quantity of mobile phase: 15 ml
9. Migration distance: 75 mm
10. Migration time: 15 min

Densitometric evaluation:

Wavelength: UV–280 nm (iso-absorption point)

Scanning mode: Reflectance/Absorbance

HRF: Nebivolol HCl—34; Valsartan—83

Linearity (ng/band): Nebivolol HCl—1200–2800; Valsartan—600–1400

Recovery (%): Nebivolol HCl—98.39–101.49; Valsartan—98.40–101.13

References: M.C. Damle, Bothara Kailash G and Topagi Kirtis, *J. Pharm. Res.*, **8(4)**, 198–200, 2009.

Comments:

- The method is validated for accuracy precision, linearity, LOD, LOQ and specificity.
- The method is stability indicating (HCl, NaOH, H_2O_2).

HPTLC : High Performance Thin Layer Chromatography
HPTLC Densitogram

No. 104

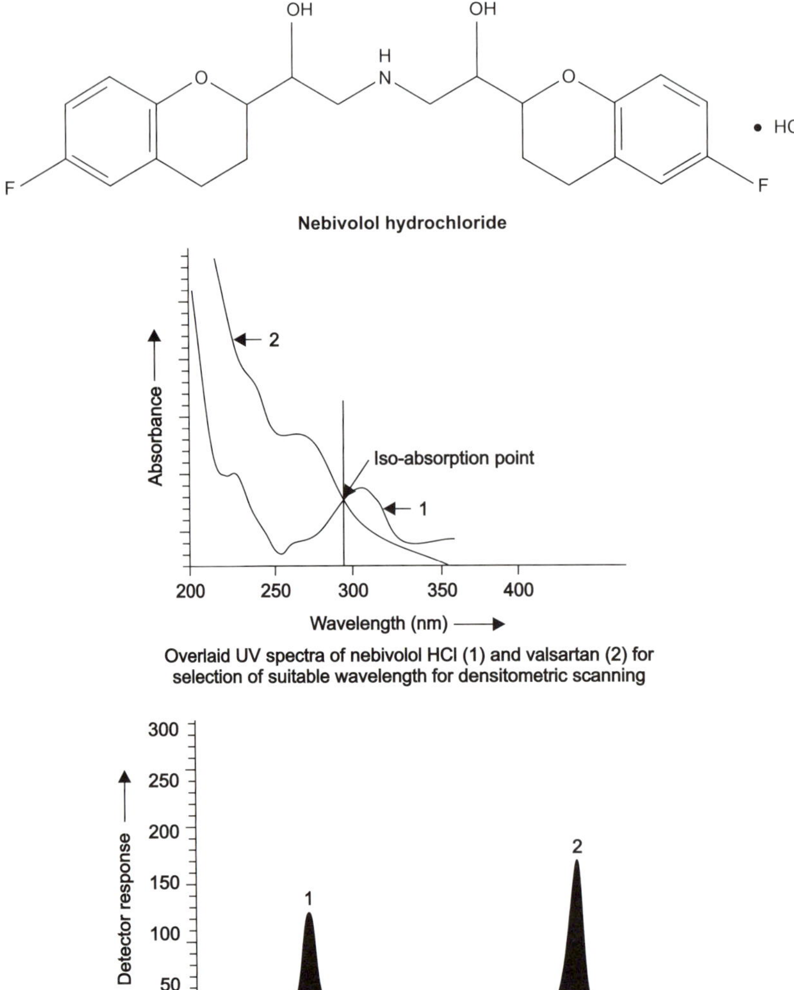

Typical densitogram of the standard containing nebivolol hydrochloride and valsartan. For detailed experimental and chromatographic conditions, refer to Protocol No. 104. Peaks identification: 1. Nebivolol HCl; 2. Valsartan.

PROTOCOL FOR HPTLC ANALYSIS OF PHARMACEUTICAL FORMULATION

Protocol No. 104

Formulation: Nebivolol hydrochloride, Valsartan

Classification: Cardiovascular System **Dosage form:** Tablets

Standard preparation: Prepare 1 mg/ml solution of each compound in methanol. Further dilutions made with methanol to get 100 µg/ml of valsartan and 200 µg/ml of nebivolol HCl. Apply 5 µl for analysis.

Sample preparation: Powdered sample equivalent to 5 mg of valsartan suspended in 5 ml of methanol, sonicated for 10 min, diluted to 10 ml with methanol, filtered and the filtrate suitably diluted for analysis.

Chromatographic equipments:

Sample applicator: Camag Linomat–V sample applicator

Development chamber: Camag twin–trough glass chamber, 10 × 10 cm

Densitometric scanner: Camag TLC Scanner–III

Chromatographic conditions:

1. Stationary phase: Silica gel $60F_{254}$ pre-coated HPTLC plates, 10 × 10 cm (200 µm) – Merck, pre-washed with methanol, dried and used
2. Mobile phase (MP): Ethyl acetate–methanol–25% ammonia (6.5 : 2.5 : 0.5 v/v)
3. Standard/Sample application:
   Band length: 10 mm Volume applied: 5 µl Spacing: 10 mm
4. Chamber saturation: 20 min (MP)
5. RH (%): 55 ± 5
6. Temperature °C: 22 ± 2
7. Separation technique: Ascending
8. Quantity of mobile phase: 10 ml
9. Migration distance: 70 mm
10. Migration time: 15 min

Densitometric evaluation:

Wavelength: UV–280 nm Scanning mode: Reflectance/Absorbance

HRF: Nebivolol HCl—22; Valsartan—78

Linearity (ng/band): Nebivolol hyrochloride—800–2400; Valsartan—200–1000

Recovery (%): Nebivolol HCl—99.48–100.10; Valsartan—98.80–100.88

References: Shradhanjali M. Singh; Kirtis Topagi and M.C. Damle, *Research J. Pharm. and Tech.*, **2(4)**, 746–748, 2009.

Comments: The method is validated for accuracy precision, linearity, LOD, LOQ, specificity and robustness as per ICH guidelines.

HPTLC : High Performance Thin Layer Chromatography
HPTLC Densitogram

No. 105

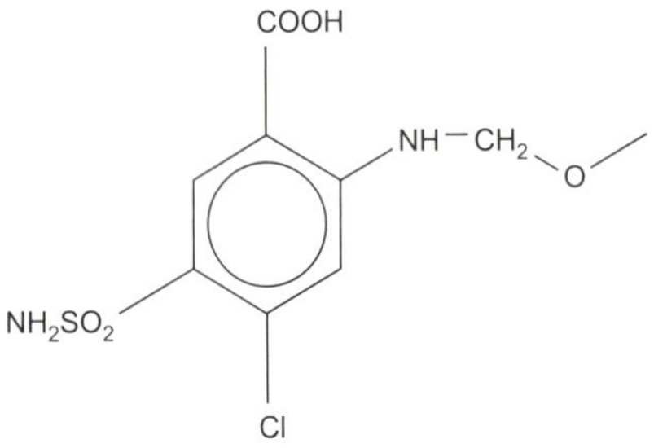

Frusemide

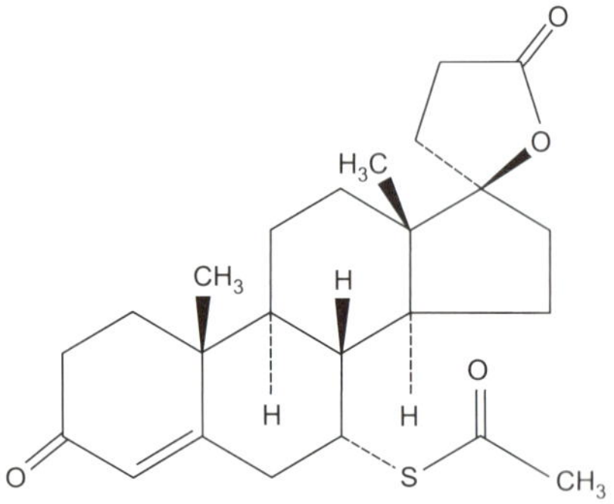

Spironolactone

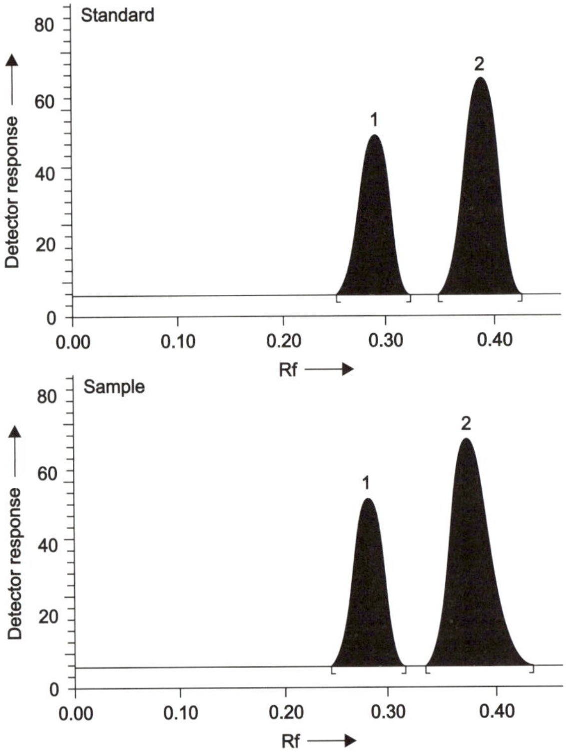

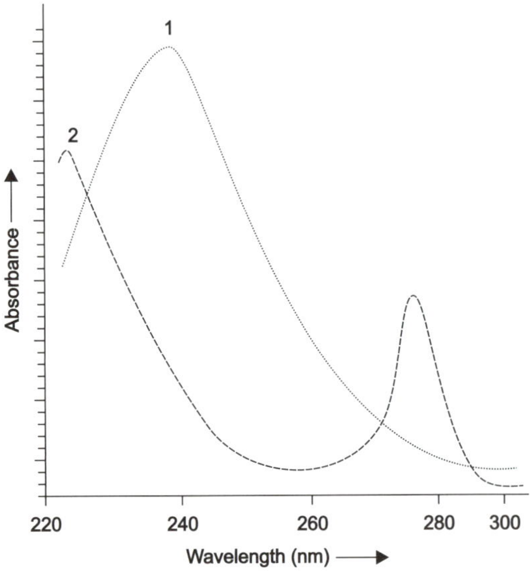

Overlaid UV spectra of spironotactone (1) and frusemide (2) for selection of suitable wavelength for densitometric scanning

Typical densitogram of the sample and standard containing frusemide and spironolactone. For detailed experimental and chromatographic conditions, refer to Protocol No. 105. Peaks identification: 1. Frusemide; 2. Spironolactone.

PROTOCOL FOR HPTLC ANALYSIS OF PHARMACEUTICAL FORMULATION

Protocol No. 105

Formulation: Spironolactone, Frusemide

Classification: Cardiovascular System **Dosage form:** Tablets

Standard preparation: Weigh accurately 10 mg of frusemide (F) and 25 mg of spironolactone (S), dissolve in methanol to make 25 ml, dilute 1 ml to 10 ml with methanol and use for chromatographic application.

Sample preparation: Weigh powdered sample equivalent to 10 mg of frusemide, add 30–40 ml of methanol, sonicate for 5 min and dilute to 25 ml, filter and dilute 1 ml to 10 ml with methanol and use for analysis.

Chromatographic equipments:

Sample applicator: Camag Linomat–IV

Development chamber: Camag twin–trough glass chamber, 10 × 10 cm

Densitometric scanner: Camag TLC Scanner–III

Chromatographic conditions:

1. Stationary phase: Silica gel $60F_{254}$ pre-coated HPTLC plates, 10 × 10 cm (200 μm) – Merck
2. Mobile phase (MP): Chloroform–methanol–glacial acetic acid (7 : 3 : 0.1 v/v) or chloroform–ethyl acetate–glacial acetic acid (7 : 3 : 0.5 v/v) or n-hexane–ethyl acetate–glacial acetic acid (4 : 6 : 0.05 v/v)
3. Standard/Sample application:
   Band length: 8 mm Volume applied: 4 μl Spacing: 22 ± 2 mm
4. Chamber saturation: 20 min (MP)
5. RH (%): 55 ± 5
6. Temperature °C: 22 ± 2
7. Separation technique: Ascending
8. Quantity of mobile phase: 10 ml
9. Migration distance: 50 mm
10. Migration time: 12 min

Densitometric evaluation:

Wavelength: UV–254 or 265 nm Scanning mode: Reflectance/Absorbance

HRF: Frusemide—27; Spironolactone—37

Linearity (ng/band): Frusemide—20–200; Spironolactone—50–500

Recovery (%): 99.40–102.0 for both the compounds

References: N.M. Tendulkar, B.S. Desai and V.M. Shinde, Abstract No. E–8, 45th IPC, 1993.

Comments:

- The method was repeated in the laboratory by the author and found to give reproducible results.
- All the three mobile-phases gave good resolution.
- The above formulation when analysed by reversed phase HPTLC using silica get $60RP\text{-}18F_{254}$ as stationary phase and mixture of acetone-water (9 : 1 v/v) as mobile phase, there was reversal of retention order.

HPTLC : High Performance Thin Layer Chromatography
HPTLC Densitogram

No. 106

COOH
NH—CH$_2$—O—
NH_2SO_2
Cl
Frusemide

H_3C
CH_3
H
S
CH_3
Spironolactone

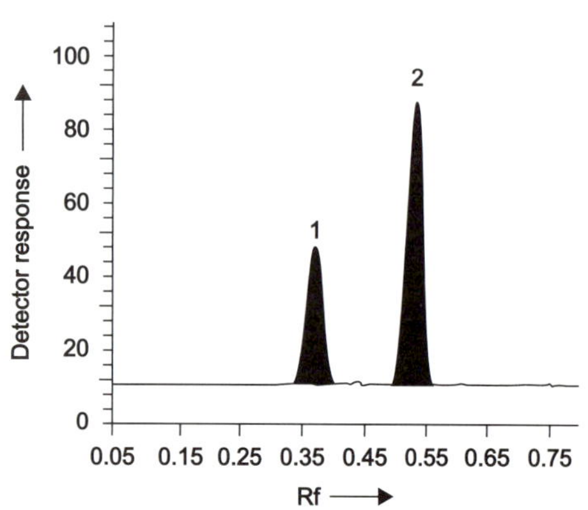

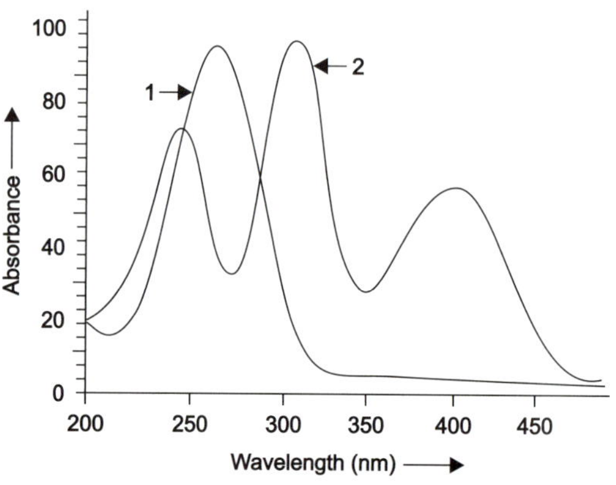

In-situ overlaid UV-spectra of frusemide (1) and spironolactone (2) selection of suitable wavelength for densitometric scanning

Typical densitogram of the standard containing frusemide and spironolactone. For detailed experimental and chromatographic conditions, refer to Protocol No. 106. Peaks identification: 1. Frusemide; 2. Spironolactone.

PROTOCOL FOR HPTLC ANALYSIS OF PHARMACEUTICAL FORMULATION

Protocol No. 106

Formulation: Spironolactone, Frusemide

Classification: Cardiovascular System **Dosage form:** Tablets

Standard preparation: Prepare 1 mg/ml solution of each compund in methanol. Further serial dilutions made with methanol to get different concentrations; 8–32 ng/μl (frusemide) and 20–80 ng/μl (spironolactone). Apply 10 μl of each solution for analysis.

Sample preparation: Powdered sample equivalent to 20 mg of frusemide suspended in 40 ml of methanol, sonicated, diluted, filtered and the filtrate further diluted to get 20 ng/μl of frusemide and 50 ng/μl of spironolactone. Apply 10 μl for assay.

Chromatographic equipments:

Sample applicator: Camag Linomat–IV

Development chamber: Camag twin–trough glass chamber, 10 × 10 cm

Densitometric scanner: Camag TLC Scanner–III

Chromatographic conditions:

1. Stationary phase: Silica gel $60F_{254}$ pre-coated HPTLC plates, 10 × 10 cm (200 μm) – Merck
2. Mobile phase (MP): Toluene–acetonitrile–glacial acetic acid (7 : 3 : 0.2 v/v)
3. Standard/Sample application:
   Band length: 70 mm Volume applied: 10 μl Spacing: 10 mm
4. Chamber saturation: 15 min (MP)
5. RH (%): 55 ± 5
6. Temperature °C: 25 ± 2
7. Separation technique: Ascending
8. Quantity of mobile phase: 10 ml
9. Migration distance: 80 mm
10. Migration time: 30 min

Densitometric evaluation:

Wavelength: UV–254 nm Scanning mode: Reflectance/Absorbance

HRF: Frusemide—38; Spironolactone—54

Linearity (ng/band): Frusemide—8–32; Spironolactone—20–80

Recovery (%): Frusemide—99.59–100.7; Spironolactone—99.72–99.40

References: M.M. Baing, V.V. Vaidya, P.A. Champanekar and Willy Shaha, *Indian Drugs*, **44(3)**, 205–208, 2007.

Comments:

- The method validated for accuracy, precision and linearity.
- The method is comparable with the RP-HPLC method.

HPTLC : High Performance Thin Layer Chromatography
HPTLC Densitogram

No. 107

Torsemide

Spironolactone

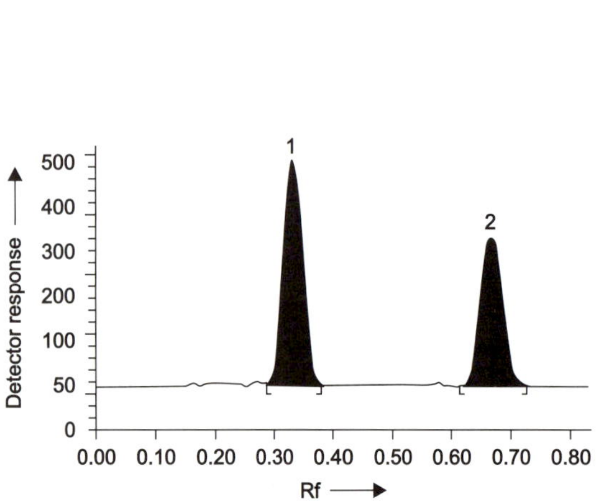

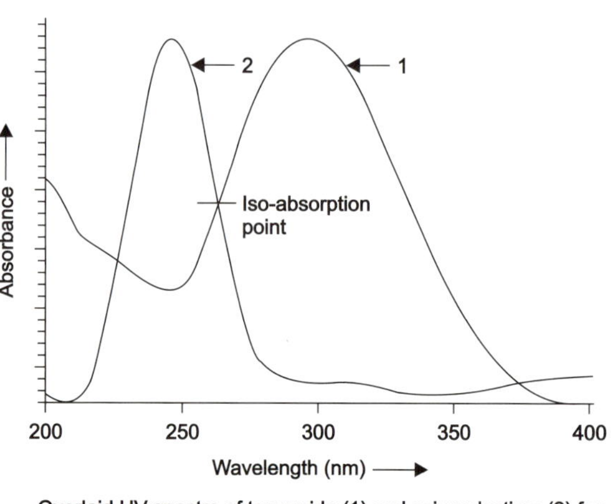

Overlaid UV-spectra of torsemide (1) and spironolactime (2) for selection of suitable wavelength for densitometric scanning

Typical densitogram of the standard containing spironolactone and torsemide. For detailed experimental and chromatographic conditions, refer to Protocol No. 107. Peaks identification: 1. Spironolactone; 2. Torsemide.

PROTOCOL FOR HPTLC ANALYSIS OF PHARMACEUTICAL FORMULATION

Protocol No. 107

Formulation: Spironolactone, Torsemide

Classification: Cardiovascular System **Dosage form:** Tablets

Standard preparation: Prepare 100 μg/ml solution of each compound separately in methanol and carry out the linearity studies by applying varying volumes (1–10 μl) for chromatographic analysis.

Sample preparation: Powdered sample equivalent to 10 mg of spironolactone suspended in methanol, sonicated, adjusted to 10 ml with methanol. Filtered through Whatman paper No. 41 and 1 ml of filtrate diluted to 10 ml with methanol. Apply 4 μl for chromatographic evaluation.

Chromatographic equipments:

Sample applicator: Camag Linomat–V

Development chamber: Camag twin–trough glass chamber, 10 × 10 cm

Densitometric scanner: Camag TLC Scanner

Chromatographic conditions:

1. Stationary phase: Silica gel 60F_{254} pre-coated TLC plates, 10 × 10 cm (250 μm) – Merck
2. Mobile phase (MP): n-hexane–ethyl acetate–methanol–glacial acetic acid (7 : 3 : 1.5 : 0.5 v/v)
3. Standard/Sample application:
   Band length: 6 mm Volume applied: 4 μl Spacing: 5 mm
4. Chamber saturation: 20 min (MP)
5. RH (%): 55 ± 5
6. Temperature °C: 22 ± 2
7. Separation technique: Ascending
8. Quantity of mobile phase: 12 ml
9. Migration distance: 90 mm
10. Migration time: 20 min

Densitometric evaluation:

Wavelength: UV–263 nm (iso-absorption point)

Scanning mode: Reflectance/Absorbance

HRF: Torsemide—34; Spironolactone—67

Linearity: 100–1000 ng/band for both the compounds

Recovery (%): 98.95–100.15 for both the compounds

References: Nilesh V. Gaikwad, Padmanabh B. Deshpande, Santosh V. Gandhi and Kapil K. Khandagale, *Res. J. Pharm and Tech.*, **3(4)**, 1106–1108, 2010.

Comments: The method validated for accuracy, precision, linearity, LOD, LOQ, specificity, robustness and ruggedness.

HPTLC : High Performance Thin Layer Chromatography
HPTLC Densitogram

No. 108

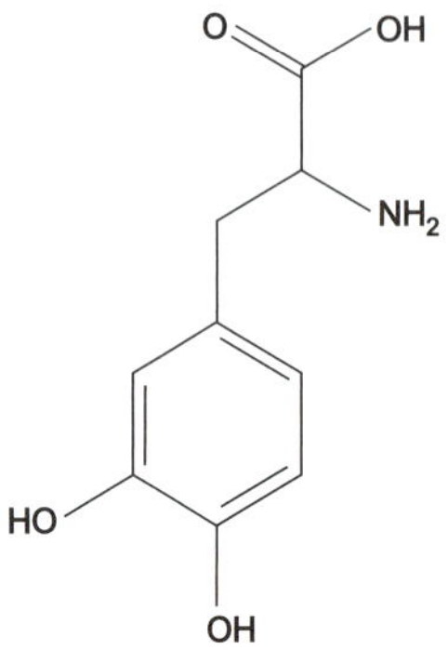

O OH NH$_2$ HO OH **Levodopa**

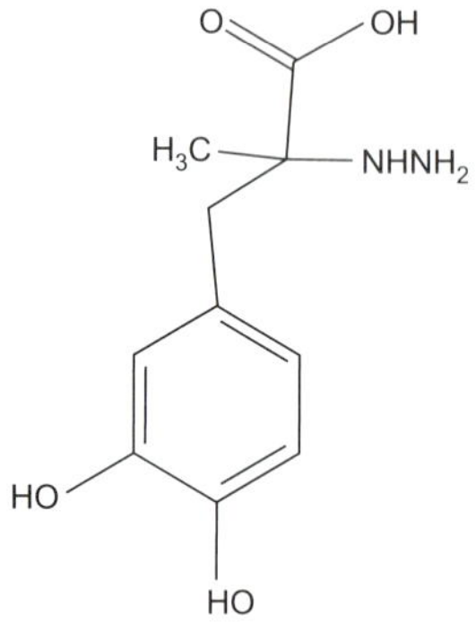

O OH H_3C NHNH$_2$ HO HO **Carbidopa**

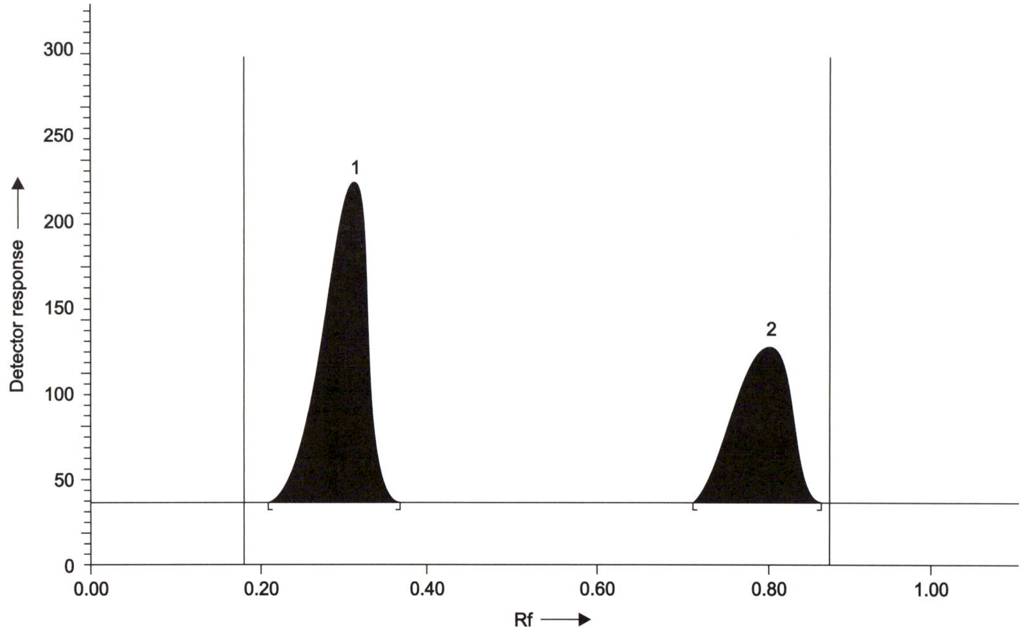

Detector response ⟶ 0 50 100 150 200 250 300

1 2

0.00 0.20 0.40 0.60 0.80 1.00

Rf ⟶

Typical densitogram of the sample containing levodopa and carbidopa. For detailed experimental and chromatographic conditions, refer to Protocol No. 108. Peaks identification: 1. Levodopa; 2. Carbidopa.

PROTOCOL FOR HPTLC ANALYSIS OF PHARMACEUTICAL FORMULATION

Protocol No. 108

Formulation: Levodopa, Carbidopa

Classification: Cardiovascular System **Dosage form:** Tablets

Standard preparation: Prepare 1 mg/ml solution of each compound in the solvent. Further dilute to get 50 μg/ml solution of each.

Solvent: Methanol–0.05 M HCl (1: 1 v/v).

Sample preparation: Powdered sample equivalent to 20 mg of carbidopa suspended in solvent, sonicated for 30 min, diluted to volume, filtered and filtrate suitably diluted with solvent and used for spotting and chromatographic evaluation.

Chromatographic equipments:

Sample applicator: Camag Linomat–V

Development chamber: Camag twin–trough glass chamber, 10 × 10 cm

Densitometric scanner: Camag TLC Scanner–III

Chromatographic conditions:

1. Stationary phase: Silica gel $60F_{254}$ pre-coated HPTLC plates, 10 × 10 cm (200 μm) – Merck, pre-washed with methanol, dried at 50°C
2. Mobile phase (MP): Acetone–chloroform–n-butanol–glacial acetic acid–water (5 : 4.5 : 4.2 : 3.5 : 2.5 v/v)
3. Standard/Sample application:
   Band length: 3.8 mm Volume applied: 5 μl Spacing: 10 mm
4. Chamber saturation: 30 min (MP)
5. RH (%): 55 ± 5
6. Temperature °C: 22 ± 2
7. Separation technique: Ascending
8. Quantity of mobile phase: 15 ml
9. Migration distance: 55 mm
10. Migration time: 18 min

Densitometric evaluation:

Wavelength: UV–283 nm Scanning mode: Reflectance/Absorbance

HRF: Levodopa—30; Carbidopa—80

Linearity (ng/band): Levodopa—200–700; Carbidopa—200–700

Recovery (%): 98.9–100.55 for both the drugs

References: D.B. Gandhi, N.J. Patel and P.J. Mehta, Personal communication, 2010.

Comments: The method validated for accuracy, precision, linearity, LOD and LOQ.

HPTLC : High Performance Thin Layer Chromatography
HPTLC Densitogram

No. 109

Entacapone

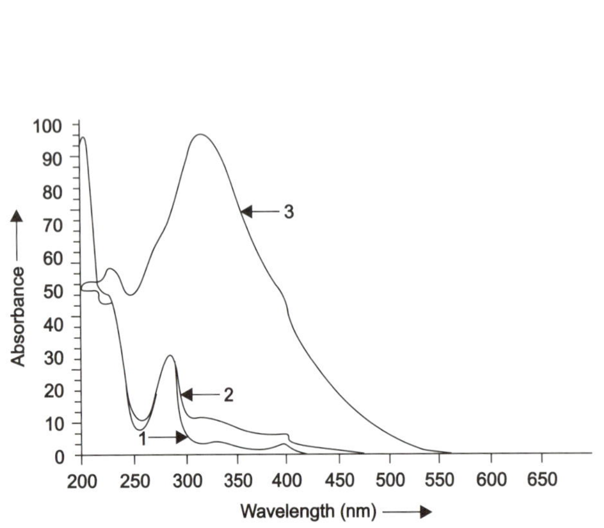

Overlaid UV-spectra of levodopa (1), carbidopa (2) and entacapone (3) for selection of suitable wavelength for densitometric scanning

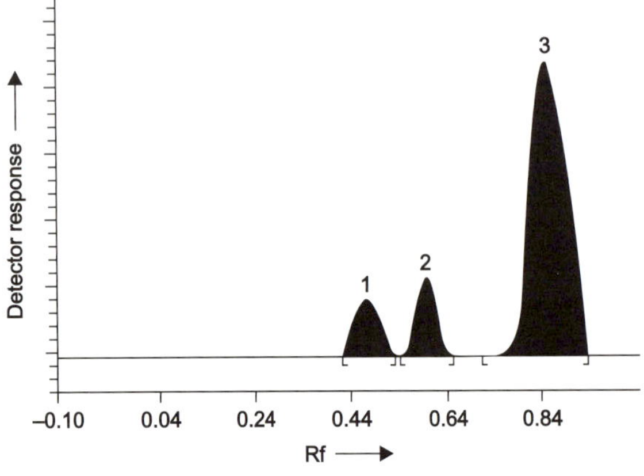

Typical densitogram of the standard containing levodopa, carbidopa and entacapone. For detailed experimental and chromatographic conditions, refer to Protocol No. 109. Peaks identification: 1. Levodopa; 2. Carbidopa; 3. Entacapone.

PROTOCOL FOR HPTLC ANALYSIS OF PHARMACEUTICAL FORMULATION

Protocol No. 109

Formulation: Levodopa, Carbidopa, Entacapone

Classification: Cardiovascular System **Dosage form:** Tablets

Standard preparation: Prepare 1 mg/ml solution of each compound in solvent. Further dilute appropriate volume of each solution with methanol to get 100 μg/ml. Apply varying volumes of each solution to study linearity profile.

Sample preparation: Powdered sample equivalent to 25 mg of carbidopa suspended in 75 ml of solvent, sonicated for 15 min, dilute to 100 ml with solvent, filter through Whatman filter No. 41 and dilute the filtrate suitably to get 50 μg/ml (LEV), 62.5 μg/ml (CAR), 100 μg/ml (ENT). Apply 13 μl of sample for chromatographic analysis.

Solvent: Methanol–0.05 M HCl (1 : 1 v/v).

Chromatographic equipments:

Sample applicator: Camag Linomat–V

Development chamber: Camag twin–trough glass chamber, 10 × 10 cm

Densitometric scanner: Camag TLC Scanner–III

Chromatographic conditions:

1. Stationary phase: Silica gel 60 RP–18F_{254s} TLC plates 5 × 7.5 cm (250 μm) – Merck, pre-washed with methanol, activated at 50°C (20 min)
2. Mobile phase (MP): Acetone–n-butanol–water–triethylamine (0.5 : 9.5 : 1 : 0.001 v/v), pH adjusted 3.6 with O-H_3PO_4
3. Standard/Sample application:
   Band length: 3 mm Volume applied: 13 μl Spacing: 7.5 mm
4. Chamber saturation: 25 min (MP)
5. RH (%): 55 ± 5
6. Temperature °C: 22 ± 2
7. Separation technique: Ascending
8. Quantity of mobile phase: 10 ml
9. Migration distance: 50 mm
10. Migration time: 22 min

Densitometric evaluation:

Wavelength: UV–282 nm Scanning mode: Reflectance/Absorbance

HRF: Levodopa (LEV)—46; Carbidopa (CAR)—60; Entacapone (ENT)—87

Linearity (ng/band): Levodopa—300–1500; Carbidopa—200–1000; Entacapone—200–2000

Recovery (%): 99.08–100.77 for all the three compounds

References: Deesha B. Gandhi and Priti J. Mehta, *J. Planar Chromatogr.*, **24(3)**, 236–241, 2011.

Comments: The method validated for accuracy, precision, linearity, LOD, LOQ and specificity.

HPTLC : High Performance Thin Layer Chromatography
HPTLC Densitogram

No. 110

Perindopril erbumine

Indapamide

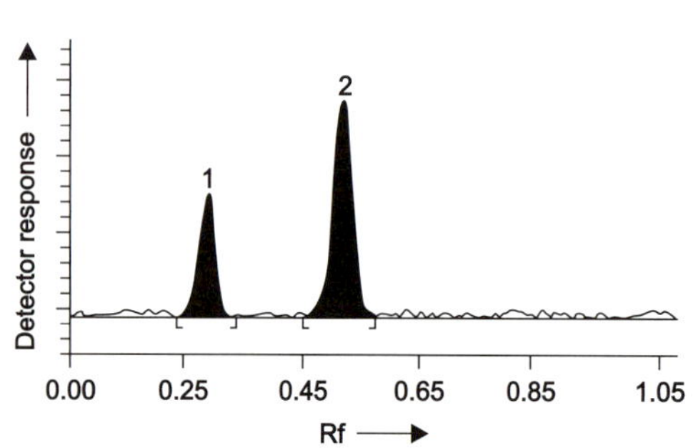

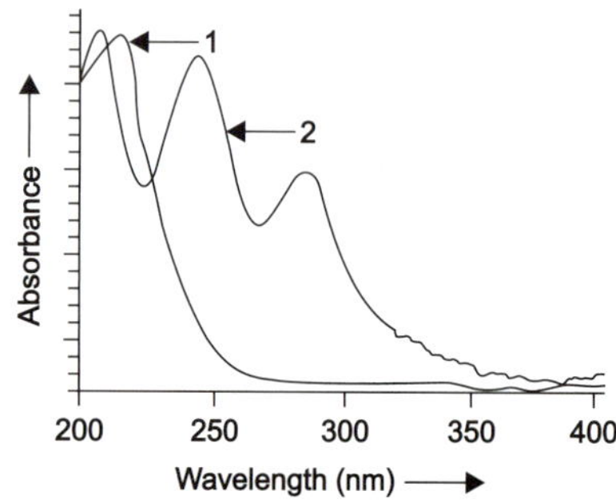

Overlaid UV-spectra of perindopril (1) and indapamide (2) for selection of suitable wavelength for densitometric scanning

Typical densitogram of the standard containing perindopril erbumine and indapamide. For detailed experimental and chromatographic conditions, refer to Protocol No. 110. Peaks identification: 1. Perindopril erbumine; 2. Indapamide.

PROTOCOL FOR HPTLC ANALYSIS OF PHARMACEUTICAL FORMULATION

Protocol No. 110

Formulation: Perindopril erbumine, Indapamide

Classification: Cardiovascular System **Dosage form:** Tablets

Standard preparation: Prepare 1 mg/ml solution of each compound separately in methanol. Further dilutions are made to get 500 μg/ml of perindopril and 100 μg/ml of indapamide. Apply 2–10 μl for linearity profile.

Sample preparation: Powdered sample equivalent to 10 mg of perindopril or 4 mg of indapamide suspended in methanol, sonicated for 10 min, diluted to 10 ml, filtered and the filtrate suitably diluted to get 400 μg/ml of perindopril and 125 μg/ml of indapamide. Apply 10 μl and 2 μl of solution for assay.

Chromatographic equipments:

Sample applicator: Camag Linomat–V

Development chamber: Camag twin–trough glass chamber, 10 × 10 cm

Densitometric scanner: Camag TLC Scanner–III

Chromatographic conditions:

1. Stationary phase: Silica gel $60F_{254}$ pre-coated TLC plates, 10 × 10 cm (250 μm) – Merck,
2. Mobile phase (MP): Dichloromethane–methanol–glacial acetic acid (9.5 : 0.5 : 0.1 v/v)
3. Standard/Sample application:
   Band length: 4 mm Volume applied: 2–10 μl Spacing: 10 mm
4. Chamber saturation: 15 min (MP)
5. RH (%): 55 ± 5
6. Temperature °C: 22 ± 2
7. Separation technique: Ascending
8. Quantity of mobile phase: 10 ml
9. Migration distance: 90 mm
10. Migration time: 25 min

Densitometric evaluation:

Wavelength: UV–215 nm Scanning mode: Reflectance/Absorbance

HRF: Perindopril erbumine—30; Indapamide—50

Linearity (ng/band): Perindopril erbumine—1000–5000; Indapamide—100–500

Recovery (%): 98.0–102.0 for both the compounds

References: Mohit G. Dewani, Kailash G. Bothara, Ashwani R. Madgulkar and M.C. Damle, *Int. J. Comprehensive Pharmacy*, **2(1)**, 1–4, 2011.

Comments: The method validated for accuracy, precision, linearity, LOD, LOQ, specificity, robustness and ruggedness.

HPTLC : High Performance Thin Layer Chromatography
HPTLC Densitogram

No. 111

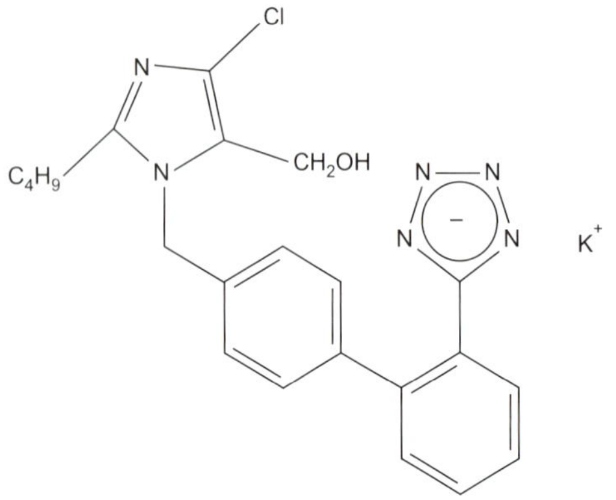

Losartan potassium

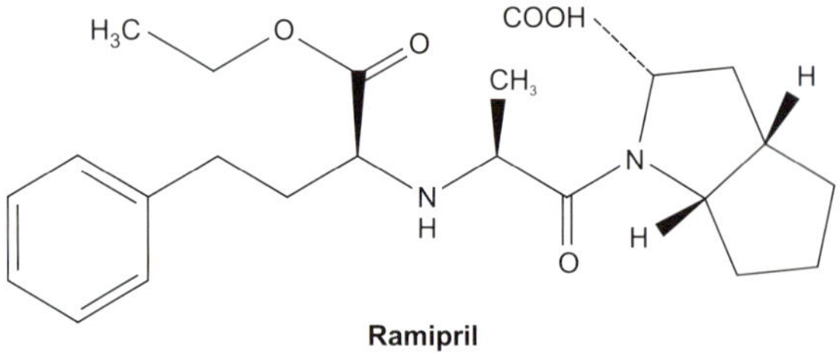

Ramipril

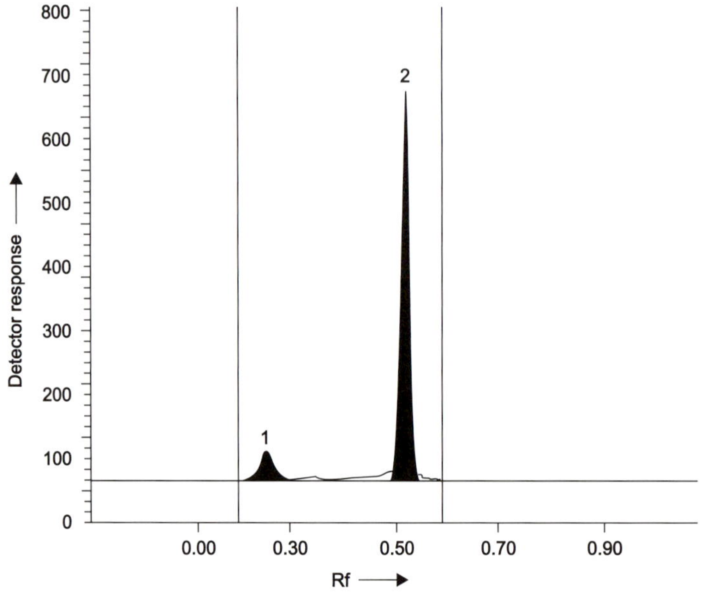

Typical densitogram of the sample containing losartan potassium and perindopril. For detailed experimental and chromatographic conditions, refer to Protocol No. 111. Peaks identification: 1. Perindopril; 2. Losartan K^+.

PROTOCOL FOR HPTLC ANALYSIS OF PHARMACEUTICAL FORMULATION

Protocol No. 111

Formulation: Losartan potassium, Perindopril

Classification: Cardiovascular System **Dosage form:** Tablets

Standard preparation: Prepare solution of both the compounds in 0.1 M sodium hydroxide to get 1 mg/ml of losartan potassium and 250 μg/ml of perindopril. Apply 1–6 μl of standard solutions for linearity profile.

Sample preparation: Powdered sample equivalent to 50 mg of losartan K^+ or 4 mg of perindopril suspended in 0.1 M NaOH, sonicated, filtered and the filtrate suitably diluted with water and used for chromatographic evaluation.

Chromatographic equipments:

Sample applicator: Camag Linomat–V

Development chamber: Camag twin–trough glass chamber, 20 × 10 cm

Densitometric scanner: Camag TLC Scanner–III

Chromatographic conditions:

1. Stationary phase: Silica gel $60F_{254}$ pre-coated HPTLC plates, 10 × 10 cm (200 μm) – Merck, pre-washed with methanol and activated at 60°C for 60 min prior to use
2. Mobile phase (MP): Toluene–acetonitrile–formic acid (5 : 5 : 0.3 v/v)
3. Standard/Sample application:
   Band length: 6 mm Volume applied: 1–6 μl Spacing: 5 mm
4. Chamber saturation: 15 min (MP)
5. RH (%): 55 ± 5
6. Temperature °C: 22 ± 2
7. Separation technique: Ascending
8. Quantity of mobile phase: 20 ml
9. Migration distance: 90 mm
10. Migration time: 25 min

Densitometric evaluation:

Wavelength: UV–215 nm Scanning mode: Reflectance/Absorbance

HRF: Perindopril—27; Losartan K^+—52

Linearity (ng/band): Losartan K^+—1000–6000; Perindopril—250–1500

Recovery (%): 98.20—99.70 for both the compounds

References: K.S. Lakshmi, Lakshmi Sivasubramanian and Ajit Kumar Pandey, *Research J. Pharm. and Tech.*, **3(2)**, 559–561, 2010.

Comments: The method validated for accuracy, precision, linearity, LOD, LOQ, specificity, robustness and ruggedness.

HPTLC : High Performance Thin Layer Chromatography
HPTLC Densitogram

No. 113

Ramipril

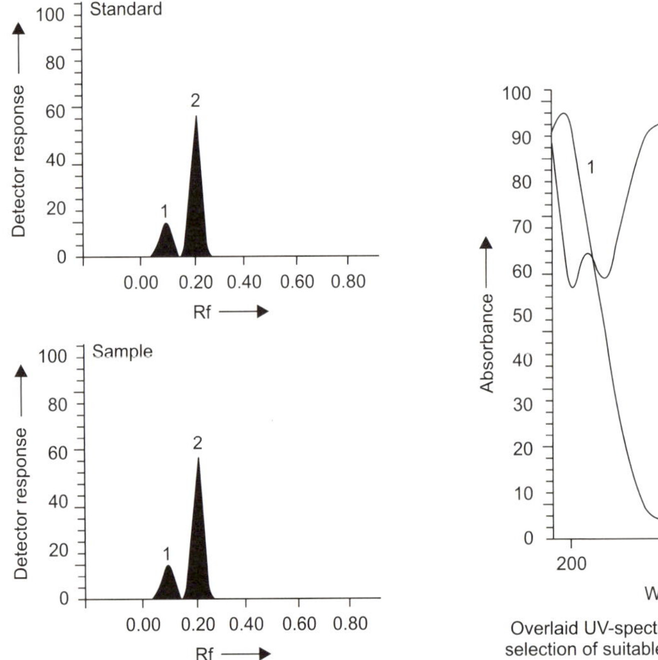

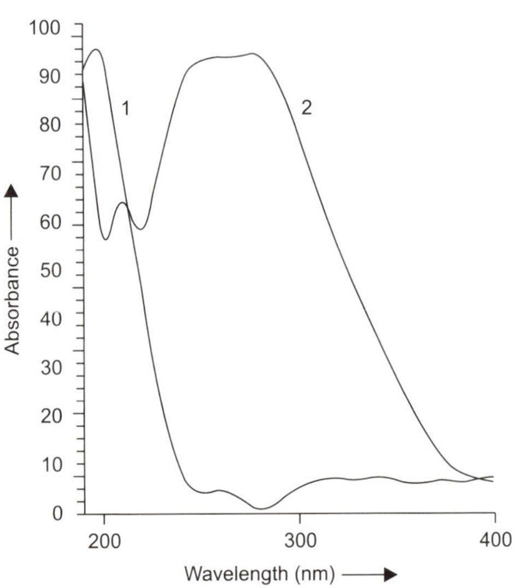

Overlaid UV-spectra of atorvastatin (2) and ramipril (1) for selection of suitable wavelength for densitometric scanning

Typical densitogram of the standard and sample containing atorvastatin and ramipril. For detailed experimental and chromatographic conditions, refer to Protocol No. 113. Peaks identification: 1. Ramipril; 2. Atorvastatin.

PROTOCOL FOR HPTLC ANALYSIS OF PHARMACEUTICAL FORMULATION

Protocol No. 113

Formulation: Ramipril, Atorvastatin calcium

Classification: Cardiovascular System **Dosage form:** Tablets

Standard preparation: Prepare 1 mg/ml solution of each compound in methanol. Further serial dilutions made with methanol for linearity studies. Apply 10 μl of each solution for chromatographic analysis.

Sample preparation: Powdered sample equivalent to 5 mg of ramipril suspended in 8 ml of methanol, sonicated for 10 min, diluted to 10 ml, filtered and 1 ml of filtrate diluted to10 ml with methanol and used for assay. Apply 10 μl of the solution for chromatographic analysis.

Chromatographic equipments:

Sample applicator: Camag Linomat–V

Development chamber: Camag automatic development chamber saturated with Camag saturation pad

Densitometric scanner: Camag TLC Scanner–III

Chromatographic conditions:

1. Stationary phase: Silica gel 60F_{254} pre-coated TLC plates glas, 20 × 10 cm (250 μm) – Merck
2. Mobile phase (MP): Toluene–ethyl acetate–methanol–glacial acetic acid (5 : 4.5 : 0.5 : 0.1 v/v)
3. Standard/Sample application:
   Band length: 8 mm Volume applied: 10 μl Spacing: 10 mm
4. Chamber saturation: 20 min (MP)
5. RH (%): 55 ± 5
6. Temperature °C: 25 ± 2
7. Separation technique: Ascending
8. Quantity of mobile phase: 20 ml
9. Migration distance: 70 mm
10. Migration time: 6 min

Densitometric evaluation:

Wavelength: UV–240 nm Scanning mode: Reflectance/Absorbance

HRF: Ramipril—11; Atorvastatin calcium—22

Linearity (ng/band): Ramipril—2.5–10; Atorvastatin calcium—2.5–20

Recovery (%): —

References: —

Comments: The method was optimized and analytical work carried out at **Anchrom's HPTLC Application Laboratory**, Mumbai, India.

HPTLC : High Performance Thin Layer Chromatography
HPTLC Densitogram

No. 114

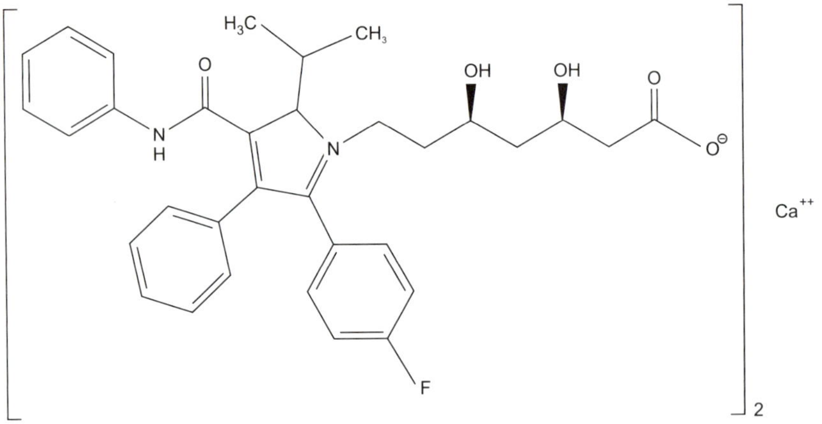

H$_3$C CH$_3$ O OH OH O N H N O$^\ominus$ Ca^{++} F 2

Atorvastatin calcium

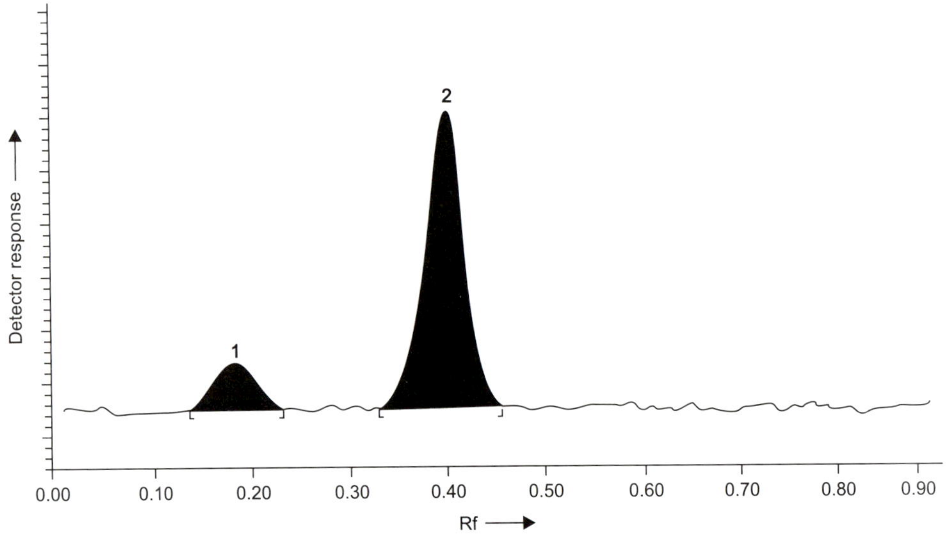

2
1
Detector response
0.00 0.10 0.20 0.30 0.40 0.50 0.60 0.70 0.80 0.90
Rf

Typical densitogram of the standard containing atorvastatin calcium and ramipril. For detailed experimental and chromatographic conditions, refer to Protocol No. 114. Peaks identification: 1. Ramipril; 2. Atorvastatin Ca^{++}.

PROTOCOL FOR HPTLC ANALYSIS OF PHARMACEUTICAL FORMULATION

Protocol No. 114

Formulation: Ramipril, Atorvastatin calcium

Classification: Cardiovascular System **Dosage form:** Capsules

Standard preparation: Prepare 200 μg/ml solution of each drug in methanol. Further dilute with methanol to get 20 μg/ml of each drug. Apply varying volumes (2–25 μl) of each for linearity profile.

Sample preparation: Weigh powdered sample equivalent to 10 mg of atorvastatin and 5 mg of ramipril, suspend in 30 ml of methanol, sonicate for 15 min, dilute to 50 ml with methanol. Filter and dilute to get 10 μg/ml of atorvastatin and 5 μg/ml of ramipril. Apply 10 μl of the solution for assay.

Chromatographic equipments:

Sample applicator: Camag Linomat–V

Development chamber: Camag twin-trough glass chamber, 10 × 10 cm

Densitometric scanner: Camag TLC Scanner–III

Chromatographic conditions:

1. Stationary phase: Silica gel $60F_{254}$ pre-coated TLC plates, 10 × 10 cm (250 μm) – Merck, pre-washed with methanol, activated at 110°C for 5 min, prior to use
2. Mobile phase (MP): Methanol–benzene–glacial acetic acid (19.6 : 80 : 0.4 v/v)
3. Standard/Sample application:
   Band length: 6 mm Volume applied: 2.5–25 μl Spacing: 6 mm
4. Chamber saturation: 20 min (MP)
5. RH (%): 55 ± 5
6. Temperature °C: 25 ± 2
7. Separation technique: Ascending
8. Quantity of mobile phase: 10 ml
9. Migration distance: 70 mm
10. Migration time: 15 min

Densitometric evaluation:

Wavelength: UV–210 nm Scanning mode: Reflectance/Absorbance

HRF: Ramipril—18; Atorvastatin Ca^{++}—40

Linearity: 50–500 ng/band for both the drugs

Recovery (%): 99.87–99.98 for both the drugs

References: Hiral J. Panchal and B.N. Suhagia, *J. AOAC. Int.*, **93(5)**, 1450–1457, 2010.

Comments: The method validated for accuracy, precision, linearity, LOD, LOQ, specificity and robustness.

HPTLC : High Performance Thin Layer Chromatography
HPTLC Densitogram

No. 115

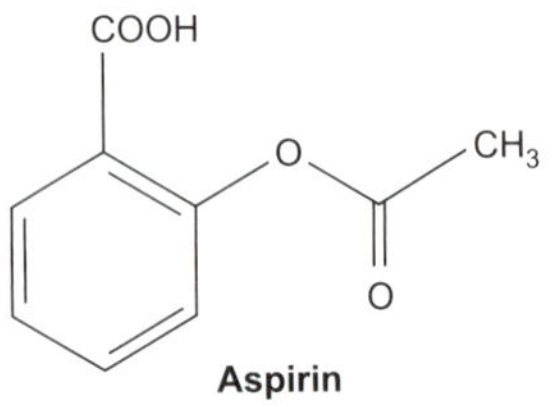

COOH
O
CH$_3$
O
Aspirin

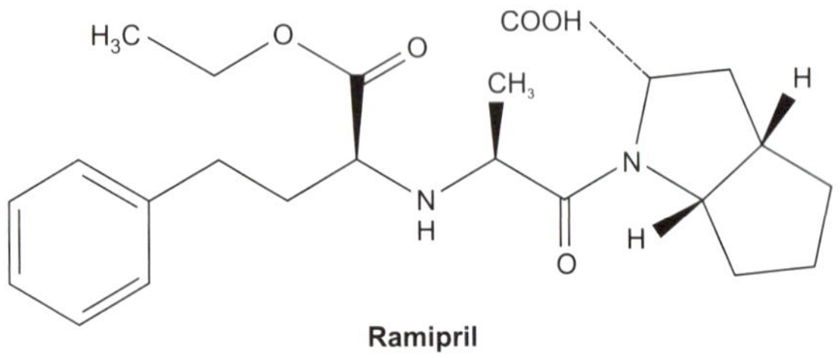

H$_3$C
O
O
COOH
CH$_3$
H
N
N
H
H
O
Ramipril

Standard
Detector response
Rf

Sample
Detector response
Rf

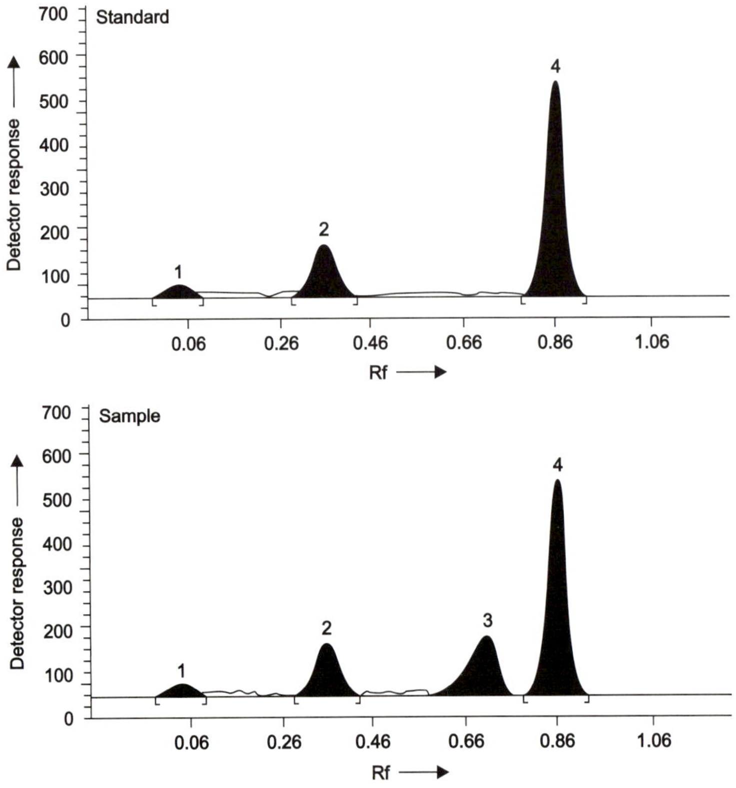

Typical densitogram of the standard and sample containing ramipril, atorvastatin and aspirin. For detailed experimental and chromatographic conditions, refer to Protocol No. 115. Peaks identification: 1. Ramipril; 2. Atorvastatin Ca^{++}; 3. Salicylic acid (decomposition product of aspirin); 4. Aspirin.

PROTOCOL FOR HPTLC ANALYSIS OF PHARMACEUTICAL FORMULATION

Protocol No. 115

Formulation: Ramipril, Atorvastatin calcium, Aspirin

Classification: Cardiovascular System **Dosage form:** Tablets

Standard preparation: Prepare stock solution of each compound in methanol to get 100 μg/ml (ramipril); 200 μg/ml (atorvastatin) and 100 μg/ml (aspirin); 2.5 ml of each stock solution diluted to 25 ml with methanol and use for application.

Sample preparation: Powdered sample equivalent to 5 mg of ramipril, 10 mg of atorvastatin calcium, 75 mg of aspirin suspended in 30 ml of methanol, sonicated for 15 min, diluted, filtered through Whatman No. 41 filter paper. 2.5 ml of filtrate diluted to 25 ml. Apply 5, 10 and 20 μl of the resulting solutions for analysis.

Chromatographic equipments:

Sample applicator: Camag Linomat–V

Development chamber: Camag twin-trough glass chamber, 10 × 10 cm, lined with filter paper

Densitometric scanner: Camag TLC Scanner–III

Chromatographic conditions:

1. Stationary phase: Silica gel $60F_{254}$ pre-coated HPTLC plates, 10 × 10 cm (200 μm) – Merck, pre-washed with methanol, dried (110°C) for 5 min, prior to use
2. Mobile phase (MP): Methanol–benzene ethyl acetate–glacial acetic acid (0.36 : 5.6 : 4.0 : 0.04 v/v)
3. Standard/Sample application:
   Band length: 5 mm Volume applied: 5, 10, 20 μl Spacing: 5 mm
4. Chamber saturation: 30 min (MP)
5. RH (%): 55 ± 5
6. Temperature °C: 25 ± 2
7. Separation technique: Ascending
8. Quantity of mobile phase: 20 ml
9. Migration distance: 70 mm
10. Migration time: 25 min

Densitometric evaluation:

Wavelength: UV–210 nm Scanning mode: Reflectance/Absorbance

HRF: Ramipril—06; Atorvastatin—38; Salicylic acid—72; Aspirin—86

Linearity (ng/band): Ramipril—50–300; Atorvastatin Ca^{++}—100–600; Aspirin—500–3000

Recovery (%): 99.97–100.92 for all three compunds

References: Hiral J. Panchal, Bhanubhai N. Suhagia and Natvarlal J. Patel, *J. Planar. Chromatogr.*, **22(4)**, 265–271, 2009.

Comments:

- The method validated for accuracy, precision, linearity, specificity, LOD, LOQ and robustness.
- Salicylic acid, the decomposition product of aspirin, was well separated in samples.

HPTLC : High Performance Thin Layer Chromatography
HPTLC Densitogram

No. 116

Atorvastatin calcium

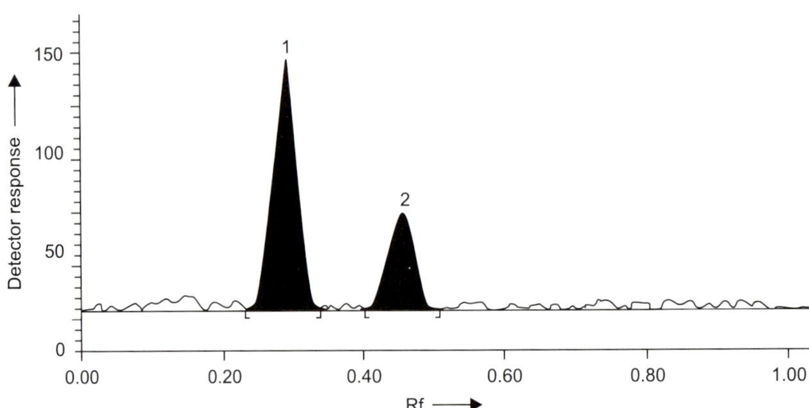

Typical densitogram of the sample containing losartan potassium and atorvastatin calcium. For detailed experimental and chromatographic conditions, refer to Protocol No. 116. Peaks identification: 1. Losartan K^{+}; 2. Atorvastatin Ca^{++}.

PROTOCOL FOR HPTLC ANALYSIS OF PHARMACEUTICAL FORMULATION

Protocol No. 116

Formulation: Losartan potassium, Atorvastatin calcium

Classification: Cardiovascular System **Dosage form:** Tablets

Standard preparation: Prepare 200 μg/ml solution of each compound in methanol. Further dilute 6.25 ml of each solution to 50 ml with methanol (25 μg/ml). Apply varying volumes for linearity profile.

Sample preparation: Powedered sample equivalent to 10 mg of atorvastatin calcium or 25 mg of losartan potassium suspended in 30 ml of methanol, sonicated for 15 min, diluted to 50 ml, filtered and further diluted suitably with methanol for assay.

Chromatographic equipments:

Sample applicator: Camag Linomat–V

Development chamber: Camag twin-trough glass chamber, 20 × 10 cm

Densitometric scanner: Camag TLC Scanner–III

Chromatographic conditions:

1. Stationary phase: Silica gel $60F_{254}$ pre-coated HPTLC plates, 10 × 10 cm (200 μm) – Merck, pre-washed with methanol and activated at 110°C for 5 min prior to use
2. Mobile phase (MP): Methanol–carbon tetrachloride–ethyl acetate–glacial acetic acid (8 : 63.6 : 28 : 0.4 v/v)
3. Standard/Sample application:
   Band length: 6 mm Volume applied: 1–10 μl Spacing: 6 mm
4. Chamber saturation: 30 min (MP)
5. RH (%): 55 ± 5
6. Temperature °C: 25 ± 2
7. Separation technique: Ascending
8. Quantity of mobile phase: 20 ml
9. Migration distance: 70 mm
10. Migration time: 14 min

Densitometric evaluation:

Wavelength: UV–238 nm Scanning mode: Reflectance/Absorbance

HRF: Losartan potassium—30; Atorvastatin calcium—45

Linearity (ng/band): 50–500 for both the compounds

Recovery (%): 100.48–100.59 for both the compounds

References: H.J. Panchal and B.N. Suhagia, *Acta Chromatographica*, **22(2)**, 173–187, 2010.

Comments:

- The method validated for accuracy, precision, linearity, specificity, LOD, LOQ and robustness.
- The method was compared with RP-HPLC method carried out simultaneously. No significant difference observed in results.

HPTLC : High Performance Thin Layer Chromatography
HPTLC Densitogram

No. 117

Telmisartan

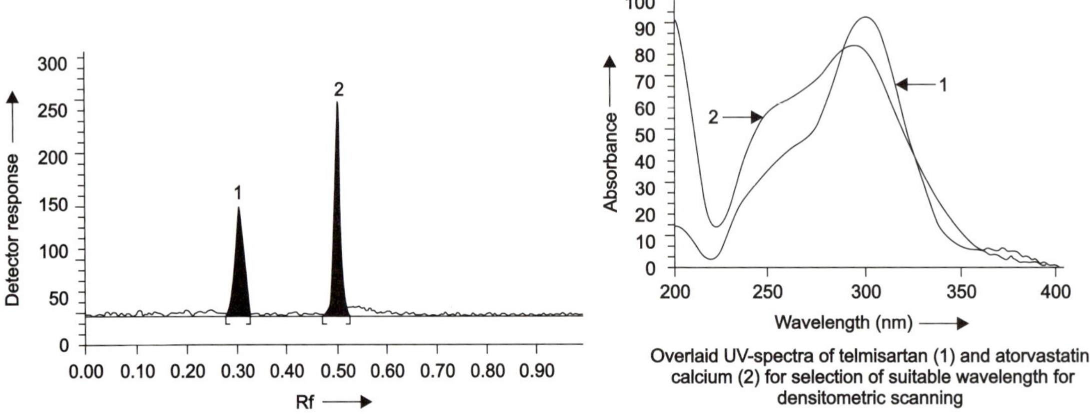

Overlaid UV-spectra of telmisartan (1) and atorvastatin calcium (2) for selection of suitable wavelength for densitometric scanning

Typical densitogram of the standard containing telmisartan and atorvastatin calcium. For detailed experimental and chromatographic conditions, refer to Protocol No. 117. Peaks identification: 1. Atorvastatin calcium; 2. Telmisartan.

PROTOCOL FOR HPTLC ANALYSIS OF PHARMACEUTICAL FORMULATION

Protocol No. 117

Formulation: **Telmisartan, Atorvastatin calcium**

Classification: Cardiovascular System **Dosage form:** Tablets

Standard preparation: Prepare 1 mg/ml solution of each compound in methanol. Further dilute with methanol to get 100 μg/ml. Apply varying volumes (1–10 μl) for linearity profile.

Sample preparation: Powdered sample equivalent to 10 mg of atorvastatin suspended in methanol, sonicated for 5 min, diluted to 10 ml with methanol, filtered and 1 ml of the filtrate diluted to 10 ml with methanol. Apply 3 μl for assay.

Chromatographic equipments:

Sample applicator: Camag Linomat–V

Development chamber: Camag twin-trough glass chamber, 20 × 10 cm

Densitometric scanner: Camag TLC Scanner–III

Chromatographic conditions:

1. Stationary phase: Silica gel $60F_{254}$ pre-coated TLC plates, 20 × 10 cm (250 μm) – Merck, pre-washed with methanol, activated at 110°C (5 min) prior to use
2. Mobile phase (MP): Toluene–methanol (7 : 3 v/v)
3. Standard/Sample application:
   Band length: 6 mm Volume applied: 3 μl Spacing: 6.8 mm
4. Chamber saturation: 30 min (MP)
5. RH (%): 55 ± 5
6. Temperature °C: Ambient
7. Separation technique: Ascending
8. Quantity of mobile phase: 20 ml
9. Migration distance: 90 mm
10. Migration time: 30 min

Densitometric evaluation:

Wavelength: UV–280 nm Scanning mode: Reflectance/Absorbance

HRF: Atorvastatin Ca^{++}—29; Telmisartan—50

Linearity (ng/band): Telmisartan—200–1000; Atorvastatin Ca^{++}—200–700

Recovery (%): Telmisartan—99.49–100.33; Atorvastatin Ca^{++}—98.92–100.5

References: U.P. Patil, S.V. Gandhi, M.R. Sengar and V.S. Rajmane, *J. Chil. Chem. Soc.*, **55(1)**, 94–96, 2010.

Comments: The method validated for accuracy, precision, linearity, LOD, LOQ, specificity, robustness and ruggedness.

HPTLC : High Performance Thin Layer Chromatography
HPTLC Densitogram

No. 118

Telmisartan

Pioglitazone

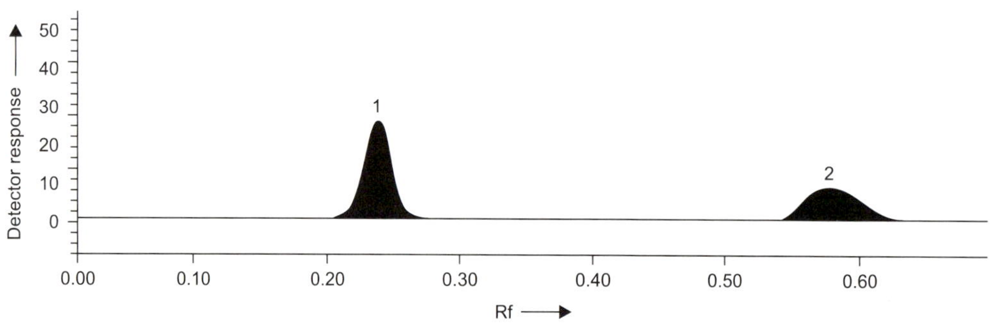

Typical densitogram of the standard containing telmisartan and pioglitazone HCl. For detailed experimental and chromatographic conditions, refer to Protocol No. 118. Peaks identification: 1. Telmisartan; 2. Pioglitazone HCl.

PROTOCOL FOR HPTLC ANALYSIS OF PHARMACEUTICAL FORMULATION

Protocol No. 118

Formulation: **Telmisartan, Pioglitazone hydrochloride**

Classification: Cardiovascular System **Dosage form:** Tablets

Standard preparation: Prepare 1500 μg/ml solution of pioglitazone and 2000 μg/ml of telmisartan separately in methanol. Carry out serial dilutions for linearity studies. Apply 10 μl of each solution for chromatographic separation and analysis.

Sample preparation: An appropriate quantity of the powdered sample suspended in methanol, sonicated for 30 min and diluted to 100 ml and used for chromatographic evaluation.

Chromatographic equipments:

Sample applicator: Camag Linomat–IV

Development chamber: Camag twin-trough glass chamber, 10 × 10 cm

Densitometric scanner: Camag TLC Scanner–II

Chromatographic conditions:

1. Stationary phase: Silica gel $60F_{254}$ pre-coated HPTLC plates, 10 × 10 cm (200 μm) – Merck
2. Mobile phase (MP): Toluene–ethyl acetate–methanol (7 : 2 : 1 v/v)
3. Standard/Sample application:
   Band length: 8 mm Volume applied: 10 μl Spacing: 10 mm
4. Chamber saturation: 30 min (MP)
5. RH (%): 55 ± 5
6. Temperature °C: 22 ± 2
7. Separation technique: Ascending
8. Quantity of mobile phase: 10 ml
9. Migration distance: 80 mm
10. Migration time: 30 min

Densitometric evaluation:

Wavelength: UV–299 nm (Telmisartan); 269 nm (Pioglitazone HCl)

Scanning mode: Reflectance/Absorbance

HRF: Telmisartan—23; Pioglitazone HCl—58

Linearity (ng/band): Telmisartan—40–200; Pioglitazone HCl—30–150

Recovery (%): 99.08–100.12 for both the compounds

References: D.C. Prem Anand, K.L. Senthikumar, B. Senthikumar, M. Saravanakumar and R. Thirumurthy, *Int. J. Pharma. Res. and Development*, **2(9)**, 185–190, 2010.

Comments:

- The method validated for accuracy, precision, linearity, LOD, LOQ, specificity, robustness and ruggedness.
- The methods is stability indicating (acid, base, oxidative, thermolytic, photolytic).

HPTLC : High Performance Thin Layer Chromatography
HPTLC Densitogram

No. 119

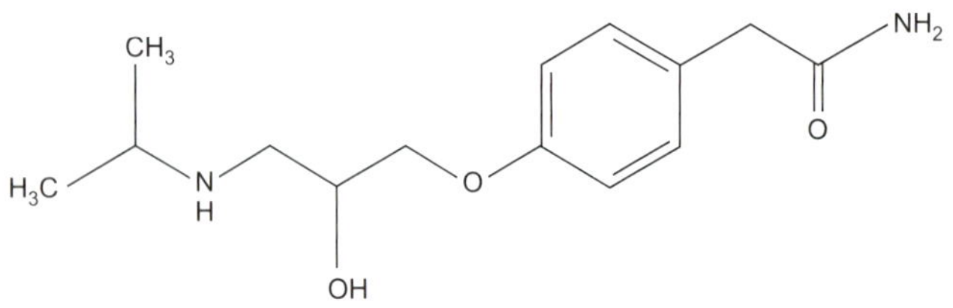

Atenolol

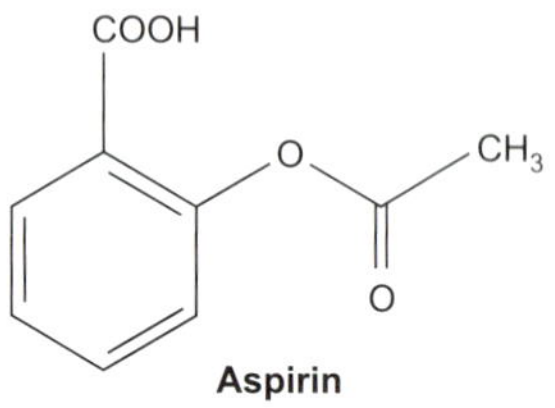

Aspirin

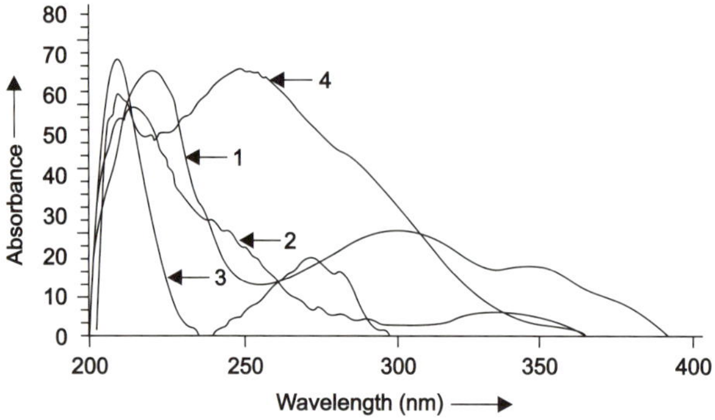

Overlaid UV-spectra of atenolol (1), losartan K^{+} (2), atorvastatin Ca^{++} (3) and aspirin (4) for selection of suitable wavelength for densitometric scanning

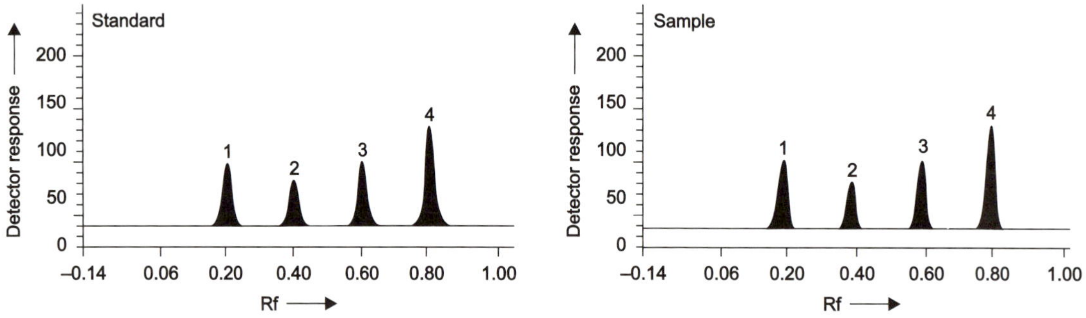

Typical densitogram of the sample and standard containing losartan K^{+}, atenolol, atorvastatin Ca^{++} and aspirin. For detailed experimental and chromatographic conditions, refer to Protocol No. 119. Peaks identification: 1. Atenolol; 2. Losartan K^{+}; 3. Aspirin; 4. Atorvastatin Ca^{++}.

PROTOCOL FOR HPTLC ANALYSIS OF PHARMACEUTICAL FORMULATION

Protocol No. 119

Formulation: Losartan potassium, Atenolol, Atorvastatin calcium, Aspirin

Classification: Cardiovascular System **Dosage form:** Tablets

Standard preparation: Prepare 1 mg/ml solution of each compound in methanol. Further serial dilutions suitably made for linearity studies. Apply 10 µl of each solution for chromatographic evaluation.

Sample preparation: An appropriate quantity of powdered sample suspended in methanol, sonicated, diluted and filtered. The filtrate suitably diluted and used for chromatographic separation and evaluation.

Chromatographic equipments:

Sample applicator: Camag Linomat–V

Development chamber: Camag twin-trough glass chamber, 20 × 10 cm

Densitometric scanner: Camag TLC Scanner–III

Chromatographic conditions:

1. Stationary phase: Silica gel $60F_{254}$ pre-coated TLC plates, 20 × 10 cm (250 µm) – Merck
2. Mobile phase (MP): n-hexane–ethyl acetate–chloroform–methanol–25% ammonia (1.5 : 4 : 1 : 4.5 : 0.1 v/v)
3. Standard/Sample application:
   Band length: 6 mm Volume applied: 10 µl Spacing: 10 mm
4. Chamber saturation: 20 min (MP)
5. RH (%): 55 ± 5
6. Temperature °C: Ambient
7. Separation technique: Ascending
8. Quantity of mobile phase: 22 ml
9. Migration distance: 80 mm
10. Migration time: 18 min

Densitometric evaluation:

Wavelength: UV–220 nm

Scanning mode: Reflectance/Absorbance

HRF: Atenolol—21; Losartan K^+—41; Aspirin—63; Atorvastatin Ca^{++}—82

Linearity (ng/band): Losartan K^+—50–500; Atenolol—100–500; Atorvastatin Ca^{++}—100–1250; Aspirin—200–1000

Recovery (%): 99.25–101.75 for all the four compounds

References: A. Manikanta Kumar et al., Personal communication with the author.

Comments: The method validated for accuracy, precision, linearity, LOD and LOQ.

HPTLC : High Performance Thin Layer Chromatography
HPTLC Densitogram

No. 120

Amlodipine besylate

Olmesartan medoxomil

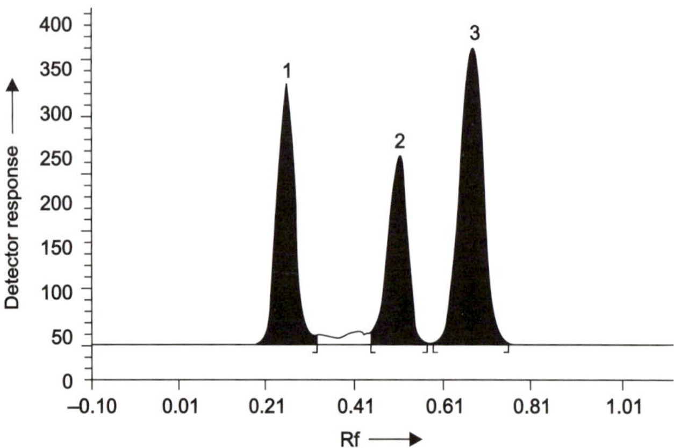

Typical densitogram of the standard containing amlodipine besylate and olmesartan medoxomil. For detailed experimental and chromatographic conditions, refer to Protocol No. 120. Peaks identification: 1. Olmesartan medoxomil; 2. Amlodipine besylate; 3. Paracetamol (IS).

PROTOCOL FOR HPTLC ANALYSIS OF PHARMACEUTICAL FORMULATION

Protocol No. 120

Formulation: Amlodipine besylate, Olmesartan medoxomil

Classification: Cardiovascular System **Dosage form:** Biological sample

Standard preparation: Prepare 1 mg/ml solution of amlodipine besylate, olmesartan medoxomil and paracetamol in methanol. Apply varying volumes of both the solutions for linearity studies.

Sample preparation: Plasma sample after protein precipitation with solvent was extracted with the same solvent, organic layer separated, evaporated to dryness and residue taken up in 1 ml of methanol. Apply 0.2 µl for chromatographic evaluation.

Solvent: Methanol–acetonitrile (3 : 0.1 v/v).

Chromatographic equipments:

Sample applicator: Camag Linomat–V

Development chamber: Camag twin-trough glass chamber, 20 × 10 cm

Densitometric scanner: Camag TLC Scanner–III

Chromatographic conditions:

1. Stationary phase: Silica gel $60F_{254}$ pre-coated TLC plates, 20 × 10 cm (250 µm) – Merck, pre-washed with methanol, activated at 120°C for 20 min prior to use
2. Mobile phase (MP): Chloroform–methanol (9 : 1 v/v)
3. Standard/Sample application:
   Band length: 8 mm Volume applied: 0.2 µl Spacing: 10 mm
4. Chamber saturation: 30 min (MP)
5. RH (%): 55 ± 5
6. Temperature °C: Ambient
7. Separation technique: Ascending
8. Quantity of mobile phase: 20 ml
9. Migration distance: 70 mm
10. Migration time: 15 min

Densitometric evaluation:

Wavelength: UV–254 nm Scanning mode: Reflectance/Absorbance

HRF: Olmesartan medoxomil—26; Amlodipine besylate—50; Paracetamol (IS)—66

Linearity (ng/band): 500–3000

Recovery (%): 90.41–90.64 for both the compounds

References: Ambadas R. Rote and Sadhana K. Kande, *J. Anal. Bioanal. Techniques*, 2–5, 2011.

Comments:

- The method validated for accuracy, precision, linearity, LOD, LOQ, selectivity and extraction efficiency.
- The method is suitable for bioequivalence studies.

Index

D

E

F

G

H

I

K

L

M

N

O

P

Q

R

S

T

V

Z